Longevity Promotion: Multidisciplinary Perspectives

ILIA STAMBLER, PHD

DEDICATION

This work is dedicated to longevity research activists around the world. Thank you for your vital effort.

CONTENTS

Notes 5
Summary 7
I. Longevity Advocacy 8
    1. The Longevity Movement Building 9
    2. Outreach Materials for Longevity Promotion 14
    3. Frequently Asked Questions on the Ethics of Lifespan and
    Healthspan Extension 28
    4. Policy Suggestions for the Promotion of Longevity Research,
    Development and Treatment 46
    5. Regulatory and Policy Frameworks for Healthy Longevity
    Promotion 77
II. Longevity History 93
    6. Introduction to "A History of Life-Extensionism in the Twentieth
    Century" 94
    7. Reductionism and Holism in the History of Aging and Longevity
    Research: Does the Whole have Parts? 114
    8. Life-extensionism as a Pursuit of Constancy 140
    9. The Legacy of Elie Metchnikoff 156
    10. The Historical Evolution of Evolutionary Theories of Aging 160
III. Longevity Philosophy 173
    11. Longevity and the Indian Tradition 174
    12. Longevity in the Ancient Middle East and the Islamic Tradition 181
    13. Longevity and the Jewish Tradition 188
    14. Longevity and the Christian Tradition 195
    15. Aristotle on Life and Long Life 205
IV. Longevity Science 238
    16. Potential Interventions to Ameliorate Degenerative Aging 239
    17. Methodological Problems of Diagnosing and Treating
    Degenerative Aging as a Medical Condition to Extend Healthy
    Lifespan 253
    18. The Use of Information Theory for the Evaluation of Biomarkers
    of Aging and Physiological Age to Predict Aging-related Diseases and
    Frailty 276
    19. Physical Means for Healthy Life Extension 292
    20. Resources for Longevity Promotion 314

NOTES

Please quote this work as:

Ilia Stambler, *Longevity Promotion: Multidisciplinary Perspectives*, Longevity History, Rison Lezion, Israel,
2017.

For more information, please visit

www.longevityhistory.com

TITLE IMAGE

"Fukurokuju"

In the traditional Chinese household pantheon, "Longevity" (Shou, 寿) is one of the three most venerated deities, alongside "Happiness" (Fu, 福) and "Prosperity" (Lu, 禄), altogether referred to as the "three lucky star gods – Fu, Lu, Shou."

The iconography of the Chinese god of longevity (Shou) is almost identical to that of the large-headed, scroll and elixir-carrying Japanese Shinto "lucky god" Fukurokuju (福禄寿) combining *fuku* – "happiness"; *roku* – "wealth"; and *ju* – "longevity" in a single person.

See: Ilia Stambler, *A History of Life-Extensionism in the Twentieth Century*, Longevity History, Rison Lezion, Israel, 2014.

.

SUMMARY

This book considers the multidisciplinary aspects of longevity promotion, from the advocacy, historical, philosophical and scientific perspectives. The first part on longevity advocacy includes examples of pro-longevity campaigns, outreach materials, frequent debates and policy suggestions and frameworks that may assist in the promotion of research and development for healthy longevity. The second part on longevity history includes analyses of the definition of life-extensionism as a social and intellectual movement, the dialectics of reductionism vs. holism and the significance of the concept of constancy in the history of life extension research, an historical overview of evolutionary theories of aging, and a tribute to one of the founding figures of modern longevity science. The third part on longevity philosophy surveys the aspirations and supportive arguments for increasing healthy longevity in the philosophical and religious traditions of ancient Greece, India, the Middle East, in particular in Islam and Judaism, and the Christian tradition. Finally, the fourth part on longevity science includes brief discussions of some of the scientific issues in life extension research, in particular regarding some potential interventions to ameliorate degenerative aging, some methodological issues with diagnosing and treating degenerative aging as a medical condition, the application of information theory for aging and longevity research, some potential physical means for life extension, and some resources for further consideration. These discussions are in no way exhaustive, but are intended to simulate additional interest, consultation and study of longevity science and its social and cultural implications. It is hoped that this book will contribute to broadening, diversifying and strengthening the academic and public deliberation on the prospects of healthy life extension for the entire population. The setting and careful consideration of a goal may be seen as a first step toward its accomplishment.

I. LONGEVITY ADVOCACY

1. The Longevity Movement Building

There is now an emerging international social advocacy movement dedicated to promotion of biomedical research and development to alleviate aging-related morbidity and improve healthy longevity for the elderly population. It is commonly referred to by the activists as the "longevity movement" or "longevity research and advocacy movement." It is a "hybrid" between the aged rights advocacy and science advocacy, as it emphasizes the need to improve health care for the elderly around the world via enhanced medical scientific research around the world. The movement is only emerging, and is not yet strongly related to other forms of health care advocacy. But a stronger relation is hoped for. The movement is also not well organized or coordinated. Many groups are united by the idea of the need to improve healthy longevity thanks to increasing biomedical research in the field of aging and aging-related diseases. But the actions of each group and even of each individual activist in the movement are mostly independent and autonomous.[1] In practice, every activist group and even every individual activist, considers the possibilities at hand – and acts accordingly autonomously. The actions may include publications, meetings, social media promotions, support of particular research projects, also by fundraising, sometimes involving "crowd-funding" and "crowd-sourcing." Some higher level advocacy initiatives were undertaken, such as the "Longevity Dividend" initiative (US, since around 2006),[2] the efforts to lobby for biomedical aging research in the US congress (2016),[3] the effort to emphasize the need to strengthen biomedical research of aging at the WHO Consultation on the Global Strategy and Action Plan on Aging and Health (GSAP) in October 2015,[4] or the advocacy for the "Law Proposal for the Establishment of the National Advisory Committee for the Promotion of Longevity and Quality of Life for the Elderly Population" in Israel (ongoing since July 2012).[5]

The main types of activities that are being organized by various groups mostly include:

1) Organizing live and online meetings and study groups, and 2) Writing and distributing advocacy and popular scientific texts - including in national languages (websites, articles, petitions, blog posts, flyers, media press releases, etc.). And the methods of their organization can be summarized as simple as the following: 1) An individual activist just thinks what he or she can organize personally in his/her area and invites friends among longevity activists to think what they can organize together, 2) The activists write and distribute texts and appeals.

The main message of these actions is also rather simple: "Increase support for biomedical research of aging to improve healthy longevity." Yet it can be scaled to almost any dimensions, from a local meeting of friends to international campaigns. The main message implies the realization that biomedical interventions into degenerative aging processes can provide the best foundations for combating aging-related ill health and for attaining healthy longevity. Yet, not enough is known about these processes and their countermeasures to provide truly effective means of combat. Hence "More Research is Needed!" This simple realization and the wish to induce this realization in others, have proven to give enough motivation for longevity research activists to step up to participate in actions, study groups and campaigns. It should be noted that the vast majority of the groups and activities so far have been entirely voluntary.

Diverse materials have been included in discussion, distribution and promotion, that could be taken from ready made resources.[6] Among many other resources, the position paper by the International Society on Aging and Disease (ISOAD) on the "Critical need to promote research of aging and aging-related diseases to improve health and longevity of the elderly population" briefly describes the rationales, technologies and policies needed to promote this research. The position paper has been translated by activists and is now available in 12 languages: with full texts in 9 languages and partial translations in 3 more languages. It has served as a "universal advocacy paper" both for the grass roots discussions and promotions and for the outreach to officials in several countries.[7] Also some frequently asked questions and topics of discussion on longevity research promotion, regarding both scientific and social aspects, have been summarized.[8]

Even though the activities are mostly autonomous, several concerted international actions, dedicated to the promotion of biomedical and biological research of aging and longevity, have been undertaken by various groups of advocates. The method of organization was straightforward – personally contacting known longevity research activists and leaders and consulting with them about what events and promotions they could organize personally as a part of the joint international action toward specific dates. The importance of taking personal responsibility for the organization and personal contacts cannot be overestimated. Massive "calls to action" are virtually useless as compared to personal engagement!

Some of the concerted actions, involving longevity activists groups from several countries, included the "Future of Longevity" campaign around the "Future Day" on March 1, 2013[9] and the "Metchnikoff Day" – around May 15, 2015, in honor of the anniversary of the founder of gerontology – Elie Metchnikoff.[10] Yet, perhaps the most successful and wide-reaching was the so-called "International Longevity Day" campaign, which has been organized since 2013, around October 1 – the UN "International Day of Older Persons."[11]

Perhaps unintentionally, "the day of older persons" may appear value-neutral and indifferent toward the "older persons," while the "longevity day," celebrating and aspiring to healthy longevity for all, may be more uplifting. Yet, as this is the officially recognized "UN International Day of Older Persons," this has provided the longevity research activists a perfect opportunity, perhaps even a perfect "excuse," to emphasize the importance of aging and longevity research for the development of effective health care for the elderly, in the wide public as well as among decision makers.

This campaign has a bit of a history. In 2013, events during or around that day – ranging from small meetings of friends to seminars and rather large conferences, alongside special publications, distributions of outreach materials (petitions and flyers) and media appearances – were held in over 30 countries, and in 2014 in over 20 countries.[11]

In 2015, record participation was attained with meetings and promotions held in over 40 countries, with outreach materials (videos, newsletters, social media) reaching out to hundreds of thousands of people. Dozens of organizations participated in the campaign. The support ranged from small emerging local groups of activists to authoritative scientific societies and associations, including the endorsements and promotions at the sites of such global organizations as the International Federation on Ageing (IFA), International Association of Gerontology and Geriatrics (IAGG), Healthspan Campaign, International Society on Aging and Disease (ISOAD) and others.

In 2016, while keeping the "longevity day" concept as would be desirable to particular groups and activists, an additional emphasis was placed on organizing the longevity promotion events through the entire month of October in the framework of "The Longevity Month" – as usually the "longevity day" events spread through the entire month. Promoting various "commemorative months" to support particular advocacy issues has been a well established and effective practice, and a dedicated "month" could give people more flexibility and space to organize events and publications. The extent of the campaign in 2016 was less than in 2015, with events and promotions held in over 20 countries.[11] This might have been at least partly due to the ebbs and flows of personal and communal enthusiasm and availability that should be always kept in consideration. Generally, the impact of any campaign ultimately depends on the strength of involvement of every individual activist, for every event and every publication of the campaign.

Despite their still rather limited extents, such campaigns may be considered as exercises for the longevity movement building. They provided a demonstration that massive grass roots actions for biomedical research of aging are possible. Yet, much remains to be aspired to even begin to think of approaching the level of public involvement and influence that has been achieved by the campaigns of other movements, such as the "green movement," or other forms of health advocacy. Hopefully, the movement for healthy longevity through scientific research may gradually approach such levels. Hopefully also, this fledging movement will become a truly integral and involved part of the global health movement.

References and notes

1. "Groups," Longevity for All, 2017, http://www.longevityforall.org/groups/; "Network of anti-aging organizations," Reddit Longevity, 2017, https://www.reddit.com/r/longevity/comments/5xl8dh/map_of_all_antia ging_organizations_i_could_find/.
2. S. Jay Olshansky, Daniel Perry, Richard A. Miller, Robert N. Butler, "In Pursuit of the Longevity Dividend: What Should We Be Doing To Prepare for the Unprecedented Aging of Humanity?" *The Scientist*, 20(3), 28-36, March 1, 2006, http://www.the-scientist.com/article/display/23191/; *Pursuing the Longevity Dividend. Scientific Goals for an Aging World*, September 12, 2006, including a full list of the campaign signatories: http://www.longevityforall.org/wp-content/uploads/2014/05/Longevity_Dividend_Signatories.pdf.)
3. "Ask Congress to Fund the First FDA-Approved Drug Trial to Prevent Cancer and Other Diseases of Aging," Global Healthspan Policy Institute, February 24, 2016, https://healthspanpolicy.org/metformin-campaign/; http://tame.healthspanpolicy.org/; "The New Age of Aging," Global Healthspan Policy Institute, March 2017, https://healthspanpolicy.org/the-new-age-of-aging/; http://www.longevityforall.org/wp-content/uploads/2014/05/The-new-age-of-aging.pdf .
4. "WHO consultation on the Global Strategy and Action Plan on Ageing and Health," Longevity for All, October 22, 2015, http://www.longevityforall.org/who-consultation-on-the-global-strategy-and-action-plan-on-ageing-and-health/; "ILA position with respect to WHO's Global Strategy and Action Plan on Ageing and Health," International Longevity Alliance, October 23, 2015, http://longevityalliance.org/?q=ila-position-respect-who-s-global-strategy-and-action-plan-ageing-and-health.
5. "Law Proposal for the Establishment of the National Advisory Committee for the Promotion of Longevity and Quality of Life for the Elderly Population," Israeli Longevity Alliance, http://www.longevityisrael.org/longevity-bill.html;

Ilia Stambler, "Political struggle against the disease of aging," Institute for Ethics and Emerging Technologies (IEET), July 17, 2012, https://ieet.org/index.php/IEET2/more/stambler201207171;
Ilia Stambler, "Longevity research program is established in Israel," IEET, September 10, 2014, https://ieet.org/index.php/IEET2/more/stambler20140910.
6. "Resources," Longevity for All, 2017, http://www.longevityforall.org/resources/.
7. Kunlin Jin, James W. Simpkins, Xunming Ji, Miriam Leis, Ilia Stambler, "The critical need to promote research of aging and aging-related diseases to improve health and longevity of the elderly population," *Aging and Disease*, 6, 1-5, 2015, http://www.aginganddisease.org/EN/10.14336/AD.2014.1210.
The text is available in full in Arabic, Chinese, English, German, Hebrew, Italian, Portuguese, Russian, Spanish, and as a partial (summary) translation in Danish, Finnish, Swedish: http://www.longevityforall.org/the-critical-need-to-promote-research-of-aging-around-the-world/.
8. "Frequently asked questions about life extension," Longevity For All, 2017, http://www.longevityforall.org/faq-of-the-ethics-of-lifespan-and-healthspan-extension/.
9. Ilia Stambler, "For the Future of Longevity - Celebrating longevity on the international 'Future Day' March 1, 2013," International Longevity Alliance, http://longevityalliance.org/?q=future-longevity; http://www.longevityforall.org/future-day-march-1-2013-theme-longevity/.
10. Ilia Stambler, "The 170th anniversary of Elie Metchnikoff – the founder of gerontology, May 15, 2015," Longevity for All, http://www.longevityforall.org/170th-anniversary-of-elie-metchnikoff-the-founder-of-gerontology-may-15-2015/; http://hplusmagazine.com/2015/05/06/may-15-2015-170th-anniversary-of-elie-metchnikoff-the-founder-of-gerontology-an-opportunity-to-promote-aging-and-longevity-research/.
11. Ilia Stambler, "International Longevity Day - October 1" (2013, 2014, 2015, 2016)
http://ieet.org/index.php/IEET/more/stambler20131029;
http://ieet.org/index.php/IEET/more/stambler20140110;
http://www.longecity.org/forum/topic/72013-promoting-longevity-research-on-october-1-%E2%80%93-the-international-day-of-older-persons/;
http://www.longevityforall.org/international-longevity-day-october-1-2015/;
http://www.longevityforall.org/longevity-day-and-longevity-month-october-2016.

2. Outreach Materials for Longevity Promotion

Introduction

For any social movement and for any advocacy cause, it is important to provide a clear explanation, both to the cause's existing and potential supporters, what the cause precisely calls for, what it plans to achieve and how it plans to achieve it. For the longevity promotion, one of the major general mission statements may be formulated as follows: "Increase support for biomedical research of aging to improve healthy longevity." But of course, "the devil is in the details." When it comes to specifying the exact research types and projects that need to be supported, and the ways of support that are required – the issue may become extremely complex and involved. Yet, as a general "primer" or "conversation starter," this simple mission statement may serve well for an initial goal setting, to advance further negotiations and elaborations. More elaborate calls to thought and to action may be formulated, from very concise manifestos and petitions to extensive monographs and roadmaps. Below are several examples of concise calls that were practically used in aging and longevity research advocacy in the past.

First, the "Longevity Manifesto" was the original credo of the International Longevity Alliance, an organization that started in 2012 (emerging from the informal international "Longevity Party" activists network) and in 2013 included emerging groups of activists in over 50 countries, altogether advocating for increasing biomedical research to achieve healthy longevity for all.[1] Thanks to the efforts of many activists, this manifesto was translated to over 30 languages. Later, it became the manifesto of the informal Longevity for All advocacy network.[2]

Secondly, the open letter to a Nordic gerontological congress is based on a short summary excerpt from the position paper of the International Society on Aging and Disease (ISOAD) entitled "The critical need to promote research of aging and aging-related diseases to improve health and longevity of the elderly population." The original position paper provides a rather detailed, but still concise overview of the rationales, scientific and technological fields, and policy suggestions that may be needed for the support of aging and longevity research.[3] The short open letter that was based on it, recapitulates the main rationales and policy action points. Besides the original English, the open letter was prepared in other Nordic languages – Finnish, Swedish and Danish (that is in addition to the 9 more languages in which the entire position paper is available).[4] Though originally directed to the audience in "Nordic" countries, similar texts may be adopted for other "developed" countries with high life-expectancy and

14

quality of life – urging people to maintain and intensify the positive trends and warning against potential adverse affects of unhealthy and unproductive aging of the population.

Thirdly, the open outreach letter to officials and policy makers in India in support of aging and longevity research was originally addressed to the Department of Biotechnology of the Indian Ministry of Science and Technology. It was signed by several leading researchers of aging and longevity advocates in India and abroad. Following the initial outreach, it was published at the Institute for Ethics and Emerging Technologies (IEET).[5] Though the letter was originally addressed to the officials and general public in India, similar texts can be adopted for other "developing countries" – encouraging people to address the problems of aging in advance, before they hit hard the still relatively young populations of those countries, advocating to close the research and development gaps with the so-called "developed countries" and strongly urging to contribute to making potential anti-aging and life-extending therapies universally available to all, including people of lesser means everywhere.

The forth outreach text is the appeal calling to participate in the "Longevity Day" campaign, in support of biomedical research of aging and longevity. This campaign has been organized, since 2013, around October 1 – the "official" UN International Day of Older Persons, emphasizing the importance of advancing biomedical research to improve healthcare for the elderly.[6] Though, usually the events and promotions of this campaign continued through the entire month of October, designating it at the "Longevity Month." These campaigns have involved longevity activists in dozens of countries worldwide. The appeal argues for the need to organize joint international actions in support of longevity research, and provides some suggestions for activities that may be undertaken during the campaign by various groups of activists, either autonomously or in cooperation with each other. Such activities may include organizing meetings and producing dedicated on-line and printed publications. Though the text was intended to simulate participation in the "Longevity Day/Month" campaign, similar calls can be produced for other joint actions and campaigns, on other dates and occasions, both locally and internationally.

The final fifth text is the law proposal suggesting the "Establishment of the National Advisory Committee for the Promotion of Longevity and Quality of Life for the Elderly Population" in Israel. The proposal argues that the stimulation of biomedical research of aging is a necessary condition for any potential attempt or program to address the problem of population aging. Therefore, it advocates that one of the primary functions of such a committee "for the Promotion of Longevity and Quality of Life for the Elderly Population" should be the development of incentives, strategic analysis and road-mapping, and the communication between governmental, scientific, industrial and public stakeholders, for the advancement of fundamental, translational and therapeutic biomedical research of aging. The short sections on the rationales and potential functions of such a committee are reproduced here (the administrative parts considering the possible committee operations are omitted). This proposal was submitted for consideration to members of the Israeli Parliament – the Knesset, and the text has been republished as an open petition. Since the proposal submission, the efforts have been ongoing to lobby Israeli decision makers about the importance of increasing financial and institutional support for biomedical research of aging to improve health and productivity not only of the elderly, but of the entire population.[7] Hopefully, this advocacy action and outreach document will help inspire and develop other similar efforts in other countries and internationally.

It must be noted that the above advocacy actions and appeals so far have produced little measurable effect in terms of actual increase of financial and institutional support for the field of aging research, or some tangible increase of professional and scientific effort in the field, or some concrete scientific or therapeutic outcomes. This may be due to their still limited scope and public involvement. Yet, it is hoped that these efforts have produced at least some minimal positive contribution for raising communal awareness about the critical importance of therapeutic biomedical research of aging for improving public health and longevity. It is hoped that thanks to such increased public awareness, there will be more civic demand for safe, effective and universally available anti-aging and life-extending therapies, which may in turn increase the actual scientific and technological offer. The results may not be seen at once, but many such small and persistent efforts may produce cumulative and ever-growing effects in time. Therefore, these documents are suggested for consideration, in the hope that they will help inspire and advance further advocacy actions. The readers are welcome to freely modify and circulate these texts, as they consider appropriate, or write advocacy outreach texts of their own, share them (or various modifications) in their social networks, forward such appeals to politicians, potential donors and media, organize discussion groups to debate the topics raised (that may later grow into grassroots longevity research and activism groups in different countries), translate such texts into native languages, reference and link to them, republish them in part or in full in available venues (such as blogs and social media, or print brochures and flyers), consult and join forces with many emerging and developing aging and longevity research and advocacy organizations.

Finally, these texts and their translations and disseminations are the result of collaborative work of many longevity advocates and researchers from around the world. As there have been many contributors and promoters, the texts are presented here as anonymous, yet some special thanks are included in the notes. Many thanks to all longevity researchers and advocates for everything they do to achieve healthy longevity for all!

1. The Longevity Manifesto

We advocate the advancement of healthy longevity for the entire population through scientific research, public health, advocacy and social activism. We emphasize and promote the struggle against the chief enemy of healthy longevity – the aging process.

The aging process is the root of most chronic diseases afflicting the world population. This process causes the largest proportion of disability and mortality, and needs to be treated accordingly. Society needs to dedicate efforts toward its treatment and correction, as for any other material disease.

The problem of aging is grave and threatening. Yet, we often witness an almost complete oblivion to its reality and severity. There is a soothing tendency to ignore the future, to distract the mind from aging and death from aging, and even to present aging and death in a misleading, apologetic and utopian light. At the same time, there is an unfounded belief that aging is a completely unmanageable, inexorable process. This disregard of the problem and this unfounded sense of impotence do not contribute to the improvement of the well-being of the aged and their healthy longevity. There is a need to present the problem in its full severity and importance and to act for its solution or mitigation to the best of our ability.

We call to raise the public awareness of the problem of aging in its full scope. We call the public to recognize this severe problem and dedicate efforts and resources – including economic, social-political, scientific, technological and media resources – to its maximal possible alleviation for the benefit of the aging population, for their healthy longevity. We promote the idea that mental and spiritual maturation and the increase in healthy longevity are not synonymous with aging and deterioration.

We advocate the reinforcement and acceleration of basic and applied biomedical research, as well as the development of technological, industrial, environmental, public health and educational measures, specifically directed for healthy longevity. If given sufficient support, such measures can increase the healthy life expectancy of the aged population, the period of their productivity, their contribution to the development of society and economy, as well as their sense of enjoyment, purpose and valuation of life.

We advocate that the development of scientific measures for healthy life extension be given the maximal possible public and political support that it deserves, not only by the professional community but also by the broad public.

17

2. The Critical Need to Promote Research of Aging and Aging-related Diseases to Improve Health and Longevity of the Elderly Population in Nordic Countries and Globally

Over the past decades, the average life expectancy has increased globally, reaching a worldwide average of about 70 years in 2014 (6 years longer than in 1990) and around 80 in the developed countries (compared to about 50 years in the developed countries in the early 20th century). In the Nordic countries – Finland, Sweden, Norway, Denmark, Iceland – the life expectancy is of the highest in the world, well over 80. Although the increasing life expectancy generally reflects positive human development, new challenges are arising. They stem from the fact that growing older is still inherently associated with biological and cognitive degeneration, although the severity and speed of cognitive decline, physical frailty and psychological impairment can vary between individuals. Degenerative aging processes are the major underlying cause for non-communicable diseases (NCDs), including cancer, ischemic heart disease, stroke, type 2 diabetes, Alzheimer's disease, obstructive lung disease, and others. Aging also increases the risk of morbidity and mortality from infectious diseases like pneumonia and influenza. Moreover, the susceptibility to injury and trauma (such as falls and concussions), due to the impairment of balance and mental state, and even falling victim to violence, are strongly increased by the aging process. Also, the processes of aging exacerbate and reinforce the effects of other risk factors of non-communicable diseases (tobacco use, unhealthy diet, physical inactivity, and harmful use of alcohol). In sum, aging-related health decline is the main cause of mortality and morbidity worldwide and should be addressed according to the severity of the problem. Because of these severe and negative effects, aging is already regarded as one of the greatest economic and societal challenges that most countries – especially in the industrialized world – will face in the coming decades.

The challenge of the aging society has been widely recognized and numerous research and development programs around the globe have been initiated to tackle age-related diseases. Yet, medical research and development efforts currently are focused mainly on single diseases, like Alzheimer's dementia, heart disease, osteoporosis, diabetes, cancer, etc. The underlying degenerative aging processes, determinative for the emergence of those diseases, are often underemphasized. New directions in research and development take a more holistic approach for tackling the degenerative processes and negative biological effects of human aging, addressing several major fundamental causes of aging and aging-related diseases at once and in an interrelated manner. Such approaches are very promising, for the following reasons:

18

- They are already supported by scientific proofs of concept, involving the evidential increase in healthy lifespan in animal models and the emerging technological capabilities to intervene into fundamental aging processes. Any reinforcement in this research can produce cumulative effects and speed up the translation from basic studies to widely available therapies.

- They can provide solutions to a number of non-communicable, age-related diseases, insofar as such diseases are strongly determined by degenerative aging processes (such as chronic inflammation, cross-linkage of macromolecules, somatic mutations, loss of stem cell populations, and others). Moreover, they are likely to decrease susceptibility of the elderly also to communicable diseases due to improvements in immunity.

- The innovative, applied results of such research and development will lead to sustainable solutions for a large array of age-related medical and social challenges, that may be globally applicable. The most important of them are the savings in healthcare costs for aging-related diseases and increase in the period of productivity of older persons. These prospective effects make this research potentially the most profitable form of general and biomedical research.

- Such research and development should be supported on ethical grounds, to provide equal health care chances for the elderly as for the young.

Therefore it is the societal duty, especially of the professionals in biology, medicine, health care, economy and socio-political organizations to strongly recommend greater investments in research and development dealing with the understanding of mechanisms associated with the human biological aging process and translating these insights into safe, affordable and universally available applied technologies and treatments.

Hence we urge you to advocate with the government, or in any institutional framework where you are active and influential, for the creation and implementation of the following policies to promote research into the biology of aging and aging-related diseases, for improving the health of the global elderly population:

1) Funding: Act to ensure a significant increase of governmental and non-governmental funding for goal-directed (translational) research in preventing the degenerative aging processes, and the associated chronic non-communicable diseases and disabilities, and for extending healthy and productive life, during the entire life course.

2) Incentives: Act to develop and adopt legal and regulatory frameworks that give incentives for goal-directed research and development designed to specifically address the development, registration, administration and accessibility of drugs, medical technologies and other therapies that will

19

ameliorate the aging processes and associated diseases and extend healthy life.

3) Institutions: Act to establish and expand national and international coordination and consultation structures, programs and institutions to advance research, development and education on the biology of aging and associated diseases and the development of clinical guidelines to modulate the aging processes and associated aging-related diseases and to extend the healthy and productive lifespan for the population.

These measures are designed to reduce the burden of the aging process on the economy and to alleviate the suffering of the aged and the grief of their loved ones. On the positive side, if granted sufficient support, these measures can increase the healthy life expectancy for the elderly, extend their period of productivity and their interaction with society, and enhance their sense of enjoyment, purpose, equality and valuation of life.

Nordic countries – building on their proven achievements in increasing healthy life expectancy, their tremendous medical, scientific, social, economic and humanitarian capabilities – can play a prominent part in achieving these goals in the region and globally. We urge to use any occasion to raise the awareness of the issue and advance the goal of achieving healthy longevity for all through the support of biomedical science of aging.

3. Support Ageing and Longevity Research in India

We write to draw the attention to the need for increased support for biological research of ageing and improving healthy longevity for the population in India. This subject is pressing and urgent for the global society, and for Indian society and economy in particular. Although it is a positive sign that the life expectancy is increasing around the globe, the rapid ageing of the world population could have grave consequences for the global society, in particular economy, which forces the society to seek solutions. On the other side, biomedical science and technology are developing rapidly as well, fostering our hope that medical and biotechnological solutions to ameliorate those problems may be found. These forces warrant increased interest and involvement in research of ageing and healthy longevity.

India has only begun this demographic transition, with an average life expectancy of about 66 years, compared to about 80 in "high-income" countries. Yet, it is rapidly advancing in the direction of population ageing. Just since 1990, the life expectancy increased by about 9 years, and further large gains can be expected soon. Hence foresight in addressing this issue, before it becomes acute in India, can be critical.

20

Furthermore, we believe India is poised to become a critically important player in the global effort to address the challenges of ageing, not only because of the tremendous potential brain power that can be dedicated to this area, but also because of the strategic ability to make biomedical and biotechnological developments in the field widely accessible for the public of lesser means, not only in India but in the entire developing and developed world.

Developed countries, including USA and UK, are facing tremendous economic burden trying to support their ageing populations. The White-House expects healthcare spending to account for almost 40% of GDP by 2040. Other countries in Europe are facing similar insurmountable economic pressures for healthcare. Advantageously, India has previously been able to avoid economic pressures in the information infrastructure domain by leap-frogging the developed countries and building the world's largest wireless communication network. Today almost every Indian has access to mobile phone. Similarly, India can leverage its enormous talent-pools, and inexpensive engineering infrastructure to get ahead of the developed countries in the healthcare arena. India can strategically fund preventive and regenerative medicine to tackle the chronic diseases of ageing, before they impair the ageing population. This will help India maintain a healthy and productive population, and avoid the economic-healthcare catastrophe faced by the developed countries. This will also ensure India's integral and prominent place in the collective bid of nations together facing this task.

In particular, strong engagement in this area can help create bi-national and international research and development programs between India and other countries, including US, EU, UK, Israel – all the countries endeavoring to address the medical problems of the ageing population.

Hence, we call to increase broad public interest in ageing and longevity research (also in the media), improve networking and collaboration among and with researchers from India and abroad, as well as to address potential decision makers in India, perhaps in a proposal to form a national ageing and longevity research program, mainly focusing on biological, biomedical and biotechnological aspects of ageing, with the establishment of dedicated centers of excellence based on existing research and development institutions.

We hope for broad support in fostering collaboration and dialogue for the advancement of the vital field of ageing and longevity research in India.

4. The Longevity Day Appeal

There has been emerging a tradition by longevity researchers and activists around the world to organize events dedicated to promotion of

21

longevity research on or around October 1 – the UN International Day of Older Persons.

This day is sometimes referred to in some parts of the longevity activists community as the "International Longevity Day." As this is the official UN Day of Older Persons, this provides the longevity research activists a perfect opportunity, perhaps even a perfect "excuse," to emphasize the importance of aging and longevity research for the development of effective health care for the elderly, in the wide public as well as among decision makers.

The critical importance and the critical need to promote biological research of aging derives from the realization that tackling the degenerative processes and negative biological effects of human aging, at once and in an interrelated manner, can provide the best foundations to find holistic and effective ways for intervention and prevention against age-related ill health. Such an approach has been supported by scientific proofs of concept, involving the evidential increase in healthy lifespan in animal models and the emerging technological capabilities to intervene into fundamental aging processes. The focus on intervention into degenerative aging processes can provide solutions to a number of non-communicable, age-related diseases (such as cancer, heart disease, type 2 diabetes, chronic obstructive lung diseases and neurodegenerative diseases), insofar as such diseases are strongly determined by degenerative aging processes (such as chronic inflammation, cross-linkage of macromolecules, somatic mutations, loss of stem cell populations, and others). This approach is likely to decrease susceptibility of the elderly also to communicable, infectious diseases due to improvements in immunity. The innovative, applied results of such research and development will lead to sustainable, economically viable solutions for a large array of age-related medical and social challenges, that may be globally applicable. Furthermore, such research and development should be supported on ethical grounds, to provide equal health care chances for the elderly as for the young.

Yet, clearly, such measures will take time and massive communal investment and effort. In contrast, the present appeal proposes an immediate and simple measure, which, however, can contribute to changing the public attitude to the problems of aging and longevity.

We propose celebrating the International Longevity Day on or around October 1 – the International Day of Older Persons – to help change public attitude to healthy longevity from negative or indifferent to positive and proactive! The events and promotions can even be extended through the entire month of October that could be designated as the "Longevity Month." This can provide the researchers and advocates an opportunity to raise these points and make these demands. Let us plan and organize a mutually reinforcing network of events worldwide. If you plan to organize an event for that day or month – either live meetings or on-line publications and promotions – please let your plans be known to encourage others. Together we can create an activism wave of strong impact.

5. Law Proposal for the Establishment of the National Advisory Committee for the Promotion of Longevity and Quality of Life for the Elderly Population in Israel

Rationale:
The longevity and quality of life of the elderly population are crucial national priorities, necessary for the normal functioning of the entire society. On the contrary, the deteriorative aging process is the root cause and main endangering factor for most chronic diseases afflicting the developed world generally and Israel in particular.

The death rate in Israel is approximately 0.52%, out of which over 90% die as a result of age-related diseases due to the aging process. In other words, each year approximately 40,000 residents of Israel die from aging, twice the number of all the casualties of war throughout the country's history, and twice the number of all deaths from traffic accidents throughout the country's history.

According to the report of the Bank of Israel, published in March 2012, both the private and public national expenditures on the senescent population in Israel (persons over 65 years old, comprising about 10% of the country's population) is NIS 9.9 billion (~$ 2.5 billion) yearly, which comprises 1.2% of the entire Gross Domestic Product.

Aging is a basic material process manifesting in the accumulation of damage, the gradual deregulation of metabolic balance, and impairment of normal functioning. This is a process causing the largest proportion of disability and mortality, and is the major endangering factor for most chronic diseases, such as cancer, heart disease, type 2 diabetes, dementia, and other diseases – and it should be treated accordingly.

Yet, medical research in Israel and other developed countries focuses on the symptoms of the deteriorative aging process and not on its prevention or treatment. Despite their immediate importance, palliative measures, such as increasing nursing care, will not drastically improve the healthy longevity of the elderly, will not resolve the economic burden and human suffering caused by the process of aging, but will only slightly relieve and postpone them. In contrast, investments and efforts in the research and development directed toward prevention and treatment of the deteriorative aging process, if given sufficient support, may be able to bring about a substantial improvement.

While the deteriorative aging process, that is the accumulation of structural damage, impairment of metabolic balance and functioning, is a

23

disabling and debilitating process that requires prevention and treatment; the rise in healthy life-expectancy is its cure. In other words, the spiritual maturation during the years and the increase in healthy life expectancy are not and should not be synonymous with degeneration and deterioration.

The trends of increasing healthy life-expectancy, as well as the results of basic research on aging, indicate the practical possibility of intervention into the aging process and the chronic diseases derived from it, and as a result demonstrate the practical possibility of healthy life extension for the elderly population.

This positive process can be reinforced and accelerated for the long term by regulated support of basic and applied research, as well as technological, industrial and environmental development directed toward delaying and treatment of the deteriorative aging process and for improving the quantity and quality of life for the elderly population.

These measures will reduce the burden of the aging process on Israeli economy and will alleviate the suffering of the aged and the grief of their close ones. On the positive side, if granted sufficient support, these measures can increase the healthy life expectancy for the elderly, extend their period of productivity and their contribution to the society, and enhance their sense of enjoyment, purpose and valuation of life.

In view of this and in accordance to the Israeli Basic Law: Human Dignity and Liberty, and in accordance to the Jewish principle: "Do not reject a soul for another soul" – there is a need to give to the Promotion of Longevity and Quality of Life for the Elderly Population the necessary support that it deserves, and hence establish the National Advisory Committee for the Promotion of Longevity and Quality of Life for the Elderly Population in Israel.

The committee functions:

The committee will determine the policy for scientific research, technological development, public and academic education and institutional coordination for the improvement of longevity and quality of life for the elderly population, so it shall become the basis for the committee activity and the government activity in this area. In case the committee determines a policy on a subject within the area of its function, the head of the committee will submit it for the government approval upon a request by the committee.

Without detracting from this general statement, the committee functions will include the following:

a) Formulating policy and acting to promote cooperation between governmental departments, national and international research institutes and other organizations active for improving longevity and quality of life for the elderly population;

b) Providing long-term planning for the implications of an increase in life-expectancy in Israel;

c) Acting for the establishment, development, management and maintenance of appropriate research and action frameworks, services and programs, for improving longevity and quality of life for the elderly population, in cooperation with relevant governmental departments.

These include:

– Providing grants and scholarships for research aimed to delay and treat the deteriorative aging process and promote longevity and quality of life for the elderly population, particularly in the fields of regenerative medicine, nano-medicine, bio-gerontology and optimal hygienic life-style for aging persons;

– Encouraging investments in biotechnology and medical technology companies, as well as in academic and public organizations for research, development and application – that will be involved in the prevention and treatment of the deterioration caused by the aging process and its derivative chronic diseases.

d) Acting for the expansion of education and raising public awareness about the damage caused by the aging process, about potential ways to minimize this damage and scientific developments in the field.

These include:

– Encouraging the collection of up-to-date, evidential scientific information regarding the optimal hygienic life-style for aging persons and providing education on the subject to the health care community and the wide public.

– Acting to create academic and communal learning frameworks and programs on basic and applied research of aging and promotion of longevity and quality of life for the elderly population, including its biological, medical and social aspects;

e) Assisting governmental and local services in providing consultation and direction for the treatment of the aged in Israel.

These include:

– Acting to improve the living conditions of the elderly, including the development of means of access and convenience in their daily life.

– Acting to create and expand social, educational and occupational frameworks involving the aged and encouraging their integration with the entire population.

References and notes

1. Maria Konovalenko, "Russians create the 'Longevity Party,'" Institute for Ethics and Emerging Technologies (IEET), July 26, 2012, https://ieet.org/index.php/IEET2/more/konovalenko201207261;

Hank Pellissier, "Who are the "Longevity Party" Co-Leaders, and What do They Want? (Part 1)," IEET, August 20, 2012, https://ieet.org/index.php/IEET2/more/pellissier20120820;
Hank Pellissier, "18 Nations Join the "Longevity Party," IEET, September 21, 2012, https://ieet.org/index.php/IEET2/more/longevityparty20120921;
Ilia Stambler, "50 countries in the International Longevity Alliance!" International Longevity Alliance, August 13, 2013, http://longevityalliance.org/News/TabId/109/ArtMID/500/ArticleID/28/50-countries-in-the-International-Longevity-Alliance.aspx;
http://www.longevityalliance.org/?q=50-countries-international-longevity-alliance;
Ilia Stambler, "International Longevity Alliance (ILA) – Annual Report for 2013 – Roadmap for 2014," IEET, January 10, 2014, http://ieet.org/index.php/IEET/more/stambler20140110.
2. "Longevity is the common language. The Longevity Manifesto," Longevity for All (in 32 languages), May 16, 2014,
http://www.longevityforall.org/longevity/;
http://longevityalliance.org/longevity-is-the-common-language/.
3. Kunlin Jin, James W. Simpkins, Xunming Ji, Miriam Leis, Ilia Stambler, "The critical need to promote research of aging and aging-related diseases to improve health and longevity of the elderly population," *Aging and Disease*, 6, 1-5, 2015, http://www.aginganddisease.org/EN/10.14336/AD.2014.1210.
The text is available in full in Arabic, Chinese, English, German, Hebrew, Italian, Portuguese, Russian, Spanish, and as a partial (summary) translation in Danish, Finnish, Swedish: http://www.longevityforall.org/the-critical-need-to-promote-research-of-aging-around-the-world/.
Special thanks go to Dr. Miriam Leis for her contribution to the policy justification and Prof. Kunlin Jin for his leadership of the International Society on Aging and Disease.
4. "The Critical Need to Promote Research of Aging and Aging-related Diseases to Improve Health and Longevity of the Elderly Population in Nordic Countries and Globally," Longevity for All, May 19, 2016, http://www.longevityforall.org/nordic-longevity-outreach-english/.
5. "Support aging and longevity research in India," Longevity for All, January 15, 2017, http://www.longevityforall.org/support-ageing-and-longevity-research-in-india/;
and IEET, January 26, 2017,
https://ieet.org/index.php/IEET2/more/Stambler20170126.
Special thanks go to Prof. Kalluri Subba Rao for inspiring and implementing this outreach effort, and Dr. Avi Roy and Dr. Miriam Leis for their contributions to the text of the petition.

See also: Kalluri Subba Rao, "Should India Promote Scientific Research of Aging," IEET, March 20, 2016 (first published in 2007)
http://ieet.org/index.php/IEET/more/rao20160320;
http://www.longevityforall.org/should-india-promote-scientific-research-on-aging/.
6. Ilia Stambler, "International Longevity Day - October 1" (2013, 2014, 2015, 2016)
http://ieet.org/index.php/IEET/more/stambler20131029;
http://www.longecity.org/forum/topic/72013-promoting-longevity-research-on-october-1-%E2%80%93-the-international-day-of-older-persons/;
http://www.longevityforall.org/international-longevity-day-october-1-2015/;
http://www.longevityforall.org/longevity-day-and-longevity-month-october-2016.
7. "Law Proposal for the Establishment of the National Advisory Committee for the Promotion of Longevity and Quality of Life for the Elderly Population," Israeli Longevity Alliance, 2012-2017, http://www.longevityisrael.org/longevity-bill.html;
Ilia Stambler, "Political struggle against the disease of aging," IEET, July 17, 2012, https://ieet.org/index.php/IEET2/more/stambler201207171;
The original of this law proposal can be found at:
http://www.singulariut.com/2012/07/601.
Regarding some other actions of Israeli longevity research activists, see:
Ilia Stambler, "Demonstration for Radical Life Extension in Tel Aviv," IEET, January 26, 2012,
https://ieet.org/index.php/IEET2/more/stambler20120126;
Ilia Stambler, "Longevity research program is established in Israel," IEET, September 10, 2014,
https://ieet.org/index.php/IEET2/more/stambler20140910.
Special thanks go to Mr. Oded Carmeli for initiating the ideas of the demonstration for life extension and of the law proposal to establish the advisory committee to combat aging-related ill health and for healthy life extension in Israel.

3. Frequently Asked Questions on the Ethics of Lifespan and Healthspan Extension

Introduction

The mission of healthy life extension, or healthy longevity promotion, raises a broad variety of questions and tasks, relating to science and technology, individual and communal ethics, and public policy, especially health and science policy. Despite the wide variety, the related questions may be classified into three groups. The first group of questions concerns the *feasibility* of the accomplishment of life extension. Is it theoretically and technologically possible? What are our grounds for optimism? What are the means to ensure that the life extension will be healthy life extension? The second group concerns the *desirability* of the accomplishment of life extension for the individual and the society, provided it will become some day possible through scientific intervention. How will then life extension affect the perception of personhood? How will it affect the availability of resources for the population? Yet, the third and final group can be termed *normative*. What actions should we take? Assuming that life extension is scientifically possible and socially desirable, and that its implications are either demonstrably positive or, in case of a negative forecast, they are amenable – what practical implications should these determinations have for public policy, in particular health policy and research policy, in a democratic society? Should we pursue the goal of life extension? If yes, then how? How can we make it an individual and social priority? Given the rapid population aging and the increasing incidence and burden of age-related diseases, on the pessimistic side, and the rapid development of medical technologies, on the optimistic side, these become vital questions of social responsibility. And indeed, these questions are often asked by almost any person thinking about the possibility of human life extension, its meaning for oneself, for the people in one's close circle, for the entire global community. Many of these questions are rather standard, and the answers to them are also often quite standard. Below some of those frequently asked questions and frequently given answers are provided, with specific reference to the possibility and desirability of healthy human life extension, and the normative actions that can be undertaken, by the individual and the society, to achieve this goal.

Q: Is human life extension possible? Why do you think so?

A: Is it possible for people to achieve a significant life extension? In other words, is it possible to achieve either a substantial increase in the

28

average human life expectancy or an increase in the maximum (or record) lifespan specific for the human species? The wide-spread belief in the impossibility of significant human life extension often relies on the notion of a "limit" to the human lifespan. Yet, it should be noted that, even when proposing a "limit" to the lifespan, it is often realized by the proponents that this "limit" is quite flexible and theoretically not very limiting. It is theoretically possible to overcome this "limit" by changes in inner biological structure and/or environmental conditions, including improvements in biomedical technology.[1] But of course, there are currently clear practical limits and constraints in our ability to greatly increase the human lifespan with the current medical technological means. And these practical constraints and limits have been realized even by the most ardent advocates of human life extension. They just do not reconcile with those limits, they desire and strive to overcome them by improving biomedical technology.

However, on the basic theoretical level, there is no law in nature that sets a strict insurmountable limit to the lifespan of any organism. As stated by the Nobel Prize winning physicist Richard Phillips Feynman, "there is nothing in biology yet found that indicates the inevitability of death."[2] This is demonstrated by the existence of non-aging, slowly aging, and even "potentially immortal" life-forms and the constant evolutionary adaptations of the lifespan even for the humans, according to particular changing environmental and genetic conditions.[3] There may be contingent limitations due to the inner biological structure and environment, but these are not "limits" in the principal physical sense (like "nothing can travel faster than the speed of light"). The existing practical limits to the human lifespan, due to internal disorder, adverse environment and imperfect medical capabilities, are "rules that can be broken."

Indeed the seemingly well-established "rules" and "limitations" of human longevity have been overcome continuously. There has been a persistent increase in life expectancy around the world. It is estimated that during the past 150 years especially, the average life expectancy at birth increased by several decades globally.[4] The rise in life expectancy continues, though currently the increases in the "developing world" are much faster and larger than in the "developed world."[5] There is no ceiling yet seen or foreseen for this increase. An ever growing proportion of the life expectancy rise is attributable to advances of biomedical technology, rather than mere hygiene.[6] Still, closing the gaps in life expectancy and in access to medical technologies, within particular societies and between societies, remains a grand challenge.[7] The rise in human life expectancy is not a "law of nature" either, it is not inevitable or to be taken for granted, it also can be negatively affected by inner disorder, adverse external environment or bad medicine. The things that can be fixed can also be broken, and vice versa. Yet, the possibility of a significant, even radical, rise in life expectancy appears to be proven beyond any doubt.

Perhaps the greatest source of hope is the rapid development of therapeutic means for life extension. The primary proofs of feasibility are based on the successful cases of life extension experimentally achieved in animal models and the development of new intervention techniques, based on the ever better elucidation of the mechanisms of aging. For example, there were proposed several arrays of presumed major determinants of aging and pathways toward their counteraction, based on empirical evidence in cell, tissue and animal models, and even some initial human indications. Some examples of such arrays include the SENS program (Strategies for Engineered Negligible Senescence),[8] the NIH Geroscience priority research areas,[9] and the "hallmarks of aging."[10] Notably, these sets of major aging determinants and countermeasures tend to focus on research and intervention at the cellular and molecular levels, with relatively little attention paid to the systemic regulatory level of aging. Addressing the regulatory mechanisms may perhaps be the next big frontier of life extension research and development.[11] That is to say, having created the necessary technological tools to tackle the basic molecular mechanisms of aging, it may then become necessary to learn to coordinate, dose and calibrate the use of those tools. Nonetheless, despite the challenges, there are now clear proofs of practical technological feasibility of intervention into aging processes and lifespan modification.

These feasibility proofs for aging modification and lifespan intervention are a part of the more general and very encouraging trend of the rapid development of biomedical technologies. This rapid general progress of biomedical science and technology gives hope, but also breeds concerns, mainly the concerns over safety, efficacy and availability of potential interventions. Hopefully the potential drawbacks can be avoided, while the benefits can be brought to fruition and enjoyed to the fullest by the largest possible number of people. But in any case, the fact of progress in scientific, technological and medical capabilities is difficult to deny. For example, consider the amount of progress made since the positing of the cellular theory of immunity by the founder of gerontology Elie Metchnikoff in the late nineteenth century (slightly more than 100 years ago) until the beginning of synthesis of the first prototypes of artificial immune cells recently.[12] Aging and longevity research has always been an integral part of this progress, and moreover, several important biomedical technologies and therapies, such as probiotic diets, hormone replacement therapy and cell therapy, were born out of aging and longevity research.[13] There are grounds to hope for a continuation of this tendency, for its reinforcement, rather than its cancellation or reversal.

In fact, the recent progress in technology (including biomedical technology) has been so vast and rapid that some authors spoke of "exponential acceleration" of technological development, due to technologies' convergence and cross-fertilization, improved communication and computational capabilities.[14] Yet, even with less optimistic and uncertain forecasts, assuming the speed of technological development to continue at least as fast as it was for the last century and a half, and at least for a comparable time in the future – we may expect dramatic improvements in biomedical technological capabilities and their distribution. Of course, reaching truly effective, safe and widely available anti-aging and life-extending capabilities may still be a long way off. Their actual achievement, as well as their safety, efficacy and affordability, especially at the initial stages of application, may remain some of the main potential problems to be overcome. Still, the principal feasibility of a significant human life expectancy and lifespan extension by scientific and technological means appears to be evident. But do we want this extension, if it were possible? Is it generally desirable? In other words, is life extension "a good thing"? What would we use it for and who would use it? The scientific and technological feasibility assessment opens the door for the ethical desirability assessment.

Q: Is healthy life extension a good thing?

A: Quite surprisingly (at least for the proponents of healthy longevity), for decades and centuries, there has been expressed strong opposition to the very idea of life extension. The opposition has been frequent among philosophers, and even among physicians and researchers of aging. There has been a strong tendency among well-established physicians and scholars to consider aging as inexorable and therefore "normal," and to see the lifespan as fixed and immutable. Accordingly, any attempts to "meddle" with the aging process or to significantly extend longevity would be considered foolish, futile and even somehow unethical. A host of ethical and societal problems contingent on life extension were hypothesized by the doubters of this pursuit.[15] Their arguments have often substituted the terms, opposing "immortality" or "indefinite life extension" as a way to imply the undesirability of *any* significant longevity extension, even healthy longevity. This implied the general undesirability of the development of medical technologies for longevity extension. Of course, it is necessary to note that the contrary view, namely that the pursuit of life extension is possible and desirable, has also been a persistent and highly respectable ethical and medical tradition. It was upheld, among others, by a founder of modern hygiene – Christoph Wilhelm Hufeland (1762-1836), the founder of therapeutic endocrinology – Charles-Édouard Brown-Séquard (1817-

31

1894), the founder of geriatrics – Ignatz Leo Nascher (1863-1944), the founder of gerontology – Elie Metchnikoff (1845-1916) and many more.[16] Yet, so far the intellectual stream purporting to oppose the possibility and desirability of a significant life extension has been by far the more dominant. The apparent weight of authority of the critics and skeptics, and the wide popularity of the skeptical views, may again emphasize the question: "Is increasing longevity, especially healthy longevity, really desirable, for the individual or the society?"

The answer that may be given by the proponents of life extension is very simple: "YES. People want to live longer and to liver healthier." Or to put it even more bluntly, "it is better to be healthy, wealthy, wise and long-lived, than otherwise." And that may conclude the discussion. Yet, some explanations and arguments are still required. Usually, the arguments against extending longevity are standard and are refutable in standard ways. Some of these "golden standards" are briefly presented below. These arguments have been adduced and countered in the relevant ethical literature.[17] Indeed, almost any person, anywhere in the world, reflecting for a short time on the possibilities of human life extension, comes up with most of these concerns, and if reflecting or debating a little longer arrives at most of the refutations. The questions and answers below may provide a short summary of such debates.

Q: Would extending longevity enhance human suffering, or conversely, is death a solution against suffering?

A: No. Death is not a solution against suffering. Suffering is not inevitable. Human beings have the ability to actively influence their fate and relieve suffering. And essentially, the desire to extend life does not imply a desire to prolong suffering, but a desire to prolong health (increase the healthspan).

Q: Would extending longevity lead to extending boredom?

A: Arguably no, as extended life also implies extended ability to learn and change. The sense of boredom does not necessarily depend on the period, and often comes and goes periodically. And generally, the feeling of boredom does not seem to be a sufficient reason to abandon the pursuit of life. And if it is (for some people) – their choices are in their hands, and should not diminish the choices and chances of others.

Q: Would extending longevity make human life meaningless?

A: Arguably no, as life may carry a meaning of its own, independent of death. It is difficult or even impossible to place a temporal limit on the meaning, love and enjoyment of life. Human beings are entitled to choose a prolonged existence, and that choice and pursuit alone may give their life meaning.

Q: Would not extending longevity stop progress, make individuals and societies stagnant?

A: Rather to the contrary, the potential for learning will be increased by longer life-spans, and such a prolonged "cultural adaptation" may be sufficient and necessary for the survival of the society. Moreover, rationally controlled development and care for the survival of the weak may be more advantageous for progress than blind and cruel Darwinian selection.

Q: Are not aging and death from aging natural and inevitable? Does not their acceptance as natural and inevitable give comfort in facing them?

A: Concerning the inexorable "natural" limit to the human life, however comforting a reconciliation with death may be, it should not replace an active quest for life preservation. Almost never is a particular cause of death completely "inevitable," but is always due to some identifiable material agent, and thus subject to prevention or amelioration. There is no limit "set in stone" to either the lifespan or the healthspan.

Q: Would not there be a problem of "identity" when extending life? In other words, would the incessant transformations of the body and mind permit us to speak of a long-term preservation of identity?

A: During a prolonged life history, there may be a continuity of human existence. Or else, some "core" personal pattern may be preserved, while various extensions and additions to it may develop in time.[18]

Q: Would not the life-extending means be made available only for the rich and powerful, or some other select groups? How can we prevent this injustice?

A: Indeed, perhaps the most frequent type of worry relates to the future availability of resources due to life extension. The common assumption is that 'there will never be enough for everybody.' This assumption has taken the form of two major related concerns: 'longevity will only be available for the rich' and 'overpopulation will happen due to extending longevity.' Referring to the availability of resources, a very strong and persistent apprehension has been about the potentially unequal and selective access to life-extending technologies. Of all the possible concerns and challenges of human life extension, this is probably one of the most likely and disturbing, seeing the present inequalities in the access to health care.[19] Would then the extension of life only be made accessible for the rich and powerful? Would such preferential access for select groups be justifiable or inevitable? Would not such a fundamental disparity in the ability to survive threaten the very fabric of social coherence, when the society will be filled with constant resentment and struggle? It has been asserted that the inability to provide a good to all people should not prevent providing it to some people.[20] Yet, such assertions may offer little consolation to people doomed to an early death by their social status. The inequality of access to medical means and technologies, and hence the unequal possibilities for lifespan and healthspan extension, appears to be a real danger. This danger is already here, manifesting in the present unequal access to health care, and is not necessarily reserved to future technologies. This danger needs to be recognized and a wide and equitable sharing of medical technologies, both the present and emerging ones, needs to become a primary social objective.

When addressing this concern, the upper class life-extensionists often reassure that the life-extending treatments will eventually be made cheaper as the technologies develop, and they will 'trickle down' to the poor from the rich. Moreover, the rich may allow such treatments to the poor as they are interested to maintain 'active and healthy workforce.' Hence, in this type of social agreement, for the poor, a chance to obtain the treatments may only be contingent on their utility as 'workforce,' and if they have no such utility (for example, if the labor needs are already fulfilled, also from robotics), there are absolutely no incentives and no obligations to provide them with the life-extending treatments. Hence, at least for the initial stages of therapy development, the following options may be available for people of lesser means: 1) Wait patiently until the therapies will 'become cheaper' and/or 'trickle down' from the rich; 2) Fight for the right of access (perhaps also violently); 3) Advocate for universal public research, development and distribution programs for life-extending and health-extending therapies, that will also give the public strong entitlement to such therapies. The third option appears preferable. Yet, in any case, the inequality of access does not seem to be a reason to hinder the emergence of new medical technologies, but only to intensify their development. The sooner they emerge, the faster they will likely become available for the people, hopefully for all.

Q: Would not extending longevity lead to shortage of resources for the society, or "overpopulation"?

34

A: It has been a persistent fear that extending longevity would lead to a shortage of resources for the global population as a whole due to its unsustainable increase. This scenario is also commonly known as 'the problem of overpopulation due to life extension.' Yet, it must be argued that the term "overpopulation" does not simply relate to the number of people on a certain territory. Rather, it indicates the degree of availability of resources, especially food, for people at that territory. And, based on the available evidence and trends of development, scarcity of resources should not be anticipated as a result of increasing longevity. It was calculated already in the 1960s by the Agricultural Economics Research Institute, Oxford, that the agricultural productivity, even at that time, would be more than sufficient to feed 45 billion people globally.[21] Since that time the agricultural capabilities in the developed countries increased dramatically, way ahead of increases in life expectancy or population.[22] The technological capabilities are here to feed the world. Then, why are there still famines? It often happens because of mismanagement or because the right technologies are not applied.[23] But technologies generally, or life-extending technologies in particular, should not be considered a cause of overpopulation or shortage of resources. On the contrary, in wealthy, technologically advanced countries, with high life expectancy, there are hardly any signs of "overpopulation" or shortage of resources. "Overpopulation" is often the problem of poorer, "developing" countries that overcompensate for high mortality (low life expectancy) with high birth rates, and that have limited access to medical and technological means to provide for the population increase. Hence, also in those countries, the way to combat overpopulation may be by increasing life expectancy, and the concomitant quality of life, medical and technological capabilities, not by decreasing them. Indeed, longevity (life expectancy) is an indispensable part of the Human Development Index, and it correlates with and synergistically reinforces its other parts, such as education and quality of life.[24] One may argue that even at diminishing resources, the prolongation of human life may be valuable and desirable. Yet, the most likely concomitant of extended longevity is rather abundance and not scarcity, as the same types of technologies that improve agricultural, technological and medical capabilities, are also instrumental for increasing the lifespan and healthspan.

Q: Would not increasing life quantity mean decreasing life quality? In other words, wouldn't we have "too many old sick people"?

A: Arguably, the perception of the life of the elderly person as a "liability" to the person or to the society is ethically questionable, and the preservation of life may be desirable even at some loss of life quality. Yet, it must be emphasized that the improvement in life quantity is commonly (though not always) inseparable from the improvement in life quality. A robust organism (similar to a robust machine) as a rule both operates efficiently and for longer periods of time. The same mechanisms that improve health, also improve longevity. A good example is centenarians, who enjoy both exceptional longevity as well as quality of life, preserved mental and physical ability, almost to the end of their lives.[25] This is a model worth attempting to imitate or even improve on. Still, there is an evidently increasing incidence of aging-related diseases, following increasing life expectancy. Yet, this increasing incidence is not a reason to stop biomedical research and development, especially for the amelioration of aging-related degeneration – the main cause of disease and disability in the aged, but to intensify this research and development. The advancement of this research and development is perhaps the only practical way to alleviate the aging-related suffering and improve healthy and productive longevity for the elderly population. Essentially, it is the extension of the human healthspan (healthy and productive lifespan) and not just of the lifespan that is pursued in the research and development of new medical means and technologies.

Q: Would the new life-extending technologies be safe and effective?

A: This is a critically important scientific question. The responsible and active research and development will help answer it. It is quite possible that the emerging anti-aging and life-extending therapies may not be as effective as anticipated or may be even unsafe, at least at their initial stages of development and application. The efficacy and safety of any new medical treatment are essential scientific and public concerns and they need to be addressed through rigorous study, through the development of and adherence to strict scientific criteria for efficacy and safety. Compliant with such criteria, new anti-aging and life-extending therapies may be highly desirable and beneficial commodities.

Q: What should be done to extend one's life? What should be done to develop the means to achieve healthy life extension?

A: Given the feasibility and desirability of the pursuit of healthy life extension, we enter the realm of normative suggestions and actions. What is it exactly that we need to do to achieve something that we desire and may have a chance to achieve, if not for ourselves then for our loved ones? What should we do to facilitate the emergence and availability of life-extending therapies? These are critical questions of public policy, in particular healthcare and science policy, and they need to be raised in the public arena. Clearly, particular regulatory, organizational and policy frameworks will yet need to be developed for the efforts to achieve healthy life extension for the population. It may be yet too early to provide detailed regulatory and policy recommendations toward this achievement. Yet, some preliminary suggestions may be offered. These may include increased funding, incentives and institutional support for research and development deliberately directed toward alleviation of the degenerative aging process and for healthy life extension.[26] More specific policies should be elaborated thanks to increased public and academic involvement and debate.[27] However, these are also questions of personal responsibility, and each person should study, think and decide for oneself and make personally feasible plans to facilitate the achievement of these goals.

Q: What are the main obstacles slowing down progress in the development of anti-aging and life-extending therapies? What would be the best way to overcome them?

A: The main obstacle is perhaps the immense scientific difficulty of the problem itself. Aging is an extremely complex process, with many uncertainties. Hence, any potential attempts at intervention will yet require a vast amount of careful thought and effort. This does not mean that such attempts should be abandoned. On the contrary – we need to tackle the problem, "not because it is easy, but because it is hard." The payoff from its solution would be too great to abandon. But we need to admit that the problem is difficult and therefore its solution will require strong efforts. People would need to make such efforts, and they are not always willing or ready to make them. Hence one of the major bottlenecks is perhaps the general deficit in the ability or willingness of many people to invest time, effort, money and thought for the development of healthspan and lifespan extending therapies and technologies. Clearly, the more people become supportive and involved for their development, the more resources are intelligently and productively invested in it, the faster the technologies will arrive and the wider will be their availability.

There may be many reasons why such massive involvement and support have not been happening as strongly as the healthy longevity enthusiasts would hope for. One reason may be a common mental or emotional block against such therapies – many people simply do not believe that ameliorating degenerative aging and healthy life extension are possible or even beneficial, and hence they are unwilling to get involved in the impossible and undesirable tasks. It is the duty of healthy longevity advocates to convince people that these tasks are scientifically feasible and humanely desirable – and they have all the necessary arguments and data to prove it. Yet, more worrying may be the people who already admit that the combat of aging and healthy life extension are feasible, but they still do not invest any (or any significant) intellectual or material resources to achieve these goals. The main reasons for this inaction may be that they do not see immediate or fast benefits or profits for themselves, or are preoccupied with making a living (why pursue some distant goals, when one and one's family need to survive tomorrow?) or are generally apathetic. Hence a major bottleneck is this transition from a theoretical "belief" or "understanding" into a practical action and support. Presumably, this transition can be facilitated by creating tangible incentives for people to get involved, such as jobs and grants for researchers, advocates and educators in the field, and improved institutional and social status for the field. These are largely issues of state-level public health and research policy, and they may be advanced by more political involvement. But these are also issues of individual persuasion, a person after a person. Even if it may be difficult or even impossible to convince most people to make longevity research and advocacy their main priority, without appropriate immediate material and social benefits and incentives, hopefully many could be convinced to dedicate at least a tiny bit of their time, effort, thought and money to this worthy long-term goal.

Q: What suggestions should be made to people who want to get involved in longevity research and advocacy, but don't know where to start?

A: The main advice for people who want to get involved in longevity research and advocacy is just: "Start getting involved" – pick yourself up and start studying, thinking and working for the cause. This may sound trivial, but this is exactly the problem of transition from theoretical "understanding" and "wishes" to practical action. Many people remain in the theoretical "wishing" stage. But if there is a sincere heart-felt "wish" – there can be many practical "ways" that can be quickly found and pursued. First of all, the person should become better acquainted with the field, study it, even at the popular level. There are now plenty of online resources. If there is sufficient motivation, one may consider an academic study course or professional carrier in the area or related areas, depending on the possibilities at hand. But for the first "acquaintance" stage, just getting some familiarity with longevity science can initiate a person into the field. Such increased interest and knowledge, combined from many people, may raise the demand for therapies that may in turn improve the offer.

Another basic way to start is to band with others. There are now extensive possibilities to join others with a similar interest, ranging from discussions with friends to more formal live and online study groups to joining networks and public associations of supporters of longevity science. Communication with like-minded people can catalyze joint focus groups, research or outreach projects. The most tangible products of such communication could be individual and joint publications (online or in print) and meetings (online or live), or even concrete research and technological outcomes – which may in turn instigate further waves of interest and involvement. There are now expanding possibilities to participate, volunteer and assist in research, donate to or join existing academic and public organizations involved in longevity research and advocacy. There are now also increasing possibilities to participate in "crowd-sourcing" and "crowd-funding" campaigns and projects. If there are no such possibilities yet in one's area or country, one may consider creating such organizations, campaigns and projects themselves, even in a small scale.

And of course, anyone could endeavor to research and practice a healthy, life-prolonging life-style (such as moderate exercise, moderate and balanced nutrition, and sufficient rest and sleep), to improve one's chances to benefit from effective, safe and accessible life-extending technologies whenever they may arrive. This may also sound trivial, but this could also be an attractive way of initiation, with immediate practical benefits, yet with an eye for the future.

These pieces of advice may not seem very specific. It seems yet impossible to more specifically state: Do this regimen, study this text, join this organization, vote to advance this legislation, or support this project – and your and everybody else's healthy longevity is guaranteed! It is unlikely that anyone can be that specific, given the current imperfect state of knowledge, and the diversity of situations and approaches. Yet anyone and everybody should be encouraged to become more interested, knowledgeable, communicative and active in the field, according to their personal wishes and possibilities. From our cumulative actions, not necessarily coordinated, we may have a better chance to create the necessary "gradient" toward our common goal of extending healthy longevity.

References and notes

1. Various historical perceptions of the lifespan limit are discussed in Ilia Stambler, *A History of Life-Extensionism in the Twentieth Century* (2014), in particular in Chapter 4, in the sections "Theories of Aging" and "Rectifying 'Discord' and conserving 'Vital Capital'" and *passim* throughout the book (Ilia Stambler, *A History of Life-Extensionism in the Twentieth Century*, Longevity History, 2014, http://www.longevityhistory.com/).

Below are some of the notable works in the relatively recent history of these debates. Interestingly, even when positing a limit to a species-specific, particularly human, maximum lifespan (under particular internal biological organization and external environmental conditions), the authors do acknowledge that these internal and environmental parameters can be modified, especially through biomedical interventions into fundamental aging processes. See:

Nathan Keyfitz, "What difference would it make if cancer were eradicated? An examination of the Taeuber Paradox," *Demography*, 14(4), 411-418, 1977; Nathan Keyfitz, "Improving life expectancy: An uphill road ahead," *American Journal of Public Health*, 68, 954-956, 1978;

Arthur Schatzkin, "How long can we live? A more optimistic view of potential gains in life expectancy," *American Journal of Public Health*, 70, 1199-1200, 1980;

James F. Fries, Lawrence M. Crapo, *Vitality and Aging. Implications of the Rectangular Curve*, W.H. Freeman and Co., New York, 1981;

James F. Fries, "Aging, Natural Death, and the Compression of Morbidity," *The New England Journal of Medicine*, 303, 130-135, 1980;

Edward L. Schneider, Jacob A. Brody, "Aging, natural death and the compression of morbidity: Another view," *The New England Journal of Medicine*, 309, 854-856, 1983;

J. Michael McGinnis, "The limits of prevention," *Public Health Reports*, 100, 255-260, 1985;

S. Jay Olshansky, Bruce A. Carnes, *The Quest for Immortality. Science at the Frontiers of Aging*, W.W. Norton and Co., New York, 2001.

2. Richard P. Feynman, "What Is and What Should be the Role of Scientific Culture in Modern Society," presented at the Galileo Symposium in Florence, Italy, in 1964, in Richard P. Feynman, *The Pleasure of Finding Things Out: The Best Short Works of Richard P. Feynman*, Perseus Books, NY, 1999, p. 100.

3. Michael R. Rose, *Evolutionary Biology of Aging*, Oxford University Press, Oxford, 1991;

Richard Cutler, "Evolution of human longevity and the genetic complexity governing aging rate," *Proceedings of the National Academy of Sciences USA*, 72(11), 4664-4668, 1975, https://www.ncbi.nlm.nih.gov/pmc/articles/PMC388784/;

Anca Iovita, *The Aging Gap Between Species*, Longevity Letter, 2015, http://longevityletter.com/.

4. James C. Riley, *Rising Life Expectancy: A Global History*, Cambridge University Press, Cambridge, 2001.

5. World Health Organization, *World Health Statistics 2014: Large gains in life expectancy*, 2014, http://www.who.int/mediacentre/news/releases/2014/world-health-statistics-2014/en/.

6. Stephen J. Kunitz, "Medicine, mortality, and morbidity," in William F. Bynum, Roy Porter (Eds.), *Companion Encyclopedia of the History of Medicine*, Routledge, London and New York, 2001, pp. 1693-1711.

7. David Ansell, *The Death Gap: How Inequality Kills*, University of Chicago Press, 2017.

8. Aubrey D.N.J. de Grey, Michael Rae, *Ending Aging. The Rejuvenation Breakthroughs That Could Reverse Human Aging in Our Lifetime*, St. Martin's Press, New York, 2007;

SENS Research Foundation, "A Reimagined Research Strategy for Aging," accessed June 2017, http://www.sens.org/research/introduction-to-sens-research/.

9. Healthspan Campaign, "NIH Geroscience Interest Group (GSIG) Releases Recommendations from the October 2013 Advances in Geroscience Summit," 2013, http://www.healthspancampaign.org/2014/02/27/nih-geroscience-interest-group-gsig-releases-recommendations-october-2013-advances-geroscience-summit/;

Brian K. Kennedy, Shelley L. Berger, Anne Brunet, Judith Campisi, Ana Maria Cuervo, Elissa S. Epel, Claudio Franceschi, Gordon J. Lithgow, Richard I. Morimoto, Jeffrey E. Pessin, Thomas A. Rando, Arlan Richardson, Eric E. Schadt, Tony Wyss-Coray, Felipe Sierra, "Geroscience: linking aging to chronic disease," *Cell*, 59(4), 709-713, 2014, http://www.cell.com/cell/fulltext/S0092-8674(14)01366-X.

10. Carlos López-Otín, Maria A. Blasco, Linda Partridge, Manuel Serrano, Guido Kroemer, "The hallmarks of aging," *Cell*, 153(6), 1194-1217, 2013, http://www.cell.com/cell/fulltext/S0092-8674(13)00645-4.

11. Alan A. Cohen, "Complex systems dynamics in aging: new evidence, continuing questions," *Biogerontology*, 17(1), 205-220, 2016, https://www.ncbi.nlm.nih.gov/pmc/articles/PMC4723638/;

David Blokh, Ilia Stambler, "The application of information theory for the research of aging and aging-related diseases," *Progress in Neurobiology*, S0301-0082(15)30059-9, 2016, doi: http://dx.doi.org/10.1016/j.pneurobio.2016.03.005.

12. Ilia Stambler, "Elie Metchnikoff – the founder of longevity science and a founder of modern medicine: In honor of the 170th anniversary," *Advances in Gerontology*, 28(2), 207-217, 2015 (Russian), 5(4), 201-208, 2015 (English).

13. Ilia Stambler, "The unexpected outcomes of anti-aging, rejuvenation, and life extension studies: an origin of modern therapies," *Rejuvenation Research*, 17(3), 297-305, 2014.

14. Ray Kurzweil, *The Singularity Is Near: When Humans Transcend Biology*, Penguin Books, New York, 2005.

15. A partial list of authors and works ostensibly opposing the idea of a significant life extension on ethical grounds, due to various hypothesized negative social and personal outcomes, includes the following. Of course, the list can be greatly expanded.

Thomas Malthus, *An Essay on the Principle of Population, as it Affects the Future Improvement of Society with Remarks on the Speculations of Mr. Godwin, M. Condorcet, and Other Writers*, J. Johnson, London, 1798, reprinted in Project Gutenberg, http://www.gutenberg.org/files/4239/4239-h/4239-h.htm;

William Osler, "Farewell address on leaving the Johns Hopkins University" (1905), *Scientific American*, March 25, 1905, reproduced in full in Stanley Hall, *Senescence, the Last Half of Life*, D. Appleton & Company, New York, 1922, pp. 3-5;

Morris Fishbein, *The Medical Follies*, Boni and Liveright, New York, 1925;

Bertrand Russell, "The Menace of Old Age" (1931), pp. 18-20, "On Euthanasia" (1934), pp. 267-268, in Bertrand Russell, *Mortals and Others, American Essays 1931-1935, Volumes I and II*, Routledge Classics, London and New York, 2009 (first published in 1975);

Bertrand Russell, "How to Grow Old" (written in 1944), in Bertrand Russell, *Portraits from Memory: And Other Essays*, Simon and Schuster, New York, 1956, pp. 50-53;

Norbert Wiener, *God and Golem, Inc. A Comment on Certain Points where Cybernetics Impinges on Religion*, The MIT Press, Cambridge, Massachusetts, 1964, pp. 66-67;

Frank Macfarlane Burnet, *The Biology of Aging*, Auckland University Press, Auckland NZ, 1974, pp. 63, 66;

Leonard Hayflick, "Address to the Select Committee on Aging, Washington, Feb, 1978," quoted in William G. Bailey, *Human Longevity from Antiquity to the Modern Lab*, Greenwood Press, Westport CN, 1987, p. ix;

Leonard Hayflick, "'Anti-aging' is an oxymoron," *Journal of Gerontology*, 59(6), B573-578, 2004;

Leonard Hayflick, *How and Why we Age*, Ballantine Books, NY, 1994, "No More Aging: Blessing or Nightmare?" pp. 336-338;

Leon Kass, "L'Chaim and Its Limits: Why Not Immortality?" *First Things*, 113, 17-24, May 2001;

Daniel Callahan, *What Price Better Health? Hazards of the Research Imperative*, University of California Press, Berkeley, 2003, Ch. 3. "Is research a moral obligation? The war against death," pp. 64-66;

Koïchiro Matsuura, "Of sheep and men," *The Daily Star*, 4(113), September 16, 2003;

Francis Fukuyama, *Our Posthuman Future. Consequences of the Biotechnological Revolution*, Picador, New York, 2002, Ch. 4. "The prolongation of life," pp. 57-71;

Michael Shermer, "The Immoralist," *Science*, 332(6025), 40, 2011;

Ezekiel J. Emanuel, "Why I hope to die at 75," *The Atlantic*, October 2014.

16. Ilia Stambler, "Has aging ever been considered healthy?" *Frontiers in Genetics*, 6, 00202, 2015, http://journal.frontiersin.org/article/10.3389/fgene.2015.00202/full;

Ilia Stambler, *A History of Life-Extensionism in the Twentieth Century*, Longevity History, 2014, http://www.longevityhistory.com/.

17. Some of the ethical works countering anti-life-extensionist arguments include:

Robert Veatch, *Death, Dying, and the Biological Revolution. Our Last Quest for Responsibility*, Yale University Press, New Haven CT, 1977, Ch. 8. "Natural death and public policy," pp. 293-305;

John Harris, "Immortal Ethics," presented at the International Association of Biogerontologists (IABG) 10th Annual Conference "Strategies for Engineered Negligible Senescence," Queens College, Cambridge, UK, September 17-24, 2003, reprinted in Aubrey de Grey (Ed.), *Strategies for Engineered Negligible Senescence: Why Genuine Control of Aging May Be Foreseeable, Annals of the New York Academy of Sciences*, 1019, 527-534, June 2004;

Christine Overall, *Aging, Death, and Human Longevity: A Philosophical Inquiry*, University of California Press, Berkeley CA, 2003;

Frida Fuchs-Simonstein, *Self-evolution: The Ethics of Redesigning Eden*, Yozmot, Tel Aviv, 2004;

Richard A. Miller, "Extending life: scientific prospects and political obstacles," *The Milbank Quarterly: A multidisciplinary journal of population health and health policy*, 80(1), 155-174, 2002;

James Hughes, *Citizen Cyborg: Why Democratic Societies Must Respond to the Redesigned Human of the Future*, Westview Press, Cambridge MA, 2004, "Living longer," pp. 23-32;

Sebastian Sethe, João Pedro de Magalhães, "Ethical Perspectives in Biogerontology," in Maartje Schermer, Wim Pinxten (Eds.), *Ethics, Health Policy and (Anti-) Aging: Mixed Blessings*, Springer, Dordrecht, 2012, pp. 173-188.

18. Ilia Stambler, "Life extension – a conservative enterprise? Some fin-de-siècle and early twentieth-century precursors of transhumanism," *Journal of Evolution and Technology*, 21, 13-26, 2010, http://jetpress.org/v21/stambler.htm, http://jetpress.org/v21/stambler.pdf;

Ilia Stambler, "Life-Extensionism as a Pursuit of Constancy," Institute for Ethics and Emerging Technologies (IEET), August 18, 2015, https://ieet.org/index.php/IEET2/more/stambler20150818;

Ilia Stambler, *A History of Life-Extensionism in the Twentieth Century*, Longevity History, 2014, http://www.longevityhistory.com/.

19. Angus Deaton, "Health, inequality, and economic development," *Journal of Economic Literature*, 41(1), 113-158, 2003.

20. John Harris, "Immortal Ethics," presented at the International Association of Biogerontologists (IABG) 10th Annual Conference "Strategies for Engineered Negligible Senescence," Queens College, Cambridge, UK, September 17-24, 2003, reprinted in Aubrey de Grey (Ed.),

Strategies for Engineered Negligible Senescence: Why Genuine Control of Aging May Be Foreseeable, Annals of the New York Academy of Sciences, 1019, 527-534, June 2004.

21. Colin Clark, "Agricultural productivity in relation to population," in Gordon Wolstenholme (Ed.), *Man and His Future: A CIBA Foundation Volume*, Gordon, Little, Brown and Co., Boston, 1963, pp. 23-35.

According to this work, the ability to feed at least 45 billion people a year globally, even with the agricultural capabilities of the 1960s, was based on the following simple assumptions and calculations:

"Our land requirements, using the best agricultural methods now available – though great further improvements will be possible" are 1800 square meters/person or 5.5 persons/hectare, when allowing for an average food requirement of "500 kilograms per person per year or 1,370 grams per person per day." Notably, in 1960, about the time *Man and His Future* was published, the yield of wheat in the UK was ~3.5 ton per hectare (3,500 kilograms dry weight grain per 10,000 square meters). Allowing for the 500 kg of food per person per year (1,370 g per person per day) to come exclusively from nutritious crops, that yield would very roughly suffice for 7 people per hectare to be fed from a single harvest, equivalent to ~1400 square meters per person. Allowing for additional milk and meat consumption would somewhat increase the land requirements, though the land resources would nonetheless be quite sufficient. According to the author's estimate, "The world has the equivalent of 6,600 million hectares of good agricultural land." With the addition of potential agricultural land in the wet tropics of Africa, Latin America and Asia, "we must have 8,200 million hectares in all, capable of giving a diet containing meat and dairy products on a North American scale to 45,000 million people."

The estimated area of usable agricultural land in the world of "8,200 million hectares" (82 million square kilometers) is approximately half of the Earth's dry land area (~148.94 million square kilometers), out of ~510.072 million square kilometers of the entire Earth surface area, including the water surface. Thus, further amelioration of the dry land, developing ocean farming, and further increases of agricultural yields and new technologies for biomass and food production – may dispel the fears of food shortage completely.

22. For example, the yield of wheat in the UK increased from 3,500 kg per hectare in 1960 to 8,000 kg per hectare in 2000 (128% increase). At the same 40 year period, the increase of population in the UK was just 15% (from 52 million to 60 million) and the increase in life expectancy was 10% (from 70.85 to 78.04 years). In 2011, the world's greatest yield of cereal grains generally was almost 19,000 kg per hectare, and was achieved in Oman.

Based on: Food and Agriculture Organization of the United Nations, FAOSTAT, 2013, http://faostat.fao.org/site/567/DesktopDefault.aspx?PageID=567#ancor; Human Mortality Database, University of California, Berkeley & Max Planck Institute for Demographic Research, 2013, http://www.mortality.org/.

23. Peter Walker, *Famine Early Warning Systems: Victims and Destitution*, Earthscan Publications Ltd, London, 1989.

24. Ilia Stambler, "The pursuit of longevity – The bringer of peace to the Middle East," *Current Aging Science*, 6, 25-31, 2014.

25. Sofiya Milman, Nir Barzilai, "Dissecting the mechanisms underlying unusually successful human health span and life span," *Cold Spring Harbor Perspectives in Medicine*, 6(1), a025098, 2015; Natalia S. Gavrilova, Leonid A. Gavrilov, "Search for mechanisms of exceptional human longevity," *Rejuvenation Research*, 13(2-3), 262-264, 2010.

26. Kunlin Jin, James W. Simpkins, Xunming Ji, Miriam Leis, Ilia Stambler, "The critical need to promote research of aging and aging-related diseases to improve health and longevity of the elderly population," *Aging and Disease*, 6, 1-5, 2015, http://www.aginganddisease.org/EN/10.14336/AD.2014.1210.

27. Ilia Stambler, "Recognizing degenerative aging as a treatable medical condition: methodology and policy," *Aging and Disease*, 8(5), 2017, http://www.aginganddisease.org/EN/10.14336/AD.2017.0130; Ilia Stambler, "Human life extension: opportunities, challenges, and implications for public health policy," in Alexander Vaiserman (Ed.), *Anti-aging Drugs: From Basic Research to Clinical Practice*, Royal Society of Chemistry, London, 2017, pp. 535-564.

4. Policy Suggestions for the Promotion of Longevity Research, Development and Treatment

The need to develop policies for healthy longevity promotion

The global society is facing the rapid population aging and the accompanying rise of aging-related ill health and the resulting social problems. This mounting challenge stares us all in the face and prompts the global community to seek remedies. At the same time, we also witness the rapid development of biotechnology and medical technology, fostering our hope to find effective therapeutic solutions to the increasing health challenges. The urgency of the problem, and the increasing possibilities for solutions, bring the issues related to population aging and the research, development and utilization of anti-aging, life-extending and healthspan-extending technologies or "longevity therapies" to the forefront of responsible social debate.[1]

Many pressing normative questions arise in this context. What should we do, as a society and as individuals, given the intensifying problems of aging and the possibility and desirability of their solution and as a result achieving a significant healthy longevity extension? How can this possibility be realized? What actions exactly should be taken? Who should undertake those actions? Who should make the decisions about the actions? And who will enjoy the results of those actions? Could there be undesirable side effects to those actions? Such normative questions translate into specific and urgent questions for public health and science policy. For example, should a greater support be given to basic, empirical, applied, engineering, environmental, or other approaches for the amelioration of degenerative aging processes and achieving healthy longevity? What should be the civic regulatory mechanisms of such support? Given the rapid population aging and the increasing incidence and burden of aging-related diseases, on the pessimistic side, and the rapid development of medical technologies, on the optimistic side, these become critical social challenges and vital questions of social responsibility.

Specific regulatory, organizational and policy frameworks will yet need to be developed to address those questions, in any deliberate effort to achieve healthy longevity for the population. It may be yet too early to provide any strictly specific regulatory and policy recommendations toward this achievement. To provide more thorough recommendations, the issue still needs to be raised more strongly in the public, academic and political discourse. Yet, some preliminary recommendations may be offered. These may include increased funding, incentives and institutional support for research and development specifically directed toward alleviation of the aging process and achieving healthy longevity. Some preliminary recommendations are given in the position paper of the International Society on Aging and Disease (ISOAD), entitled "The Critical Need to Promote Research of Aging and Aging-related Diseases to Improve Health and Longevity of the Elderly Population" (2015).[2] Below some of the suggestions of that position paper are quoted and briefly commented on, with specific reference to funding, incentives and institutional support. It must be emphasized that this list and comments are only preliminary, and are intended to stimulate further discussion, encouraging the academic community, the general public and policy makers to elaborate on the present points and add new ones.

According to the ISOAD position paper, *"Governments should ensure the creation and implementation of the following policies to promote research into the biology of aging and aging-related diseases, for improving the health of the global elderly population."* The following discussion is organized according to the main policy suggestions and their specific points.

Policy suggestion 1: "Funding: Ensuring a significant increase of governmental and non-governmental funding for goal-directed (translational) research in preventing the degenerative aging processes, and the associated chronic non-communicable diseases and disabilities, and for extending healthy and productive life, during the entire life course."

Commentary: The importance of increasing funding for biomedical research to increase its produce should be obvious. The soil should be fertile to bear fruit. Yet, sometimes the fruits (longevity therapies) are expected without infrastructure, investment and labor. One often hears from the critics and bystanders of longevity science: "When will we see the results of this research?" or "When will it become relevant to humans?" To which the longevity research advocate can answer: "Right after the research is given more time, care and support."

Unfortunately, it is often tacitly implied, and sometimes even openly stated, by lay persons and policy makers, that fundamental and translational biological research of aging is somehow wasteful or inherently dangerous, or that the scientists already have 'more than enough' and should not ask for more, or that the research money should be better spent on causes other than "aging-related" ill health (as if there are such "aging-unrelated" causes).[3] Likely as a result of such a dismissive attitude, the funding for aging-related issues generally, and biomedical aging research in particular, has been rather scarce in major international and national health and science support frameworks.[4] This attitude should change if the scientific research of aging is to advance and produce positive results. Increasing research funding should become an explicit and emphatic point of advocacy.

Specific point 1: "Dedicating a designated percentage of budget within relevant ministries, such as ministries of health and/or science, particularly in the divisions concerning research and treatment of non-communicable chronic diseases."

Commentary: Ministries of health and science may seem the natural candidates to provide such funding, but are not the only possible candidates. A thorough search for and outreach to possible providers of funding will be needed. In practical terms, such increases in funding would necessitate painstaking work of research advocates with the relevant decision-makers and stakeholders, also engaging the support of the broader community. In principle, the need to fund medical research of aging *should* be obvious, so obvious that the relevant agencies (such as the ministries of health and science) simply *should* make it a part of their policy. Unfortunately, it is very far from being obvious to many in those agencies. In many cases, the relevant decision-makers are simply not aware of the current research and its capabilities. And even if they are aware, there are quite a few obstacles for making the support of aging research a priority within those agencies, especially if it means shifting some other priorities. It is thus the duty and the task of longevity research advocates, first to explain to the relevant decision-makers the need for research support and then continue pushing for the actual achievement of such support.

The advocates would need to determine the agencies from which funding could be allocated to aging research, find out the possible procedural means to achieve these allocations, and establish contacts to negotiate and eventually achieve them. Presently, most aging research institutions are hardly in the position to hire professional lobbyists or materially support advocacy and public education organizations. The scientists are often simply not aware or dismissive of the benefits of targeted advocacy, and if they are aware of those benefits, they seldom have the time or resources to dedicate to advocacy or public education. But somebody has to do this work.

This work should include *both* "high level advocacy" with professional stakeholders and decision-makers, *and at the same time* also the work at the "grassroots" levels, convincing the "lay public" about the importance of this research. The arguments for increasing support for aging research should be clear and compelling on the professional level. Yet, professionals in various agencies may have priorities of their own even to pay any attention to the convincing arguments. They may need some encouragement to pay attention "from below," from the people for whom the new prospective therapies are eventually intended, in order to intensify the research and development for their sake.

Specific point 2: "Dedicating a specific percentage of the profits of commercial pharmacological, biotechnology and medical technology companies to such research and development."

Commentary: Pharma, biotech and medtech companies may be often reluctant to invest considerable (or any) resources into R&D for the amelioration of degenerative aging processes to extend healthy longevity for the population. There may be several reasons for this reluctance. For one, the companies' management may be often not familiar enough with the current state of aging research, even to consider involvement. And when some familiarity is gained, the investment into developing biomedical treatments of aging may appear to them too high-risk and too long-term to undertake. Anti-aging and healthspan-improving therapies are preventive by their nature, attempting to postpone chronic age-related diseases before they become debilitating. And evidential predictive diagnosis and preventive medicine may appear "bad business" to many in the management – with returns of profits too uncertain. Seeking costly "silver bullets" against chronic diseases, when they are already devastating and therefore create eager demand, may seem more lucrative for the companies – they are "businesses" after all. ("Evidential" is emphasized here, as quackery may appear to some people profitable under any circumstances. It should also be noted that here the term "anti-aging" is used in the sense of "therapeutic amelioration of aging" and not in the sense of any purely cosmetic contrivances or futile struggle against the passage of time.)

Thus, commonly, as cynical as it may sound, the companies may have little incentive and interest to develop evidence-based preventive anti-aging public health measures. They are not the only ones to blame. People's readiness to embark on and adhere to preventive health regimens may be quite low (as experience often teaches). And, in fairness, the anti-aging regimens and methodologies may not yet be validated enough to justify compliance. So it would really make little sense, "business" or otherwise, to invest in developing remedies that will likely not work, and that many people would not use even if they worked.

Nonetheless, the feasibility of developing such preventive means does exist. And a considerable proportion of people (probably including ourselves) may indeed be willing to use such means, when they are proven effective, to diminish suffering from aging-related ill health at an early stage. So "the market" does exist for the companies to become interested. Still, they may not be too quick to rush to invest into the related R&D, but would prefer to pick up and capitalize on ready or nearly ready products, after most of the burden of high risk research and development had already been borne by publicly funded institutions. This does not seem a "fair" attitude, in a sense maximizing profit from bad public health, while not willing to strongly contribute to developing solutions against it. There may be no bad intent, but that is what the lack of investments into preventive health entails.

Is there a way to encourage companies to more responsibly "carry the burden" of anti-aging research and development, for the common benefit? A mandatory obligation for biomedical, biotechnological and pharmaceutical companies to invest some portion of their profits to advance biomedical therapeutic aging research could contribute to a solution. It could help to leverage the enormous material, intellectual and logistic resources of the industry for the healing of humanity's common predicament and for the benefit of all. This would be a kind of a tax on the health industry to facilitate aging-related research and development, either to be performed by the industry itself or in qualified academic, medical and public institutions. The results from such mandatory R&D investment could be partly owned by the companies, and party stipulated to be shared with the public (the exact specifics can be debated and elaborated).

Of course, the terrible specter of "state interference" into "free market" may be raised by such a proposal. Yet, it may be argued that great value may accrue to pharma, biomed and biotech companies from such investment in biomedical aging R&D, as it would allow them: 1) early entrance into a new, untrampled niche; 2) vast potential markets, including early detection and prevention for broad populations; 3) vast demand by the governments and people; 4) fulfilling a social mission; 5) multiple opportunities for developing new products and services, in pharmaceuticals, diagnostics, analytics, early detection, biomedical technology, etc.; 6) providing wellness benefits for the workforce and life insurance companies. The management of some of the health companies may not yet realize those benefits, sticking with the old "silver bullet" quest. The mandatory obligation to dedicate a part of the profits to biomedical aging research and development, may help "initialize" them into the potential benefits of the field, in a sense "lead the horse to the water."

Some authors have argued that regulatory recognition of "aging as a disease" (a treatable medical condition) would almost automatically induce pharma, biomed and biotech industry to develop treatments against this indication.[5] Such an argument seems to be rather simplistic. Even if recognizing "aging as a disease," the development of treatments to "cure it" would still require massive investments of resources that the industry may be unwilling to spend for some of the above reasons. Even evidence-based clinical diagnostic criteria for this "disease" are still lacking,[6] and their very formulation would also require massive research that the industry may not

50

be willing to undertake on its own. On the other hand, mandating the investment of a portion of the profits into such R&D, even a small portion (or with a stipulated minimum), would gently encourage them to take interest in the issue.

Of course, if such a proposition were ever to be discussed in the political and public arena, it would require strong advocacy and public involvement, as such a measure would be unlikely to be initiated by the industry itself, or to fit the current common political agendas. In any case, whether the proposition is ever discussed or not, the increased public interest in developing effective anti-aging and healthspan-improving treatments may, nonetheless, influence the pharma, biotech and biomed in a less direct, but perhaps even a more forceful way. Increasing the expectant and intelligent "customers' base" for effective, safe and affordable preventive aging-ameliorating therapies may leave the industry no choice but to start developing relevant products for them.

Specific point 3: "Establishing relevant research grant programs on a competitive as well as goal-directed basis."

Commentary: The field of biomedical aging research is a prime example of an emerging and converging scientific and technological field, undergoing rapid growth of capabilities thanks to improved communication and interaction between diverse agencies and entities. It combines "competition" when specific agencies "race" to rapidly achieve the highly advantageous healthspan-improving capabilities, as well as "cooperation" as these capabilities are unlikely to be achieved by any separate research entity alone, but only thanks to mutual catalysis and joining forces with others. This combination has been sometimes termed "coopetition" – comprising "cooperation" and "competition." If substantial funding is to be provided by governments to the field of biomedical aging research, it should probably be directed in such a way as to strengthen the "coopetition" capabilities, to encourage both the spirit of excellence and achievement as well as mutual aid and support. Such an inclusive approach should involve as many relevant entities as possible, in order to achieve the fastest beneficial results for the widest community as possible.

Encouraging competition between research institutes will be indispensable, for example through open and competitive R&D tenders and calls for proposals. But cooperation should also be encouraged, for example by issuing calls and tenders to form consortia, specifically for the field of biomedical aging research and development. Such calls and consortia are still rather rare. Alongside the traditional consortia of research institutions, there should also be support for the more novel forms of cooperation, such as "crowd-sourcing" – distributing the research and development tasks among many participants, including "citizen scientists."

While allowing the free competition of ideas, it is also important to understand what we actually want to achieve thanks to the support. Hence, the calls should be goal-directed, with the overarching goal of effective and safe therapeutic intervention into degenerative aging processes and achieving healthy longevity, yet possibly including more specific goals, such as developing evidential clinical diagnostic criteria for degenerative aging, or devising regenerative medicine interventions for age-related tissue degeneration, or designing and testing pharmacological or physical geroprotective medications, or enhancing data-sharing, or improving education in biomedical aging research – altogether furthering the overarching goal.

Of course, "consortia," "goal orientation," "cooperation" and "synergy" should not become synonyms with monopolistic "cartels." Research and development programs, especially governmental programs, may be too often prone to "cronyism" and "favoritism," blocking the development of competing alternative ideas. The vital task of developing aging-ameliorating and healthspan-improving therapies should not fall victim to narrow bureaucratic "exceptionalism" and "selectionism." It is yet unknown which approach may be the most beneficial, fast and effective to achieve the goal of healthy longevity for all. Therefore it appears yet too early to favor any particular approach very strongly. On the other hand, without strong collaborative work to develop specific research approaches and projects, significant advancement may be unlikely. Instead, many entities would each pull resources to themselves, altogether creating teeming chaotic "Brownian" motion, yet without much noticeable gradient of progress. Balanced support of "coopetition" may be needed to encourage both the plurality of ideas and unity of efforts.

The general support for cooperation and competition in biomedical research of aging should also include support for strategic analysis and consultation, to evaluate the promise and judge the evidence of success of various approaches, ideas and efforts, and their combinations. It should also include support for creative education to foster the emergence of new approaches, ideas and efforts, and their combinations.

Specific point 4: "Mandating incremental or factorial increases of such funding."

Commentary: It is necessary to guarantee continuous increase of support for biomedical aging research. The demand for aging therapies will likely grow with the population aging, and it is important to ensure that the funding for their development is not suddenly stopped, or depleted, or

52

redirected, but intensifies in time to supply the growing need. Such a mandated continuous increase could mean, for example, doubling the funding for the field, say, every 2 or 5 years, or negotiating incremental and/or indexed increases of funding at defined periods of time. Such mandated long-term increases would, first of all, require the knowledge or establishment of the baseline for such funding. Such a baseline is often absent and needs to be determined for the very first time, at the country and agency levels. Secondly, it would posit the commitment to continued investments in this research and development.

The exact definition of the field for which such funding should be dedicated can be problematic and a subject of active debate. But as a preliminary guiding principle, the funding should be broadly devoted to biomedical research of aging, specifically directed toward therapeutic intervention into degenerative aging processes to prevent aging-related diseases and to increase healthy longevity. And of course, creating such a specific budget item and ensuring its survival and growth, should not detract from funding other important health research and health care issues.

Policy suggestion 2: "Incentives: Developing and adopting legal and regulatory frameworks that give incentives for goal-directed research and development designed to specifically address the development, registration, administration and accessibility of drugs, medical technologies and other therapies that will ameliorate the aging processes and associated diseases and extend healthy life."

Commentary: Part of the promotion of healthy longevity research could be accomplished not merely by increasing the amounts of financial investments put into the research, but by optimally effective and productive management of the financial investments, combining financial and non-financial rewards for the advancement of the field. This optimization would necessitate the developing and adopting of legal and regulatory frameworks that give incentives for the relevant goal-directed biomedical research and development. Such incentives should accelerate the development, registration, administration and accessibility of drugs, medical technologies and other therapies that will effectively and evidentially ameliorate the aging processes and associated diseases and extend healthy life for the individuals and for the population.

Specific point 1: "Developing criteria for efficacy and safety of geroprotective therapies."

One of the primary specific requirements to develop the incentives for biomedical aging research would be to establish the criteria for the efficacy and safety of geroprotective (anti-aging) therapies. Such commonly agreed criteria are presently lacking. Yet, they appear to be absolutely necessary in order to set up the goals and define the merits that should be rewarded or incentivized. In other words, we need to incentivize and promote treatments that "wok." But what are the signs or criteria that the anti-aging treatments "work" or "can work" successfully? These are not yet established, but they need to be.

There has been recently an intensifying discussion among longevity researchers and advocates about the need to recognize *the degenerative aging process as a treatable medical condition*.[5,6] That would involve recognizing as pathology the systemic aging-related factors that contribute to diseases and frailty. It is assumed that the common recognition of the problem would drive people and resources toward its solution. Yet, it appears that the primary necessary condition for the degenerative aging process to be recognized as a diagnosable and treatable medical condition and therefore an indication for research, development and treatment, is to develop evidence-based diagnostic criteria and definitions for degenerative aging and for the efficacy and safety of potential means against it. Without such scientifically grounded and clinically applicable criteria, the discussions about "treating" or even "curing" degenerative aging will be mere slogans. How can we "treat" or "cure" something that we cannot diagnose?

Interestingly, the clinical definitions of degenerative aging process and the use of drugs and other treatments specifically directed against it, can be fitted, after some reinterpretations, into major existing regulatory and policy frameworks. Thus, WHO's *International Classification of Diseases (ICD-10)* currently already includes the category called "senility," synonymous with "old age" and "senescence" (carrying the code R54).[7] But there are not yet any general symptoms, clinical definitions or test cases of this condition. These may still need to be developed. Furthermore, WHO's *Global Strategy and Action Plan on Ageing and Health (GSAP) - 2016-2020* (November 2015) includes "Strategic objective 5: Improving measurement, monitoring and research on Healthy Ageing," with a clause "5.1: Agree on ways to measure, analyse, describe and monitor Healthy Ageing" (Section 95), which recognizes the need for such agreed measures.[8] Also major regulatory authorities, such as the US Food and Drug Administration (FDA) and the EU European Medicines Agency (EMA) have struggled for the inclusion of elderly subjects in all clinical trials that may be relevant for them, and are beginning to search for clinically applicable definitions of the aging process and its concomitants. Thus, the EMA has been continuously searching for a consensus definition of age-related "frailty" and for criteria for effective and safe interventions against frailty, as well as for the accurate general assessment of medication needs of older persons.[9] The direction at the US FDA appears to be similar. Here too the need for the inclusion of older subjects in all clinical trials that may be relevant for them and the necessity for devising specific criteria for their diagnostic and therapeutic assessment are recognized,[10] including the assessment of therapeutic interventions against aging-related "multi-morbidity."[11] Yet, apparently, these needs have not yet been addressed satisfactorily. There is still no mandatory inclusion of elderly subjects in clinical trials, and no agreed criteria for their diagnostic and therapeutic evaluation, either in the EU or the US, or elsewhere.

Massive and profound consultation of scientists, physicians, policy-makers and other stake-holders will yet be required to develop such diagnostic criteria, as a necessary condition for incentivizing and advancing aging-ameliorating therapy. The consultation should encompass as many authoritative forums as possible. For example, in June 2017, the WHO started a consultation on the development of "essential diagnostics" as a necessary companion for the "essential medicines."[12] It must be realized that both "medicines" and "diagnostics" of degenerative aging are "essential" for global population health. Other authoritative discussion and implementation frameworks may be utilized.

Specific point 2: "Facilitating in silico and animal testing, and ethical safety-enhanced human testing of such therapies."

Commentary: Integrally related to the issue of devising diagnostic criteria for degenerative aging and for the efficacy and safety of anti-aging and healthspan-extending interventions is the facilitation of various modes of testing of such interventions. Indeed, in order to infer formal general criteria of the "effectiveness" of anti-aging therapy, we need to be able to measure the aging processes, and to find out what effects the various interventions actually produce in each particular case and process, in order to make generalizations.

The testing modes may include *in vivo* testing, i.e. testing in the living organism, e.g. in model animals, but also human testing falls under this category. Of special importance for anti-aging and healthspan experiments are long-term tests and tests on old animals and elderly human subjects. Further testing modes may comprise *in vitro* testing, that is, experiments "in glass" or "in a test tube," i.e. outside the living organism, including cell and tissue experiments, with various techniques such as "lab-on-a-chip." There is also *in situ* testing, i.e. in the original condition or place, for example, in the true conditions and place of a biological process (e.g. an *in vitro* test under conditions identical with or closely approximating a living organism, or an *in vivo* test under conditions that are the same or very close with the real living environment), that should be also kept in mind, as often inferences are made between biologically irrelevant or incompatible model systems. And yet another critically important form of testing is *in silico*, that is, using computer modeling of the system behavior, specifically modeling the aging processes and their modifications. Various testing modalities should be advanced simultaneously, feeding back to each other. Unfortunately, each form of testing has its impediments, both scientific and regulatory, that need to be addressed, within ethical bounds.

Thus, among such impediments, *in silico* testing is not yet commonly practiced in biogerontology. There is often a deficit of cross-talk between the fields of gerontology and bioinformatics, often due to deficit of relevant training of specialists in respective fields, even though the dialogue between these fields is constantly increasing. The various *in vitro* testing modes often suffer from logistic obstacles in supply, transportation and utilization of test materials, and deficit of appropriate equipment. Animal testing also frequently faces logistic difficulties and deficits of facilities and equipment. In addition, there are often unfavorable public perceptions and regulatory hurdles for animal trials, and not just in relation to anti-aging research. The perceptions and policies may need to improve for the benefit of aging health research. There is also a demand to develop and disseminate the guidelines for the ethical safety-enhanced human testing of anti-aging, life-extending and healthspan-improving therapies. Such authoritative guidelines are currently rather absent. A further set of incentives may need to be conceived to attract test subjects to participate in anti-aging studies, while protecting their safety, privacy and other benefits.

It should be additionally noted that all the forms and modes of testing are skilled-labor-consuming, time-consuming and cost-consuming. Hence, increased funding is a necessary and primary condition to facilitate any form of testing.

Specific point 3: "Deploying and ensuring geroprotective therapies in the status of adjuvant and life-extending therapies."

Commentary: Drugs and other medical treatments specifically directed against the degenerative aging process are not yet an accepted category in any official pharmacopoeia or regulatory registry. Their inclusion in pharmacopoeias and registries may be possible after the development of scientifically grounded and commonly accepted clinical definitions of degenerative aging, which are currently absent and need to be devised. Yet, after the necessary consultation and development of diagnostic criteria, such treatments can become recognized as a common part of pharmacopoeias and medical regulatory frameworks. In fact, several major regulatory frameworks already have some preliminary conceptual bases for such a recognition, e.g. the recommendation to evaluate drug efficacy specifically for the elderly by the FDA, or the programs to define and treat old-age frailty by the EMA.[9,10] Thus, the development and application of treatments directed against degenerative aging would not require an extraordinary conceptual or administrative leap. Attempts to include specifically anti-aging drugs as common medicines are already under way, with several notable precedents. In the absence of specific regulatory categories for "anti-aging," they "adopt" existing cognate conceptual frameworks. Such preliminary efforts could be intensified and expanded.

A primary example is the approval by the FDA in 2015 of the clinical testing of Metformin, a well known anti-diabetic drug, as the first drug to treat degenerative aging processes, rather than particular diseases or symptoms. This prospective study was called "TAME" – "Targeting Aging with Metformin." Such a therapeutic targeting of the underlying aging processes is envisioned as a plausible way to prevent general age-associated multimorbidity, i.e. to postpone the emergence of several age-related diseases and dysfunctions at once.[11] The effects on the basic aging processes would be evaluated by changes in specific biomarkers of aging, while the clinical effects would be estimated by the postponement of clinical signs of several known age-related diseases (multimorbidity), as well as reduced mortality and a reduction of functional decline. There is yet no common agreement on the most informative biomarkers of aging, and no consensus about the evaluation of multimorbidity and functional decline. Still, such a general evaluation and intervention framework – combining putative biomarkers of aging, recognized clinical age-related disease symptoms and syndromes, and demonstrable functional abilities – seems to provide a fruitful direction to follow and develop. Such and similar general combined evaluation and intervention frameworks could be easily understood and adopted both by biologists and physicians. Even though, as of this writing in 2017, funding for this specific large-scope study has not been secured, the study concept may be seminal.

Another example also stems from 2015, when the FDA approved an adjuvant therapy (the adjuvant MF59, made with squalene oil, developed by Novartis) for a flu vaccine to boost immune response in older persons. This development goes beyond "a drug against a disease" model, but seeks an appropriate regulatory framework to support the underlying health of older persons, using "adjuvant" (i.e. "supportive" or "additional") therapy.[13]

Another approach to develop and advance anti-aging and healthspan and lifespan-extending therapies may be by adopting the concepts of "life-saving therapies" and "life-extending therapies," that are already well established in major regulatory environments, mainly in relation to life-threatening conditions.[14] Logically, the lifespan-extending therapies are indeed "life-extending" and "life-saving."

The adoption of the existing regulatory frameworks and concepts, such as "age-related multimorbidity," "old-age frailty" and "functional decline" to describe the indication, and "adjuvant therapy," "life-extending therapy" and "prevention of frailty and functional decline" to describe the intervention, may be more acceptable psychologically and better grounded in existing policy than speaking about diagnosis and treatment of "aging" itself. Such an adoption of existing frameworks may be so far the most productive and fast way to develop, test and disseminate anti-aging and healthspan-improving therapies. But eventually it may yet be possible to develop and adopt clinical diagnosis and therapeutic interventions specifically for "degenerative aging" proper, provided the necessary clinical evaluation, efficacy and safety criteria. The development and adoption of such criteria will yet require considerable time, intellectual efforts and material resources. Still, we can state the eventual goal of these efforts clearly and emphatically, without hiding, equivocating or circumventing: we do wish to develop evidence-based, safe, effective and available diagnosis and treatment for degenerative aging to increase healthy lifespan.

Specific point 4: "Providing a shortened approval pathway for therapies with high level of efficacy evidence in preclinical and early clinical trials, as well as in cases of advanced degenerative and seemingly futile conditions."

Commentary: There is a special need to give priority to the clinical trials and applications of therapies that had provided excellent evidence for their efficacy and safety in preclinical and early clinical trials. Such a prioritizing and fast-tracking of well-evidenced approaches may help bring effective life-saving therapies and improve the quality of life for as many people as possible, as fast as possible. This requirement for good evidence may hold true for any therapies generally, and for anti-aging and healthspan-improving therapies in particular. Yet, regarding the latter, the question remains what constitutes "evidence" of efficacy and safety for anti-aging and healthspan-improving interventions, when there is yet no formal and agreed clinical definition of aging and of its modification. Hence, the need to prioritize the best evidence-based treatments goes hand in hand with the need to develop criteria to evaluate the evidence. Together these tasks may represent critical strategic areas for scientific and policy research.

The clinical approval and application may also need to be facilitated for cases of advanced degenerative and seemingly futile conditions. It seems ethically justifiable to give people a preferential chance of healing when all other hope is taken from them. But here again, there is the problem of the deficit of consensus criteria for defining "enhanced efficacy and safety," as well as criteria for "advanced degeneration" and "*seemingly* futile" conditions. For the "seemingly futile conditions," apparently, the criteria, methodology and terminology from critical and intensive care medicine may need to be reexamined.[15] The existing legal frameworks governing the conditions whose treatment is considered "futile" may be reconsidered in order to allow for the use of novel, less well-tested therapies in severe cases, to give the patients, and potentially others suffering from the same conditions, an improved chance to "live with dignity" rather than to "die with dignity." Such preferential administration may be advocated for any potentially life-saving and disability-eliminating therapy for the elderly.

Yet, with regard to anti-aging and healthspan-improving therapies, additional complications may arise. In a sense, presently degenerative aging is a universal, inevitable human condition, hence interventions into it may appear generally "futile" for every person on earth. Then when does the futility become "seeming," i.e. under which conditions some amelioration is possible? The priority treatment of "advanced degeneration" is also not unproblematic. On the one hand, such treatments may be more ethically justifiable, as they would give the patients in this state a unique hope. Any possible clinical benefits in such a state may be most desirable and significant. On the other, it may be very difficult to produce and show clinical benefits in such frail subjects, when the diseases are already highly complicated and hardly tractable (this is often the tacit and rather cynical reason why such subjects are frequently and unjustifiably excluded from clinical trials). Moreover, in principle, anti-aging and healthspan-improving therapies are supposed to be "preventive" – precisely in order to postpone the emergence of such advanced degeneration. Hence intervention at a younger age should be preferable as a preventive measure. The younger subjects may also show stronger responses to therapy (any therapy). But in the case of testing anti-aging therapies in the younger and healthier subjects, there may be little evidence that the intervention will actually produce any benefits for the old age (the presumably desirable outcome). These are complex scientific issues that will yet require a long and resourceful investigation.

One of the more immediate suggestions may be once again to intensify the development of clinical criteria to evaluate degenerative aging, including the evaluation of degrees of "degeneration" and "futility of interventions" – for example, measuring resources available for recovery, or potential resilience, or stability and the speed of return to baseline, or the organism's complexity, or homeostatic capacity, or others.[16] Such advanced scientific measures of degenerative aging may help gauge and prioritize the therapies, and will help inform further policy and ethical discussion.

Specific point 5: "Granting a special recognition, status and benefits to commercial and public entities engaged in such research and development."

Commentary: A clear distinction between means of support for public and commercial entities involved in biomedical aging R&D should be made. Public entities should receive substantial tokens of appreciation and support, both symbolic and material, both from the state and from the public, for doing this important research and development. Such support should stimulate them to continue on their path, not let them starve or feel abandoned, not allow the adverse living conditions and lack of status force them to relinquish their scientific and humanitarian mission. The credit they earned and the effort they made should not be taken from them, but should be rewarded.

But what benefits should be provided to commercial organizations to encourage them to enter and remain in the field? After all, as commercial organizations, their primary purpose is to make profits, to pay employees their salaries, to produce valuable products and services, to continue and expand the operations. How may it be possible to make it more worth their while to engage in the subject of biomedical aging research and development, in order for them to produce an even greater value for the entire population's health? The issue is involved. Benefits for commercial organizations have been often understood to include less regulation and less taxation. It has been a commonly voiced opinion that in order to accelerate biomedical progress generally, and the progress of anti-aging and healthspan and life-extending therapies in particular, regulation on the development and use of such therapies should be generally softened, to allow for the proliferation of new ideas and methods.[17] The concept of "conditional approval" of therapies has been advanced, that would presumably make it easier for new therapies to enter the market and would reserve a greater share of research for the "post-market analysis" (i.e. after the medicines have already been sold and used).[18] A considerable number of patients, mainly the wealthy ones, now seek to try new therapies in countries with particularly permissive regulatory requirements, as a form of "medical tourism."[19] Moreover, personal ("do-it-yourself") testing is becoming increasingly popular.[20] These customer bases demand more permissive regulation. Thus, diminished regulation is supposed to help health companies to flourish and increase delivery of health products and services, including healthy longevity products and services.

There may be some logic in the argument for easy regulation. The developing and making available of new therapies has become notoriously costly and lengthy, in a considerable measure due to regulatory obstacles, among other reasons.[21] And in many cases, there is a need to try for a chance. On the other hand, we may not wish people (including ourselves) to assume the role of mishandled guinea pigs. Some patients may become privileged gullible test subjects for their own money (if they have money). And others may become expendable unprotected test subjects (when they have no money). Both situations appear ethnically undesirable and may involve a considerable and unjustified risk to the patients' health and well-being, though possibly with a good "profit margin" and "development potential" for the producers and suppliers of the new medications. Some balanced position needs to be found. Part of the answer may again lie in the development of strict scientific criteria for the diagnosis of the aging process and for the effectiveness and safety of interventions against it. Following the development of such evidence-based criteria, it may be easier to stall the dissemination of quack nostrums as well as to facilitate the availability of truly promising therapies. In other words, such criteria may help improve regulation, not discard it. This issue too should become a subject of broad academic and political discussion.

What about taxation? In a "market-oriented" view, less taxation for companies means more investments, innovation and growth. In a more "social-safety-net-oriented" view, less taxation could also mean larger bonuses for companies' high management, not necessarily related to better products and services, but with a reduction of social benefits. Could these views be reconciled for the particular benefit of rapid development and universal application of longevity therapies? In an earlier commentary, it was suggested to consider obliging (taxing) health companies to support biomedical aging research. Could it be possible to both reduce taxes for health companies that already develop longevity therapies to encourage their continued R&D in the area, and tax those that do not yet conduct such R&D to encourage them to start? In any case, with a proper balanced consideration of the interests of all the stakeholders, taxation could become a powerful incentive to facilitate the research, development and application of healthspan-improving therapies.

Additional recognition tokens, status improvements and material benefits to encourage the entities involved in the field can and should be thought of.

Specific point 6: "Ensuring affordability of aging-ameliorating and life and healthspan-extending therapies."

Commentary: Another issue that apparently needs to be given much thought in advance is a normative procedure to make potential anti-aging and lifespan and healthspan-extending therapies universally accessible, rather than preferentially available only to the rich or to some other privileged social categories (unrelated to their medical indications). There may be several approaches to the issue of affordability. Some believe the issue will dissolve almost automatically by itself, as the healthspan-extending technologies and treatments will gradually become cheaper thanks to advancements of the underlying science and enhancing production capabilities. The means of production that could lead to cheaper prices could involve mass production and cheaper customized production, including "do-it-yourself" manufacturing. This scenario may be plausible. The question is: "When will this happen and for whom?" In other words, "How fast can the healthspan and lifespan-extending technologies become affordable enough to become universally available to all?" Until this happens, large masses of people will likely be left out of reach of these therapies. This would mean early death and suffering from aging-related ill health for the largest part of the world population for a foreseeable time in the future, while a small portion enjoys the extended health and lifespan. It has been sometimes argued that the inability to provide longevity therapies to all people (mainly implying the poor ones) should not prevent providing them to some people (implicitly the rich and powerful).[22] Yet, such an argument may offer little consolation to people of lesser means doomed to an early death by their social status, even when proven longevity therapies already exist. (Many readers of this work, and the author, may well find themselves in this group, if no special action is taken.) Such an inequality in healthcare is of course not new. But with the emergence of effective, yet likely initially highly costly lifespan and healthspan-extending therapies, the social divides may become atrocious.

Under such conditions, at least for the initial stages of therapy development, the following options may be available for people of lesser means to make the therapies accessible for them: 1) Wait patiently until the therapies will 'become cheaper' and/or 'trickle down' from the rich; 2) Fight for the right of access (perhaps also violently); 3) Through advocacy and political action, ensure the establishment of universal public research, development and distribution programs for life-extending and health-extending therapies, that will also give the public strong entitlement to such therapies.

The third option of strengthening public R&D and distribution programs appears preferable, as it would place a large degree of power for the development and application of healthy longevity therapies in the hands of the general public, who are not necessarily related to the scientific, medical or industrial establishment. The first option of resting and waiting until the therapies "trickle down" from the rich may not be very productive (especially if there is no real incentive for the wealthy to provide such therapies to the poor, and also remembering that the decades-long efforts to beg donations for longevity research from the rich have been largely unsuccessful). The second option of "fighting for the right" (of access) may be rather unpleasant, painful and even dangerous for many. Therefore, the third option, establishing programs of public support for therapy research and development, coupled with public entitlement to those therapies, should be more strongly considered and advanced, also by political means.

In any case, the concern over affordability and unequal access should not stop the emergence of new healthspan and lifespan-extending medical technologies, but only to intensify their development. The sooner they emerge, the faster they will likely become available for the people, hopefully for all. Yet, addressing the issue of affordability and accessibility is critical for maximizing public benefits from longevity therapies, and avoiding possible social disruption as their potential side effect. Hence, any effort to develop such therapies should proactively and consciously include plans and provisions to make them maximally affordable and accessible, both through scientific and technological cost-saving contrivances as well as improving the means of equitable social support and distribution.

Policy suggestion 3: "Institutions: Establishing and expanding national and international coordination and consultation structures, programs and institutions to steer promotion of research, development and education on the biology of aging and associated diseases and the development of clinical guidelines to modulate the aging processes and associated aging-related diseases and to extend the healthy and productive lifespan for the population."

Commentary: In any discussion of healthcare research and development, necessarily involving funding and regulation, aging-ameliorating and healthspan and lifespan-extending therapies must be included as an integral part. Enhanced support needs to be granted to the entities engaged in therapeutic aging and longevity research and development, on a par with any other branch of innovative biomedical science, or perhaps even higher due to the great importance and promise of the field. This essentially means strengthening the institutional basis of aging and longevity science, in all of its aspects, from fundamental science, through translation to clinical practice, to distribution of the results, to public education on the use of the results. And this simply means that we need to have more institutions explicitly dedicated to these subjects, and stronger agendas on these subjects in already existing institutions – on all levels, from small local organizations, to large associations and corporations, to state-level institutions and ministries, to supra-national and inter-national agencies and organizations. Such institutional support is yet insufficient and must be expanded.

Specific point 1: "Establishing Biogerontology specialty and courses in Biogerontology as a common part of university curriculum."

Commentary: As a part of the stronger institutional support, aging research also needs a better place in academia and other educational frameworks. Good education may be considered a primary condition for progress. There is a need to address the large deficit of knowledge and training on the subject of biological aging, its biomedical improvement and healthy longevity, in most existing institutions of learning. The need should be obvious. It should be clear that prior to any research, development and application on biological aging, there is a need to educate specialists who will be able to contribute to the various aspects of the field. There is an even prior need to educate the broader public on the importance of such research to prepare the ground for further involvement.

Such education is currently very limited. In practical terms, there are presently rather few dedicated structures around the world to promote and coordinate knowledge exchange and dissemination on biological aging and healthy longevity extension. There is an urgent necessity for such structures to make the narrative on biology of aging and healthy longevity globally prevalent.

Dissemination of knowledge in various national languages may be particularly important, as it could dramatically expand global academic and public involvement and cooperation in the field. Indeed, many disconnected chunks of knowledge on aging and longevity extension are scattered around the world. There is much information in various national languages which is not always easily accessible to speakers of English. Conversely, much information is available only in English, while it also needs to be made accessible in other languages. Hence, cross-fertilization of information in different languages could help the entire field to expand globally.

Even in particular languages, the field could benefit from better knowledge communication and data-sharing, specifically within the field of aging and longevity studies, as well as with adjacent fields. It may be argued that virtually any field of science and technology can be related to the problem of aging, and enlisted for its amelioration. Hence the stronger inclusion of biomedical research of aging into the general scientific communication and education could be beneficial for the field of aging, as well as for the allied fields.

To improve the communication and integration, it appears to be crucially important to commonly include biogerontology (or biology of aging and longevity) as one of the central parts of learning curricula, and not only in universities, but in every learning and teaching framework, especially those related to biology, medicine or natural sciences generally. Unfortunately, and strangely enough, the study of the biology of aging and longevity extension is rarely a part of university curriculum and virtually never a part of high school or community education curriculum. Thus, there is a huge range of opportunities to develop educational and training materials and courses, including materials and courses of professional interest, from undergraduate to postgraduate levels, as well as of general interest, presenting recent advances in aging and longevity science. There is a special need for developing courses and other educational materials in national languages, beside English, and in countries and areas in which information on the field is particularly scarce.

Unfortunately, these desires are yet far from fulfillment. The current curricula in life and health sciences around the world, very often, simply omit aging and longevity from processes of biological development. Furthermore, many biology textbooks do not include aging and dying, not to mention longevity, among the processes of life. The science of aging and longevity, and adjacent areas of study, need to become an entrenched part of education at every level, not just because of the scientific value of this subject, but also because of its great practical significance for the society. In fact, the World Health Organization's *Global Strategy and Action Plan on Ageing and Health (GSAP)* (2015) directly requests member states to "ensure competencies on ageing and health are included in the curricula of all health professionals."[23] Of course, it should be stressed that knowledge of the biology of aging is one of such indispensable gerontological competencies. Yet, this requirement is very far from implementation, even as relates to "competencies on ageing" generally, not to mention biology of aging. There is an urgent need to address the problem, to strengthen the standing of biogerontology in academia and other educational frameworks, to cultivate the ground of knowledge necessary for aging research, development and treatment to grow and bear fruit.

Specific point 2: "Developing and disseminating geroprotective regimens, based on the best available evidence, as part of authoritative health recommendations."

Commentary: Part of the knowledge dissemination and exchange should include actionable recommendations for ordinary people to achieve healthy longevity. It is indeed important to disseminate and popularize the knowledge of fundamental research and its long-term goals. But some more immediate practical outcomes could greatly benefit the public and increase general interest in the field, though never losing sight of the need for long-term fundamental biomedical research and development. The researchers of aging and longevity need to have a say in the development and dissemination of regimens for the extension of healthy longevity for the community, based on the best available evidence, as a part of authoritative health recommendations. Such guidelines for healthy longevity for the public are commonly lacking. There are some examples of limited materials of this kind from major research institutions.[24] But generally such educational activity can be greatly expanded globally.

Specific point 3: "Establishing cooperative centers of excellence for fundamental, translational and applied studies, alongside centers for strategic analysis, forecast, education and policy development on aging and longevity research, at academic institutes and various governmental and supra-governmental agencies."

Commentary: This is probably the most important and desirable policy recommendation that can be currently made. In fact, it encompasses and engages most of the other recommendations, including increased funding, incentives and institutional support for the field. Simply put, researchers of aging and longevity need places to do their work at. Such work places, that would be involved primarily and not tangentially with biomedical aging research, are quite few even in the "developed" world, and are almost absent in the "developing" or "low income" world.[25] There is a vital need to establish more and more cooperative centers of excellence of different kinds: for fundamental, translational and applied studies. Beside scientific research and development centers proper, there is also a need for supportive intellectual infrastructure, including centers for strategic analysis, forecast, education and policy development on aging and longevity research. Such centers, or at least dedicated thought and task forces, could be desired for virtually all large academic institutes, as the subject has critical academic and public value. Such centers and/or task forces and/or organizational structures should also be present in various governmental and supra-governmental agencies, including virtually all the agencies related to public health and science, but also possible additional entities, such as those dealing with education, social services, or aging generally.

Though the relevance of the topic of biomedical aging research, development and application should be obvious for such agencies and institutions, they still seldom have this subject on their agenda and often not at all. A strong dedicated effort still has to be made to place the subject on the agenda of those organizations. There may be many agencies that may be approached to establish such centers and structures, and the means of approaching and influencing them should yet be studied and perfected.

Conclusion: Normative discussions and recommendations should grow into actions

As a general conclusion, the common rationale for all these tentative policy recommendations is to reduce the burden of the aging process on the economy and to alleviate the suffering of the aged and the grief of their loved ones. It may be hoped that, if granted sufficient support, these measures can improve the healthy longevity for the elderly, extend their period of productivity and their interaction with society, and enhance their sense of enjoyment, purpose, equality and valuation of life. In the light of the great need and promise of healthy human longevity, it may be considered the societal duty, especially of the professionals in biology, medicine, health care, economy and socio-political organizations to strongly recommend greater funding, incentives and institutional support for research and development dealing with the understanding of mechanisms of human biological aging and translating these insights into effective, safe, affordable and universally available life-extending and healthspan-extending technologies and treatments.

We can return to the question asked at the beginning of this work: "What should be normatively done to promote longevity science and the actual achievement of healthy longevity for the population?" Given the feasibility and desirability of healthy human longevity, the normative "thing to do" would be simply "to do," to become proactive for the advancement of the field, to study and support the field, to realize the challenges facing the field, as well as its vital promises, and to contribute to overcoming the challenges and fulfilling the promises. It may be hoped that the present work will contribute to the realization of this duty. It may be further hoped that the suggestions and comments made in this work will stimulate more consultations to help find solutions for some of the literally "life-and-death" scientific and policy questions of the aging society, to achieve healthy longevity for all.

References and notes

1. Michael J. Rae, Robert N. Butler, Judith Campisi, Aubrey D.N.J. de Grey, Caleb E. Finch, Michael Gough, George M. Martin, Jan Vijg, Kevin M. Perrott, Barbara J. Logan, "The demographic and biomedical case for late-life interventions in aging," *Science Translational Medicine*, 2, 40cm21, 2010, http://stm.sciencemag.org/content/2/40/40cm21.full;
Luigi Fontana, Brian K. Kennedy, Valter D. Longo, Douglas Seals, Simon Melov, "Medical research: treat ageing," *Nature*, 511(7510), 405-407, 2014, http://www.nature.com/news/medical-research-treat-ageing-1.15585;
Dana P. Goldman, David M. Cutler, John W. Rowe, Pierre-Carl Michaud, Jeffrey Sullivan, Jay S. Olshansky, Desi Peneva, "Substantial health and economic returns from delayed aging may warrant a new focus for medical research," *Health Affairs*, 32(10), 1698-1705, 2013, https://www.ncbi.nlm.nih.gov/pmc/articles/PMC3938188/;
Ilia Stambler, "Recognizing degenerative aging as a treatable medical condition: methodology and policy," *Aging and Disease*, 8(5), 2017, http://www.aginganddisease.org/EN/10.14336/AD.2017.0130;

Ilia Stambler, "Human life extension: opportunities, challenges, and implications for public health policy," in Alexander Vaiserman (Ed.), *Anti-aging Drugs: From Basic Research to Clinical Practice*, Royal Society of Chemistry, London, 2017, pp. 535-564.

2. Kunlin Jin, James W. Simpkins, Xunming Ji, Miriam Leis, Ilia Stambler, "The critical need to promote research of aging and aging-related diseases to improve health and longevity of the elderly population," *Aging and Disease*, 6, 1-5, 2015, http://www.aginganddisease.org/EN/10.14336/AD.2014.1210.

Thanks to the translations by longevity research activists from around the world, the text of this position paper became available in full or in part in 12 languages. It is available in full in Arabic, Chinese, English, German, Hebrew, Italian, Portuguese, Russian, Spanish, and as a partial (summary) translation in Danish, Finnish, Swedish. See: http://www.longevityforall.org/the-critical-need-to-promote-research-of-aging-around-the-world/. As of June 2017, this paper was quoted over 40 times in academic literature.

3. Below are some examples of the works openly disparaging of anti-aging and pro-longevity research, including works by influential state health policy and bioethics advisors and officials, in particular in the US:

Leon Kass, "L'Chaim and Its Limits: Why Not Immortality?" *First Things*, 113, 17-24, May 2001;

Daniel Callahan, *What Price Better Health? Hazards of the Research Imperative*, University of California Press, Berkeley, 2003, Ch. 3. "Is research a moral obligation? The war against death," pp. 64-66;

Koïchiro Matsuura, "Of sheep and men," *The Daily Star*, 4(113), September 16, 2003;

Francis Fukuyama, *Our Posthuman Future. Consequences of the Biotechnological Revolution*, Picador, New York, 2002, Ch. 4. "The prolongation of life," pp. 57-71;

Ezekiel J. Emanuel, "Why I hope to die at 75," *The Atlantic*, October 2014.

4. Indicatively, as of 2016, the entire proposed budget for the Word Health Organization's "Ageing and Health" program was $13.5M, out of about $4.4 billion total WHO budget (0.3%). No budget portion is specified for anything indicative of "ageing research."

(World Health Organization, *Sixty-Eighth World Health Assembly: Proposed Programme Budget 2016-2017*, 2015, http://apps.who.int/gb/ebwha/pdf_files/WHA68/A68_7-en.pdf.)

For the United States (so far the world's largest spender on health, including aging-related issues), the investments to solve the aging challenge generally and for medical aging research particularly are rather small, despite the urgency of the problem.

Thus, in the US, as of 2014, it was estimated that the total national health expenditures were ~$3.0 trillion, representing 17.5% of the Gross Domestic Product, with yearly per capita health expenditures of $9,523. In 2015, these values respectively grew to $3.2 trillion, 17.8%, and $9,990. All these values are world records. (All the websites quoted here were accessed in June 2017.)

(US National Center for Health Statistics, CDC Centers for Disease Control and Prevention, "Health Expenditures" (2014), https://www.cdc.gov/nchs/fastats/health-expenditures.htm;

US Centers for Medicare and Medicaid Services, "National Health Expenditure Data" (2015), https://www.cms.gov/research-statistics-data-and-systems/statistics-trends-and-reports/nationalhealthexpenddata/nhe-fact-sheet.html.)

These "health expenditures" should perhaps be better designated as "sickness expenditures" – in a great measure due to the rising aging-related ill health. Yet, the expenditures on biomedical research of aging, to find clinically effective and cost-effective means to curb the aging plague are comparatively miniscule.

Thus, as of 2016, the budget of the US National Institutes of Health (NIH) – the largest medical research funding agency in the country (and in the world) – was ~$32.3 billion. Out of this general budget, in 2016, the National Institute on Aging (NIA) received about $1.6 billion (~5% of the NIH budget) and about the same in 2017.

According to the NIA budget specifications, "The FY 2017 President's Budget request is $1,598.246 million, the same as for the FY 2016 Enacted Level." Within the National Institute of Aging, the program "Biology of Aging" doing fundamental research of mechanisms of aging and intervention into aging processes underlying aging-related diseases, received in 2016 the budget of ~$184 million (~11.5% of the NIA, and 0.57% of the NIH budget). For 2017 "The FY 2017 President's Budget request is $183.174 million, a decrease of $0.736 million or 0.4 percent compared to the FY 2016 Enacted level."

Radical cuts are apparently expected in 2018: the overall NIH budget is expected to decrease to $26.9B in 2018 from $32.6B annualized budget in 2017 ($5.7B or ~17.5% reduction). The NIA expects a similar proportional reduction from $1,598.246 in 2017 to $1,303.541 in 2018 (~18% decrease). The cut appears to be even more drastic, if compared to the Fiscal Year 2017 Congressional Continuing Resolution (CR) Level: "The FY 2018 President's Budget request is $1,303.541 million which is $745.069 million below the FY 2017 Annualized CR Level. These reductions are distributed across all programmatic areas and basic, epidemiology, or clinical research" – i.e. ~36% (over one third) reduction. For 2018, allocations for specific NIA programs were not shown in the open NIA budget presentation.

(US Department of Health and Human Services, National Institutes of Health, National Institute on Aging, "Budget & Testimony," accessed June 2017, https://www.nia.nih.gov/about/budget; https://www.nia.nih.gov/sites/default/files/fy2018-budget-national-institute-on-aging.pdf; https://www.nia.nih.gov/sites/default/files/nia-fy2017-budget-2.pdf;

US Department of Health and Human Services, National Institutes of Health, NIH Office of Budget, "History," accessed June 2017, https://officeofbudget.od.nih.gov/history.html; https://officeofbudget.od.nih.gov/pdfs/FY16/Approp%20History%20by%20IC%20FY%202000%20-%20FY%202016.pdf; https://www.nih.gov/about-nih/what-we-do/budget.)

For the European Union, though the health expenditures are lower than for the US (€1723 bln or $1940 bln total, and $2,900 per capita as of 2014), the expenditures on biomedical research, and aging research in particular, appear to be lower as well, in both absolute and relative terms.

(Eurostat, "Healthcare Expenditure Statistics," accessed June 2017, http://ec.europa.eu/eurostat/statistics-explained/index.php/Healthcare_expenditure_statistics.)

Thus, in the EU, in May 2014, the Council of the European Union adopted a €22 billion Innovation Investment Package – for 7 years. It included a program to address the aging challenge in Europe, namely the renewed Active Assisted Joint Programme (AAL JP2). The AAL JP2 Programme received €175 million from the European Commission under the new Horizon 2020 (H2020) research framework programme, €350 million from industrial partners and at least €175 million from Member States: altogether more than €700 million for 7 years. Yet, notably, the emphasis of this investment package is to "to help Europe address the challenges and opportunities of the rapidly ageing population by supporting industry, and in particular SMEs [small and medium enterprises], to bring innovative digital products and services for ageing well to the European market" rather than developing and applying therapeutic solutions for aging-related ill health. That is, annually, ~€100 mln ($112 mln) a year would be expended on the Active Assisted Joint Programme (AAL JP2) which is about 3.1% of the Innovation Investment Package of €3.3 bln ($3.71 bln) yearly. Yet, even within the program, the part of actual biomedical research of aging is rather imperceptible.

(European Commission, Digital Single Market, "€700 million to meet European ageing population's needs," Projects News and Results, 06/05/2014, https://ec.europa.eu/digital-single-market/news/%E2%82%AC700-million-meet-european-ageing-population%E2%80%99s-needs.)

This relative neglect of biomedical aging R&D may be explained by the common perception that assistive technologies, "digital products and services for ageing well," may be easier to "bring to the market" than biomedical technologies and therapies that yet require long, costly and careful investigation. The commercial rationale for valorizing ready or nearly ready products is quire clear, but the critical need to research and develop effective therapies for the aged should be clear as well. Unfortunately, this need does not appear to be strongly realized within the EU research programs.

Thus, within the main current European R&D funding framework – the EU Framework Programme for Research and Innovation – Horizon 2020, the challenge on "Health, Demographic Change and Wellbeing" places a great emphasis on improving health of the aging European population. Yet, the portion of this challenge, among all the seven societal challenges of the Horizon 2020 funding program, is not very large. The Horizon 2020 program makes available for EU research and innovation nearly €80 billion (~$90 billion) of funding over 7 years (2014 to 2020), or about €11.4 Billion ($12.8 billion) yearly. During the first four years of Horizon 2020 (Work Programmes for 2014/15 and 2016/2017), the EU invested more than €2 billion in the "Health, Demographic Change and Wellbeing" Challenge, in calls for proposals or actions. That is about €500 mln ($563 mln) yearly, or €3.5 billion for the 7 years – about 4.4% of the entire Horizon 2020 budget. The portion dedicated to actual biomedical research aimed to provide internal health benefits for the elderly, and not just seeking to develop assistive technologies or information and communication technologies (ICT) for them, is smaller still. And the proportion of therapeutic research of aging processes appears to be virtually imperceptible.

It appears there are few programs within the "Health, demographic change and wellbeing" challenge that could be related, even indirectly, to biomedical therapeutic research of aging. These include the research and innovation actions "SC1-PM-09-2016: New therapies for chronic diseases" with the budget of €60 mln for 2016, and "SC1-PM-11-2016-2017: Clinical research on regenerative medicine" with the budget of €30 mln for 2016. Together these two actions comprise €90 mln ($101 mln) for the year 2016, or ~18% of the ~€510 mln total 2016 budget for the "Health, demographic change and wellbeing" challenge, or about 0.78% of the yearly Horizon 2020 budget.

Some other programs in this challenge could also be related to biomedical aging research, but only very indirectly.

Interestingly enough, within this challenge, the programs under the heading "Active ageing and self-management of health" such as the action "SC1-PM-12-2016: PCP [pre-commercial procurement] – eHealth innovation in empowering the patient" and "SC1-PM-13-2016: PPI [public procurement of innovative solutions] for deployment and scaling up of ICT solutions for active and healthy ageing," as well as "SC1-PM-14-2016: EU-Japan cooperation on Novel Robotics based solutions for active and healthy ageing at home or in care facilities" and "SC1-PM-15-2017: Personalised coaching for well-being and care of people as they age" – altogether receiving ~€40 mln for 2016 – do not seem to be interested in therapeutic research of aging at all, but only in developing electronic devices and information services for the elderly. This emphasis is understandable, insofar as such electronic and software products could be brought to the market quickly and can provide immediate assistive services for the elderly. However, it must be emphasized that such devices and services provide no direct internal health benefits for the elderly that are urgently desired and needed. Nowhere does the challenge seem to mention the need for biomedical research of the aging process directly, to enable such health benefits.

(HORIZON 2020, The EU Framework Programme for Research and Innovation, "Health, Demographic Change and Wellbeing," accessed June 2017, http://ec.europa.eu/programmes/horizon2020/en/h2020-section/health-demographic-change-and-wellbeing;
https://ec.europa.eu/programmes/horizon2020/en/h2020-section/societal-challenges;
Horizon 2020, The EU Framework Programme for Research and Innovation, "What is Horizon 2020," accessed June 2017, https://ec.europa.eu/programmes/horizon2020/en/what-horizon-2020;
Horizon 2020, Work Programme 2016 - 2017, "8. Health, demographic change and well-being," http://ec.europa.eu/research/participants/data/ref/h2020/wp/2016_2017/main/h2020-wp1617-health_en.pdf.)

It should be additionally noted that the expenditures on aging-related biomedical research (as we have seen roughly in the range of a few hundred millions of dollars per year at most for the major superpowers) are really tiny as compared to general R&D expenditures. Thus, as of 2014, for the US the total R&D expenditures were estimated to be $485 bln or 2.78% of the country's Gross Domestic Product (GDP), and for the EU, for 2014, the estimates were respectively €283 bln (~$320 bln) or 2.03% of the EU GDP.

The proportion should hopefully change in favor of enhancing the state budget for biomedical aging research and development.

It should be further added that the main part of the general estimated R&D expenditures is the industrial and commercial R&D, seemingly without direct governmental involvement and budget support. Yet, arguably, governmental recognition and raising public awareness for the importance of the problems of aging and the R&D dedicated to address these

72

problems, and the establishment of relevant R&D programs with governmental support, can encourage public demand and consequently the commercial R&D as well.

(Industrial Research Institute, "2016 GLOBAL R&D," Winter 2016, http://www.iriweb.org/; https://www.iriweb.org/sites/default/files/2016GlobalR%26DFundingFo recast_2.pdf;
Eurostat – News Release, "R&D expenditure in the EU stable at slightly over 2% of GDP in 2014. Almost two thirds spent in the business sector," 30 November 2015, http://ec.europa.eu/eurostat/documents/2995521/7092226/9-30112015-AP-EN.pdf/29eeaa3d-29c8-496d-9302-77056be6d586;
Eurostat, "R&D Expenditure," accessed June 2017, http://ec.europa.eu/eurostat/statistics-explained/index.php/R_%26_D_expenditure.)
5. Alex Zhavoronkov, Bhupinder Bhullar, "Classifying aging as a disease in the context of ICD-11," *Frontiers in Genetics*, 6, 326, 2015, http://journal.frontiersin.org/article/10.3389/fgene.2015.00326/full;
Sven Bulterijs, Raphaella S. Hull, Victor C.E. Björk, Avi G. Roy, "It is time to classify biological aging as a disease," *Frontiers in Genetics*, 6, 205, 2015, http://journal.frontiersin.org/article/10.3389/fgene.2015.00205/full;
Ilia Stambler, "Has aging ever been considered healthy?" *Frontiers in Genetics*, 6, 202, 2015, http://journal.frontiersin.org/article/10.3389/fgene.2015.00202/full.
6. Ilia Stambler, "Recognizing degenerative aging as a treatable medical condition: methodology and policy," *Aging and Disease*, 8(5), 2017, http://www.aginganddisease.org/EN/10.14336/AD.2017.0130.
7. World Health Organization, *International Statistical Classification of Diseases and Related Health Problems*, 10th Revision (ICD-10)-WHO Version for 2016, Geneva, 2016, http://apps.who.int/classifications/icd10/browse/2016/en#R54;
2017 ICD-10-CM, Diagnosis Code R54, Age-related physical debility, 2017, http://www.icd10data.com/ICD10CM/Codes/R00-R99/R50-R69/R54-/R54;
World Health Organization, *ICD-11 Beta Draft (Joint Linearization for Mortality and Morbidity Statistics)*, MJ35 Old Age, accessed June 2017, http://apps.who.int/classifications/icd11/browse/l-m/en#/http://id.who.int/icd/entity/835503193.
8. World Health Organization, *Global Strategy and Action Plan on Ageing and Health (GSAP) – 2016-2020*, November 2015, http://www.who.int/ageing/global-strategy/en/; http://apps.who.int/gb/ebwha/pdf_files/WHA69/A69_17-en.pdf?ua=1.

9. European Medicines Agency, *Medicines for older people*, London, accessed June 2017, http://www.ema.europa.eu/ema/index.jsp?curl=pages/special_topics/gen eral/general_content_000249.jsp.
Some of the major relevant EMA documents on geriatric evaluation and treatment that are available from this site, include:
European Medicines Agency, *EMA geriatric medicines strategy*, EMA/CHMP/137793/2011;
European Medicines Agency, *EMA geriatric medicines strategy: Report analysis on product information*, EMA/352652/2013;
European Medicines Agency, *Concept paper on the need for a reflection paper on quality aspects of medicines for older people*, EMA/165974/2013;
European Medicines Agency, *Proposal for the development of a points to consider for baseline characterisation of frailty status*, EMA/335158/2013.
See also:
Cesari M., Fielding R., Bénichou O., Bernabei R., Bhasin S., Guralnik J.M., et al., "Pharmacological interventions in frailty and sarcopenia: Report by the International Conference on Frailty and Sarcopenia Task Force," *The Journal of Frailty & Aging*, 4(3), 114-120, 2015, https://www.ncbi.nlm.nih.gov/pmc/articles/PMC4563815/.
10. US Department of Health and Human Services. Food and Drug Administration (FDA), *Guidance for industry. E7 studies in support of special populations: Geriatrics. Questions and answers*, Food and Drug Administration, Silver Spring, Maryland, 2012, http://www.fda.gov/downloads/drugs/guidancecomplianceregulatoryinfor mation/guidances/ucm189544.pdf;
US Department of Health and Human Services. Food and Drug Administration (FDA), *ICH Guidance Documents*, accessed June 2017, http://www.fda.gov/ScienceResearch/SpecialTopics/RunningClinicalTrial s/GuidancesInformationSheetsandNotices/ucm219488.htm.
11. Healthspan Campaign, "Dr. Nir Barzilai on the TAME Study," April 28, 2015, http://www.healthspancampaign.org/2015/04/28/dr-nir-barzilai-on-the-tame-study/;
Stephen S. Hall, "A trial for the ages," *Science*, 349(6254), 1275-1278, 2015, http://www.sciencemag.org/news/2015/09/feature-man-who-wants-beat-back-aging;
John C. Newman, Sofiya Milman, Shahrukh K. Hashmi, Steve N. Austad, James L. Kirkland, Jeffrey B. Halter, Nir Barzilai, "Strategies and Challenges in Clinical Trials Targeting Human Aging," *Journal of Gerontology: Biological Sciences*, 71(11), 1424-1434, 2016, https://academic.oup.com/biomedgerontology/article/71/11/1424/25771 75/Strategies-and-Challenges-in-Clinical-Trials.

12. Madhukar Pai, "Essential medicines require essential diagnostics," *Huffington Post*, June 12, 2017, http://www.huffingtonpost.ca/dr-madhukar-pai/essential-medicines-diagnostics_b_17047540.html; WHO Technical Report Series, *Report of the WHO Expert Committee on Selection and Use of Essential Medicines, 2017 (including the 20th WHO Model List of Essential Medicines and the 6th WHO Model List of Essential Medicines for Children)*, 2017, http://www.who.int/medicines/publications/essentialmedicines/EML_20 17_EC21_Unedited_Full_Report.pdf?ua=1.

13. Robert Preidt, "FDA Approves Flu Shot to Boost Immune Response. Vaccine can be used in seniors, who are often hit hardest by illness," *WebMD News from HealthDay*, November 25, 2015, http://www.webmd.com/cold-and-flu/news/20151125/fda-approves-first-flu-shot-with-added-ingredient-to-boost-immune-response.

14. Natalia Olchanski, Yue Zhong, Joshua T. Cohen, Cayla Saret, Mohan Bala, Peter J. Neumann, "The peculiar economics of life-extending therapies: a review of costing methods in health economic evaluations in oncology," *Expert Review of Pharmacoeconomics & Outcomes Research*, 15(6), 931-940, 2015.

15. James L. Bernat, "Medical futility: definition, determination, and disputes in critical care," *Neurocritical Care*, 2(2), 198-205, 2005.

16. Alan A. Cohen, "Complex systems dynamics in aging: new evidence, continuing questions," *Biogerontology*, 17(1), 205-220, 2016, https://www.ncbi.nlm.nih.gov/pmc/articles/PMC4723638/; David Blokh, Ilia Stambler, "The application of information theory for the research of aging and aging-related diseases," *Progress in Neurobiology*, S0301-0082(15)30059-9, 2016, doi: http://dx.doi.org/10.1016/j.pneurobio.2016.03.005; Alexey Moskalev, Elizaveta Chernyagina, Vasily Tsvetkov, Alexander Fedintsev, Mikhail Shaposhnikov, Vyacheslav Krut'ko, Alex Zhavoronkov, Brian K. Kennedy, "Developing criteria for evaluation of geroprotectors as a key stage toward translation to the clinic," *Aging Cell*, 15(3), 407-415, 2016, http://onlinelibrary.wiley.com/wol1/doi/10.1111/acel.12463/full; Alexey Moskalev, Elizaveta Chernyagina, Anna Kudryavtseva, Mikhail Shaposhnikov, "Geroprotectors: a unified concept and screening approaches," *Aging and Disease*, 8(3), 354-363, 2017, http://www.aginganddisease.org/EN/10.14336/AD.2016.1022; Vasilij N. Novoseltsev, Janna Novoseltseva, Anatoli I. Yashin, "A homeostatic model of oxidative damage explains paradoxes observed in earlier aging experiments: a fusion and extension of older theories of aging," *Biogerontology*, 2(2), 127-138, 2001, https://link.springer.com/article/10.1023/A:1011511100472.

17. Reason, "Envisaging a World Without the FDA," *Fight Aging*, May 26, 2008, https://www.fightaging.org/archives/2008/05/envisaging-a-world-without-the-fda/;

Yu Luo, Garud Iyengar, Venkat Venkatasubramanian, "Soft regulation with crowd recommendation: coordinating self-interested agents in sociotechnical systems under imperfect information," *PLoS One*, 11(3), e0150343, 2016.

18. Fujita Y., Kawamoto A., "Regenerative medicine legislation in Japan for fast provision of cell therapy products," *Clinical Pharmacology & Therapeutics*, 99(1), 26-29, 2016.

19. R. Alta Charo, "On the Road (to a Cure?) – Stem-Cell Tourism and Lessons for Gene Editing," *New England Journal of Medicine*, 374(10), 901-903, 2016, http://www.nejm.org/doi/full/10.1056/NEJMp1600891#t=article.

20. Jeremy A. Greene, "Do-It-Yourself Medical Devices – Technology and Empowerment in American Health Care," *New England Journal of Medicine*, 374(4), 305-308, 2016, http://www.nejm.org/doi/full/10.1056/NEJMp1511363#t=article.

21. United States Government Accountability Office, *New Drug Development: Science, Business, Regulatory and Intellectual Property Issues Cited as Hampering Drug Development Efforts*, 2006, http://www.gao.gov/products/GAO-07-49;

Steve Morgan, Paul Grootendorst, Joel Lexchin, Colleen Cunningham, Devon Greyson, "The cost of drug development: a systematic review," *Health Policy*, 100(1), 4-17, 2011, http://www.sciencedirect.com/science/article/pii/S0168851010003659.

22. John Harris, "Immortal Ethics," presented at the International Association of Biogerontologists (IABG) 10th Annual Conference "Strategies for Engineered Negligible Senescence," Queens College, Cambridge, UK, September 17-24, 2003, reprinted in Aubrey de Grey (Ed.), *Strategies for Engineered Negligible Senescence: Why Genuine Control of Aging May Be Foreseeable, Annals of the New York Academy of Sciences*, 1019, 527-534, June 2004.

23. World Health Organization, *Global Strategy and Action Plan on Ageing and Health (GSAP) - 2016-2020*, November 2015, "Plan of Action, 2016-2020, 3.3. Member States," http://www.who.int/ageing/global-strategy/en/; http://apps.who.int/gb/ebwha/pdf_files/WHA69/A69_17-en.pdf?ua=1.

24. US National Institute on Aging (NIA), "Featured Health Topic: Healthy Aging/Longevity," accessed June 2017, https://www.nia.nih.gov/health/featured/healthy-aging-longevity.

25. Aftab Ahmad, Shoji Komai, "Geriatrics and gerontology: neglected areas of research in most developing countries," *Journal of the American Geriatrics Society*, 63(6), 1283-1284, 2015, doi: http://dx.doi.org/10.1111/jgs.13521.

5. Regulatory and Policy Frameworks for Healthy Longevity Promotion

Introduction: Seeking policy support for biomedical aging research

The combat of the rising aging-related ill health, and the extension of healthy and productive longevity for the entire population are critically important, urgent global tasks. Unfortunately, their urgency has not yet been universally recognized by the global scientific, medical and policy-making communities. The extension of healthy longevity, for oneself, for the close ones, or for the entire society, would probably not raise too many objections. Unfortunately, few people or organizations consciously, explicitly and proactively make it their main priority. Indeed, even though the combat of aging-related ill health and the tasks of healthy longevity extension are relevant for every nation and for the entire world – these goals are seldom specifically posited in major national or international programmatic or policy documents. Such programmatic and policy recognition is needed to "authorize" increased investments of intellectual and material resources for aging amelioration and healthy life extension by the governments, large institutions, and eventually by individuals around the world. A part of this need would be even to recognize degenerative aging, causing age-related ill health, as a problem that needs to be addressed by medical means. How can we invest efforts and resources to solve a problem that is not even explicitly recognized? Even more critically needed is the recognition of the vital role biomedical research must play in developing effective means for healthy longevity, beside and beyond the well known healthy lifestyle regimens. These means are not yet a given, they still need to be researched, developed and applied, and for that purpose dedicated efforts and resources are required. This necessary requirement is too seldom recognized in policies and programs.

Despite such a relative deficit of specific programmatic and political goal-setting for the amelioration of degenerative aging and extension of healthy longevity, via enhanced biomedical research – there are nonetheless some regulatory and policy frameworks that can be interpreted as supportive of these goals. Elaborately specific programs and policies for aging amelioration and healthspan extension may still need to be developed and adopted by national and international authorities. But in their absence, a good strategy for longevity research advocates may be to justify their advocacy from the existing policy and programmatic foundations.[1] Below is a brief review of some of those existing regulatory and policy frameworks that can be leveraged for anti-aging and longevity advocacy. As we shall see, sometimes those regulatory and policy frameworks may even appear explicit about the requirements to research and develop effective diagnostic and therapeutic interventions for healthy longevity. Unfortunately, these requirements may not be explicit to everyone, they may be glossed over, simply ignored, or given conflicting interpretations. The present work presents such supportive points highlighted and adaptable for the benefit of longevity advocacy.

WHO Global Strategy and Action Plan on Ageing and Health (GSAP)

The World Health Organization's *Global Strategy and Action Plan (GSAP) on Ageing and Health for 2016-2020* (adopted in November 2015) clearly strives to improve the health of the elderly population globally.[2] Yet, within this overarching goal, there are several specific elements that lend authority to the scientific quest to find effective diagnostic and therapeutic solutions for aging-related ill health. Thus the plan implies quite clearly the need to develop diagnostic criteria for degenerative aging, including evidential biomarkers, as well as functional and clinical end points for interventions aimed to achieve "healthy ageing." In particular, the plan includes "Strategic objective 5: Improving measurement, monitoring and research on Healthy Ageing." This strategic objective incorporates clause "5.1: Agree on ways to measure, analyse, describe and monitor Healthy Ageing" (Section 95), which states:

"The current metrics and methods used in the field of ageing are limited, preventing a comprehensive understanding of the health issues experienced by older people and the usefulness of interventions to address them. Transparent discussions on values and priorities are needed, involving older people and other stakeholders, to inform how operational definitions and metrics on a long and healthy life can be constructed and implemented within monitoring, surveillance and research. *Consensus should be reached on common terminology and on which metrics, biological or other markers, data collection measures and reporting approaches are most appropriate.* Improvements will draw on a range of disciplines and fields, and should meet clear criteria." (Emphasis added)

Thus, WHO generally articulated the need to devise scientifically grounded and clinically applicable definitions, criteria and measures for aging and its improvement.

Moreover, WHO even appears to begin to recognize the modifiable nature of aging, and the need to increase research in the field. Thus according to GSAP clause "5.3: Research and synthesize evidence on Healthy Ageing" (section 105):

"Finally, better clinical research is urgently needed on the etiology of, and treatments for, the key health conditions of older age, including musculoskeletal and sensory impairments, cardiovascular disease and risk factors such as hypertension and diabetes, mental disorders, dementia and cognitive declines, cancer, and geriatric syndromes such as frailty. This must include much better consideration of the specific physiological differences of older men and women and the high likelihood that they will be experiencing mutimorbidities. *This could also be extended to include possible interventions to modify the underlying physiological and psychological changes associated with ageing.*" (Emphasis added)

Still, this emerging recognition has not yet reached the level of practicable clinical and research guidelines, apparently in a large measure due to the deficit of agreement on the main definitions, criteria and targets for intervention. Nonetheless, these statements by the WHO GSAP directly suggest the need to support biomedical diagnostic and therapeutic research of aging. In fact, in this document, the WHO member states are explicitly requested to "promote and support research to identify the determinants of Healthy Ageing and to evaluate interventions that can foster functional ability" (Plan of Action, 2016-2020, 5.3. Member States). Of course, it may be yet a long road from this recommendation to its adoption and implementation by member states as a priority. However, based on the GSAP authority, longevity research activists can have an opportunity to emphasize the importance of biological and biomedical research of aging to develop effective health care for older persons, at all levels of government.

It must be noted, however, that all these objectives and actions can be interpreted to support biomedical research of aging *if* emphasizing the correct biological/biomedical aspects. For example, "national healthy ageing policies and plans" desired by the GSAP (Plan of Action, 2016-2020, 3.1. WHO Secretariat) must be understood to include biomedical research. And the need to "ensure competencies on ageing and health are included in the curricula of all health professionals" (Plan of Action, 2016-2020, 3.3. Member States) should also be understood to include biogerontology. Otherwise the biological and biomedical interpretation of these objectives can be overwhelmed by conventional social, psychological, assistive technological or lifestyle approaches. The latter approaches are important, but need not exclude the biomedical therapeutic approaches. Still, the basis for a biomedical interpretation exists in this document, but needs to be emphasized and made more explicit by longevity research advocates, when promoting the GSAP implementation. It should be also kept in mind that the Global Strategy and Action Plan on Ageing and Health is envisioned by the WHO as a preparation for the "Decade of Healthy Ageing from 2020 to 2030." Thus the emphases that are placed now will determine policies for many years to come.

WHO World Report on Ageing and Health

At about the same time as the GSAP, The World Health Organization also issued its *World Report on Ageing and Health* (October 1, 2015).[3] It too can be construed as supportive of diagnostic and therapeutic research, development and interventions against degenerative aging. Thus, the document provides the following working definition of aging which implies its plastic modifiable nature (the original references are included in the quotes):

"The changes that constitute and influence ageing are complex.[4] At a biological level, ageing is associated with the gradual accumulation of a wide variety of molecular and cellular damage.[5,6] Over time, this damage leads to a gradual decrease in physiological reserves, an increased risk of many diseases, and a general decline in the capacity of the individual. Ultimately, it will result in death. But these changes are neither linear nor consistent, and they are only loosely associated with age in years."

Furthermore, according to WHO's report, "healthy ageing" is determined by "intrinsic capacity" that is (somewhat vaguely) defined as "the composite of all the physical and mental capacities that an individual can draw on" and that needs to be "improved." Such general definitions may fit a large number of working programs on aging. Even though there seems to be insufficient clarity regarding the definitions of "intrinsic capacity" or its evidential improvement, the proactive therapeutic approach to aging is implied. The very vagueness of the definitions suggests the need for more research and development to arrive at more practicable clinical evaluation criteria of the capabilities of the aging organism and their evidence-based enhancement.

The document is quite supportive of therapeutic biomedical aging research generally. For example the report includes a section entitled "Reframing medical research," with such encouraging statements as the following. As it can be seen, the WHO report strongly suggests that the research of the multifactorial aging process and of the actual aging patients is vital to provide effective healthcare for the elderly:

"Much medical research is focused on disease. This prevents a better understanding of the subtle changes in intrinsic function that occur both before and after the onset of disease and the factors that influence these changes. Underlying changes in capacity and body functions, and the frequent presence of comorbidities, mean that older people have physiological responses that can be quite different from those of other age groups. Yet clinical trials routinely exclude older participants or those with comorbidities, meaning that findings may not be directly applicable to older populations.[7,8] The design of clinical trials needs to be revisited to better identify how older people respond to various medications and combinations of medications.[9] Specifically, more research is needed that looks at how commonly prescribed medications affect people with multimorbidity, which is a departure from the typical default assumption that the optimal treatment of someone with more than one health issue is to add together different interventions.[9] And outcomes need to be considered not only in terms of disease markers but also in terms of intrinsic capacity."

Furthermore, the report acknowledges that such research would require funding: "This will require the reallocation of budgets, which are currently relatively small in ageing-related research.[10]" In support of this statement the WHO report quotes one of the best known aging research advocacy papers: by Luigi Fontana, Brian Kennedy and others, entitled "Medical research: Treat ageing" published in *Nature* in 2014. In its agreement with the need to enhance aging research, development and treatment, the WHO report testifies that aging research advocacy can have tangible influence on the perception of international governing bodies.

Still, the biological and proactive therapeutic interpretation of medical research of aging will need to be emphasized by aging and longevity research advocates, in every country. Otherwise, there may be a risk it will be ignored, or pushed aside or even suppressed by non-biological and non-therapeutic approaches. For example that "intrinsic function" or "intrinsic capacity" that needs to be "improved" can be given to all kinds of functionalist, psychological or even downright non-rigorous and unscientific interpretations. But it can also be given more scientific content based on biomarkers of aging and formal clinical definitions of aging. This scientific content may need to be stronger emphasized in any discussion or implementation action, invoking WHO's programmatic *World Report on Ageing and Health.*

WHO International Classification of Diseases (ICD)

The need to medically address degenerative aging and thereby extend healthy longevity can be directly inferred from the world's most authoritative disease classification system – WHO's *International Classification of Diseases (ICD)*. Interestingly enough, "senility," a term characteristic of unhealthy or degenerative aging, is already a part of the current ICD-10 listing, carrying the code R54. In the ICD-10-CM (Clinical Modification) system used in the US for billing and reimbursement purposes, the clinical term is "age-related physical debility," also applicable to "frailty," "old age," "senescence," "senile asthenia" and "senile debility," while excluding "age-related cognitive decline" (code R41.81), "sarcopenia" (M62.84), "senile psychosis" (F03) and "senility not otherwise specified" (R41.81).[11] In the main current WHO ICD-10 classification (code R54), the term is "old age," also applicable to "senescence" and "senile asthenia," as well as "senile debility," while excluding "senile psychosis" (F03).[12] And in the draft ICD-11 version (to be finalized in 2018[13]), the code is MJ35 "Old age" (without mention of psychosis), synonymous with "senescence" and "senile debility," while excluding "senile dementia" (code 6C30-6C3Z).[14] The nearly 40 associated "index terms" in the ICD-11 draft also include "ageing" itself, "senility" (not otherwise specified), "senile degeneration," "senile decay," "frailty of old age" and others.[14]

Still the current definitions, such as "senility" defined in an ICD-11 draft as "failure of function of otherwise normal physiological mental or physical process(es) by aging. Not to be used under the age of 70 years" seem to be rather deficient in terms of their clinical utility. Furthermore, a comprehensive, scientifically and clinically usable list of general symptoms for "old age" in the ICD is still lacking. This may be the reason why "senility" has been commonly considered a "garbage code" in the Global Burden of Disease (GBD) studies.[15] The reason "senility" has been considered a "garbage code" is likely because there have been no reliable, clinically applicable and scientifically grounded criteria for diagnosis of "old age" or of "senile degeneration." Consequently, there could be no official case finding lists. Hence, in order to successfully use this code in practice, it appears to be necessary to be able to develop formal and measurable, biomarkers-based and function-based diagnostic criteria for "senility" or "senile degeneration," as well as measurable agreed means to test the effectiveness of interventions against this condition. Yet, the conceptual basis to seek such diagnostic criteria and interventions is present in the International Classification of Diseases.

WHO International Classification of Functioning, Disability and Health (ICF)

Further programmatic, regulatory and policy frameworks and documents can be enlisted to support biomedical aging research. For example, alongside the *International Classification of Diseases (ICD)*, there is also WHO's *International Classification of Functioning, Disability and Health (ICF)*.[16] It appears to exist in parallel, and apparently not strongly related to either ICD or GSAP, and hardly even mentions aging as such or the "intrinsic capacity" in aging which is the focus of the GSAP.

Thus, the ICF hypothesizes that "it is possible to see if people with similar levels of difficulty are receiving similar levels of support services irrespective of age such as when there are separate systems for aged or younger individuals with disabilities."[17] But the evaluation of aging-related disability is lacking. The addition of a scientifically grounded biomedical classification of aging-related disability and function may greatly increase the utility of the ICF. The addition of biomedical tests on aging to the ICF may be parallel to an addition of some clinically applicable, science-based and practical definitions, criteria or classification of aging or senility within the ICD or GSAP or other frameworks. The addition of debilitating aging to the ICF as an impairment of biological function may be actually easier than outright defining aging as a disease (or a system of syndromes) within the ICD framework. Though, perhaps it may be most desirable to emphasize the clinical significance of the aging process on all the fronts, in all the relevant policy frameworks, at once.

UN Sustainable Development Goals (SDG) - until 2030

Some international policy documents and programs are less supportive of medical research and intervention into degenerative aging, or it may be more difficult to derive support from them. Still, with some charitable interpretation and persuasion, they can be helpful and supportive of aging research and development. Thus, within the *UN Sustainable Development Goals (SDG) - until 2030* (adopted in September 2015),[18] the Sustainable Development Goal - SDG 3 "Ensure healthy lives and promote well-being for all at all ages" mandates: "By 2030, reduce by one third *premature* mortality from non-communicable diseases through prevention and treatment" (3.4., emphasis added). This implies that "mature" mortality is somehow acceptable, as well as suggests the need to provide diagnostic criteria for the discrimination of "premature" mortality. This clause omits or does not explicitly mention the aged and the processes of aging (the formulation "for all ages" itself makes the aging problem rather inconspicuous, not prioritized). Yet it may be argued that it is only by prevention and treatment of the underlying aging processes, thanks to biomedical research and development, that the goal of a significant reduction of mortality from non-communicable age-related diseases could ever be achieved.

The SDG3 Clause 3.b mandates that the global community should "Support the research and development of vaccines and medicines for the communicable and non-communicable diseases that primarily affect developing countries, provide access to affordable essential medicines and vaccines." This statement may be interpreted to undervalue the support for research of aging-related diseases that presumably primarily affect the "developed" (also known as "high income") countries. It may seem to imply both that the aging plagues of the developed countries are not a research priority and that those plagues are irrelevant for the "developing" ("low income") countries. This is far from being the case. In fact, aging-related morbidity is an ever increasing concern for the developing countries, while their gerontological and geriatric infrastructure is far less advanced and capable of handling the aging challenge than in the developed countries.[19] The attitude of the SDG may appear dismissive of degenerative aging as a medical problem and of the need of its research and treatment. It may be that as a result of similar dismissive attitudes, biomedical research of aging is seldom even considered as a specific field of study or as a budget item, either at the international, national or institutional levels. Nonetheless, the SDG does offer some possibilities for positive interpretation in favor of biomedical aging research. In particular, the introduction of science-based evaluation criteria for the aged may contribute to the development of gerontological research and practice capabilities in the developing countries, also as a part of the SDG framework.

The International Conference on Harmonisation of Technical Requirements for Registration of Pharmaceuticals for Human Use (ICH)

Going from the international to the national level, for over two decades, the regulatory authorities of the EU, US and Japan have struggled to grant special consideration for older patients in the research, development and application of medical treatments, to involve elderly subjects in all clinical trials, and to establish criteria for treatment efficacy and safety specifically for the elderly. Thus, in 1993, The International Conference on Harmonisation of Technical Requirements for Registration of Pharmaceuticals for Human Use (ICH) issued the *Harmonized Tripartite Quideline E7. Studies in Support of Special Populations: Geriatrics* (recommended for adoption in the EU, US and Japan). This guideline posited the general principle that "Drugs should be studied in all age groups, including the elderly, for which they will have significant utility."[20] Still, this basic requirement has not yet become an overwhelming practice, while comprehensive criteria for the special medication needs of older patients, in particular the efficacy and safety criteria for the elderly, are still deficient or even lacking in many studies. Nonetheless, the need to enhance biomedical research and treatment of the elderly is suggested by this authoritative international programmatic document, which can be leveraged for aging research advocacy.

The fact that older persons are too often excluded from clinical research may be due to some rather unflattering reasons. Quite often academic or pharma researchers may be unwilling to risk confounding their study results by including the complicated, increasingly dysregulated and disbalanced, multi-morbid and frail elderly patients, undergoing multiple, often antagonistic treatments.[21] Cynically put, the confounding of research results by the elderly subjects could jeopardize the chance to publish the research, or in case of pharma research, could cast doubts on the drug efficacy and value. More charitably put, the researchers may be simply unable to handle the complexities that may be involved in including the old subjects in their investigations. Moreover, the clinical trials may even endanger the frail, high-risk elderly patients (who nonetheless do receive the potentially dangerous treatments that are not evidence-based for them). Trying to change this exclusion practice would go against quite a few odds. Still, for the benefit of the elderly patients and for the sake of scientific honesty, it may be highly beneficial to determine whether drugs and other treatments actually "work" or "should work" in the elderly patients in whom they are applied, to know the exact conditions, dosages and regimens under which they "work" in those patients. The "Harmonisation of Technical Requirements" may provide an additional authoritative justification to advocate for such research. This argument for aging research may apply not only for clinical trials on the entire aging organism, but also exploring manifestations of aging on all levels of organization, such as aging cells, tissues and organs.

European Medicines Agency (EMA)

In the EU, in the past years, the European Medicines Agency (EMA) has undertaken several programmatic initiatives to include the elderly into clinical trials and to develop the relevant diagnostic, inclusion, efficacy and safety criteria.[22] Thus, in February 2011, the EMA issued the *EMA Geriatric Medicines Strategy* that would "ensure that the needs of older people are taken into account in the development and evaluation of new medicines."[23] Yet, subsequent reports revealed that those needs, in many cases, are not sufficiently addressed.[24] There have been also continuous efforts by the EMA to develop the specific diagnostic criteria for general age-related frailty as a common determinant of age-related diseases and disabilities. Thus, in March 2013, the EMA issued the brief "Concept paper on the need for a reflection paper on quality aspects of medicines for older people." The paper urged to reflect on the fact that "there is no specific legal requirement for the development of medicines for geriatric use."[25] Also about the same time, in May 2013, the EMA issued the "Proposal for the development of a points to consider for baseline characterisation of frailty status" including physical frailty, comorbidity status and mental frailty.[26] Apparently, these documents are still in preparation.[27] Even though much work yet remains to be done to formalize the diagnostic and therapeutic criteria and guidelines for intervention into old-age frailty, old-age multimorbidity or even degenerative aging itself, the EMA appears to be open to explore their development and application.

US Food and Drug Administration (FDA)

The situation at the US Food and Drug Administration (FDA) appears to be similar. The need for the inclusion of older subjects in all clinical trials and the necessity for devising specific criteria for their diagnostic and therapeutic assessment are recognized. Thus, following the *ICH Guidance E7 Studies in Support of Special Populations: Geriatrics,* in 2012, similarly to the EMA, also the FDA expressed the hope that "certain specific adverse events and age-related efficacy endpoints should be actively sought in the geriatric population, e.g., effects on cognitive function, balance and falls, urinary incontinence or retention, weight loss, and sarcopenia."[28] Yet, apparently, this directive has not been satisfactorily accomplished. For example, there is no mandatory inclusion of elderly subjects in the US National Institutes of Health (NIH) trials, unlike children, women and minorities.[29] Still, the desire for their inclusion is clearly expressed in the FDA strategy and can be utilized for advocacy.

Another major encouragement for aging research was recently created within the FDA. In November 2015, the FDA approved the "TAME" study – "Targeting Aging with Metformin," testing the ability of metformin (a well known anti-diabetic medication) to reduce or postpone multiple age-related diseases and dysfunctions.[30] Apparently this is the first time that a regulatory agency approved a trial to intervene into the basic aging process (predominantly glycation) with the aim of reducing aging-related multimorbidity. Yet, it must be emphasized that the study does not test the effects on *"aging"* as such (for which there is presently no agreed formal or clinical definition or criteria), but on various age-related diseases and dysfunctions (which can be diagnosed in the clinic and which together are named "multimorbidity" or "comorbidity"). Yet, essentially, there is no agreed formal or clinical definition and criteria for multimorbidity either.[31] Some agreed and strict methodologies to evaluate either aging itself or age-related multimorbidity or frailty, as treatable medical conditions, still appear to be desirable tasks for the future, either for the EMA or FDA or other national regulatory agencies.

Advocates as policy makers

86

As we have seen, several major international and national programmatic, policy and regulatory frameworks and documents are either explicitly or implicitly supportive of enhanced biomedical research of aging, for the development of science-based clinical diagnostic criteria for morbid aging as opposed to "healthy aging," and for the effectiveness and safety of therapeutic interventions for healthy aging. Essentially, they are either explicitly or implicitly supportive of a pro-active therapeutic approach to aging-related ill health, in its various aspects.

Clearly, those supportive statements will yet require additional discussion and elaboration in academic, public and policy consultations. Still, even in the present form, they provide a good deal of encouragement for aging science. Yet, critically, all that expressed or implied support may remain on paper or in the minds of the interpreters, unless it is backed up by some actual local involvement, both at the grass roots and professional level, at the stage of the policy implementation. For several frameworks, it is rather unclear how this implementation could or should work at the level of countries and institutions. But apparently it is at that "lower" level where the real action will need to take place.

The WHO seems to acknowledge this need for taking topical responsibility and local involvement. During its public web based consultation on Draft 0 of The *Global Strategy and Action Plan on Ageing and Health* (conducted in August through October 2015), the WHO stated:[32]

"Contributions aligned to the GSAP from countries, non-state actors including older adults, civil society organizations, multilateral agencies, development partners and those who develop, manufacture and distribute aids, equipment or pharmaceuticals to improve intrinsic capacity or functional ability, can transform the action plan from a document to a movement."

So, in a sense, the implementation and interpretation of whatever is written in those policy documents will largely depend on "us" – on the individual and organizational involvements. If the longevity advocates are vocal, active and influential, the WHO and other policy-making authorities will need to "come to us" for the implementation of their plans. There is little doubt that, if active enough, the longevity advocates can emphasize the importance of biomedical research of aging. It will be the duty and the task of longevity advocates around the world to emphasize that, in order to make healthy longevity a reality for all, we will need the scientific "know-how."

References and notes

1. Ilia Stambler, "Recognizing degenerative aging as a treatable medical condition: methodology and policy," *Aging and Disease*, 8(5), 2017, http://www.aginganddisease.org/EN/10.14336/AD.2017.0130;
Ilia Stambler, "Human life extension: opportunities, challenges, and implications for public health policy," in Alexander Vaiserman (Ed.), *Anti-aging Drugs: From Basic Research to Clinical Practice*, Royal Society of Chemistry, London, 2017, pp. 535-564.
2. World Health Organization, *Global Strategy and Action Plan on Ageing and Health (GSAP) – 2016-2020*, November 2015, http://www.who.int/ageing/global-strategy/en/;
http://apps.who.int/gb/ebwha/pdf_files/WHA69/A69_17-en.pdf?ua=1.
3. World Health Organization, *World Report on Aging and Health*, Geneva, October 1, 2015, http://www.who.int/ageing/events/world-report-2015-launch/en/;
http://apps.who.int/iris/bitstream/10665/186463/1/9789240694811_eng.pdf?ua=1.
4. Thomas B.L. Kirkwood, "A systematic look at an old problem," *Nature*, 451(7179), 644-647, 2008.
5. Claire Joanne Steves, Timothy D. Spector, Stephen H.D. Jackson, "Ageing, genes, environment and epigenetics: what twin studies tell us now, and in the future," *Age and Ageing*, 41(5), 581-586, 2012.
6. Sonya Vasto, Giovanni Scapagnini, Matteo Bulati, Giuseppina Candore, Laura Castiglia, Giuseppina Colonna-Romano, Domenico Lio, Domenico Nuzzo, Mariavaleria Pellicano, Claudia Rizzo, Nicola Ferrara, Calogero Caruso, "Biomarkes of aging," *Frontiers in Bioscience*, 2(1), 392-402, 2010.
7. Jerry H. Gurwitz, Robert J. Goldberg, "Age-based exclusions from cardiovascular clinical trials: implications for elderly individuals (and for all of us). Comment on "the persistent exclusion of older patients from ongoing clinical trials regarding heart failure," *Archives of Internal Medicine*, 171(6), 557-558, 2011, doi: http://dx.doi.org/10.1001/archinternmed.2011.33.
8. Cynthia M. Boyd, Daniela Vollenweider, Milo A. Puhan, "Informing evidence-based decision-making for patients with comorbidity: availability of necessary information in clinical trials for chronic diseases," *PLOS ONE*, 7(8), e41601, 2012, doi: https://doi.org/10.1371/journal.pone.0041601.
9. Sube Banerjee, "Multimorbidity – older adults need health care that can count past one," *Lancet*, 385(9968), 587-589, 2015, http://dx.doi.org/10.1016/S0140-6736(14)61596-8.
10. Luigi Fontana, Brian K. Kennedy, Valter D. Longo, Douglas Seals, Simon Melov, "Medical research: treat ageing," *Nature*, 511(7510), 405-407, 2014, http://www.nature.com/news/medical-research-treat-ageing-1.15585.

11. 2017 ICD-10-CM, Diagnosis Code R54, Age-related physical debility, 2017, http://www.icd10data.com/ICD10CM/Codes/R00-R99/R50-R69/R54-/R54.
In the American ICD-10-CM (Clinical Modification) system, "R54" is a billable/specific ICD-10-CM code that can be used to indicate a diagnosis for reimbursement purposes. It is applicable to: Frailty, Old age, Senescence, Senile asthenia, Senile debility. The following ICD-10-CM Index entries contain back-references to ICD-10-CM R54 [and thus can be used as indirect clinical indications for this condition, in the absence of agreed direct clinical indications of "Old age"]:

Senile asthenia, senile atrophia or senile atrophy, senile cachexia, senile catabolism, senile (chronic) (general) (nervous) debility, senile decay, senile degeneration, senile deterioration, senile dysfunction, senile exhaustion (physical, not elsewhere classified), senile failure (general), senile fatigue, senile fibrosis, frailty, senile infirmity, senile marasmus, presbycardia, senile prostration, senectus, old age (without mention of debility), senescence (without mention of psychosis), senility (also condition), senile heart failure, tremor(s) senilis, senile weakness (generalized).

12. World Health Organization, *International Statistical Classification of Diseases and Related Health Problems*, 10th Revision (ICD-10)-WHO Version for 2016, Geneva, 2016, http://apps.who.int/classifications/icd10/browse/2016/en#R54.

13. World Health Organization, *The International Classification of Diseases*, 11th Revision (due by 2018), accessed June 2017, http://www.who.int/classifications/icd/revision/en/.

14. World Health Organization, *ICD-11 Beta Draft (Joint Linearization for Mortality and Morbidity Statistics)*, MJ35 Old Age, accessed June 2017, http://apps.who.int/classifications/icd11/browse/l-m/en#/http://id.who.int/icd/entity/835503193.
The full inclusions into the ICD-11 draft category MJ35 "Old Age" are: old age without mention of psychosis, senescence without mention of psychosis, senile debility. Exclusions: Senile dementia (6C30-6C3Z).

For the record, all the 38 Index Terms listed are: Old age, senescence, senile state, senile dysfunction, senility (not otherwise specified), general debility of old age, old age atrophy, old age, cachexia, old age debility, old age exhaustion, presbycardia, senectus, senile, senile atrophy, senile cachexia, senile catabolism, senile decay, senile degeneration, senile deterioration, senile exhaustion, senile failure, senile fibrosis, senile infirmity, senile marasmus, senile weakness, senilis atrophia, senile prostration, frailty of old age, old age without mention of psychosis, senescence without mention of psychosis, senile asthenia, tremor senilis, senile fatigue, senile change, senile debility, geriatric fraility, frail aged, age related fraility.

These codes are as they appear at the WHO ICD-11 Beta Draft, as of June 2017. Notably, the code numbers in this category have been changing continuously. The earlier codes for "Old Age" were MA20, followed by MJ43, and presently MJ35.

15. Rafael Lozano, Mohsen Naghavi, Kyle Foreman, Stephen Lim, Kenji Shibuya, Victor Aboyans, et al., "Global and regional mortality from 235 causes of death for 20 age groups in 1990 and 2010: a systematic analysis for the Global Burden of Disease Study 2010," *Lancet*, 380, 2095-2128, 2012, doi: http://dx.doi.org/10.1016/S0140-6736(12)61728-0.

16. World Health Organization, *International Classification of Functioning, Disability and Health (ICF)*, accessed June 2017, http://www.who.int/classifications/icf/en/.

17. World Health Organization, *A Practical Manual for using the International Classification of Functioning, Disability and Health (ICF)*, 2013, http://www.who.int/classifications/drafticfpracticalmanual2.pdf?ua=1.

18. United Nations, *Transforming Our World: The 2030 Agenda for Sustainable Development*, New York, September 2015, https://sustainabledevelopment.un.org/; https://sustainabledevelopment.un.org/content/documents/21252030%20 Agenda%20for%20Sustainable%20Development%20web.pdf

19. Aftab Ahmad, Shoji Komai, "Geriatrics and gerontology: neglected areas of research in most developing countries," *Journal of the American Geriatrics Society*, 63(6), 1283-1284, 2015, doi: http://dx.doi.org/10.1111/jgs.13521.

20. The International Conference on Harmonisation of Technical Requirements for Registration of Pharmaceuticals for Human Use, *ICH Harmonized Tripartite Guideline E7, Studies in Support of Special Populations: Geriatrics*, ICH, Brussels, June 24, 1993, http://www.ich.org/fileadmin/Public_Web_Site/ICH_Products/Guidelin es/Efficacy/E7/Step4/E7_Guideline.pdf.

21. Jerry H. Gurwitz, Robert J. Goldberg, "Age-based exclusions from cardiovascular clinical trials: implications for elderly individuals (and for all of us). Comment on "the persistent exclusion of older patients from ongoing clinical trials regarding heart failure," *Archives of Internal Medicine*, 171(6), 557-558, 2011, doi: http://dx.doi.org/10.1001/archinternmed.2011.33; Cynthia M. Boyd, Daniela Vollenweider, Milo A. Puhan, "Informing evidence-based decision-making for patients with comorbidity: availability of necessary information in clinical trials for chronic diseases," *PLOS ONE*, 7(8), e41601, 2012, doi: https://doi.org/10.1371/journal.pone.0041601.

22. European Medicines Agency, *Medicines for older people*, London, accessed June 2017,

http://www.ema.europa.eu/ema/index.jsp?curl=pages/special_topics/gen eral/general_content_000249.jsp.
The EMA documents cited here are available at this site.
23. European Medicines Agency, *EMA geriatric medicines strategy*, EMA/CHMP/137793/2011.
24. European Medicines Agency, *EMA geriatric medicines strategy: Report analysis on product Information*, EMA/352652/2013.
25. European Medicines Agency, *Concept paper on the need for a reflection paper on quality aspects of medicines for older people*, EMA/165974/2013.
26. European Medicines Agency, *Proposal for the development of a points to consider for baseline characterisation of frailty status*, EMA/335158/2013.
27. Cesari M., Fielding R., Bénichou O., Bernabei R., Bhasin S., Guralnik J.M., et al., "Pharmacological interventions in frailty and sarcopenia: Report by the International Conference on Frailty and Sarcopenia Task Force," *The Journal of Frailty & Aging*, 4(3), 114-120, 2015, https://www.ncbi.nlm.nih.gov/pmc/articles/PMC4563815/.
28. US Department of Health and Human Services. Food and Drug Administration (FDA), *Guidance for industry. E7 studies in support of special populations: Geriatrics. Questions and answers*, Food and Drug Administration, Silver Spring, Maryland, 2012, http://www.fda.gov/downloads/drugs/guidancecomplianceregulatoryinfor mation/guidances/ucm189544.pdf.
29. National Institutes of Health (NIH), *Inclusion of women and minorities as participants in research involving human subjects – Policy implementation page*, Bethesda, Maryland, accessed June 2017, https://grants.nih.gov/grants/funding/women_min/women_min.htm;
National Institutes of Health (NIH), *NIH inclusion of children as participants in research involving human subjects*, Bethesda, Maryland, accessed June 2017, https://grants.nih.gov/grants/funding/children/children.htm.
30. Stephen S. Hall, "A trial for the ages," *Science*, 349(6254), 1275-1278, 2015, http://www.sciencemag.org/news/2015/09/feature-man-who-wants-beat-back-aging;
John C. Newman, Sofiya Milman, Shahrukh K. Hashmi, Steve N. Austad, James L. Kirkland, Jeffrey B. Halter, Nir Barzilai, "Strategies and Challenges in Clinical Trials Targeting Human Aging," *Journal of Gerontology: Biological Sciences*, 71(11), 1424-1434, 2016, https://academic.oup.com/biomedgerontology/article/71/11/1424/25771 75/Strategies-and-Challenges-in-Clinical-Trials.
31. Marcel E. Salive, "Multimorbidity in Older Adults," *Epidemiological Reviews*, 35(1), 75-83, 2013, https://academic.oup.com/epirev/article-lookup/doi/10.1093/epirev/mxs009;
David Blokh, Ilia Stambler, "The application of information theory for the research of aging and aging-related diseases," *Progress in Neurobiology*, S0301-

0082(15)30059-9, 2016, doi: http://dx.doi.org/10.1016/j.pneurobio.2016.03.005;

Alexey Moskalev, Elizaveta Chernyagina, Vasily Tsvetkov, Alexander Fedintsev, Mikhail Shaposhnikov, Vyacheslav Krut'ko, Alex Zhavoronkov, Brian K. Kennedy, "Developing criteria for evaluation of geroprotectors as a key stage toward translation to the clinic," *Aging Cell*, 15(3), 407-415, 2016, http://onlinelibrary.wiley.com/wol1/doi/10.1111/acel.12463/full;

Alexey Moskalev, Elizaveta Chernyagina, Anna Kudryavtseva, Mikhail Shaposhnikov, "Geroprotectors: a unified concept and screening approaches," *Aging and Disease*, 8(3), 354-363, 2017, http://www.aginganddisease.org/EN/10.14336/AD.2016.1022.

32. World Health Organization, *Draft 0: The Global Strategy and Action Plan on Ageing and Health*, August-October 2015, http://www.who.int/ageing/global-strategy/GSAP-ageing-health-draft.pdf; http://www.longevityforall.org/who-consultation-on-the-global-strategy-and-action-plan-on-ageing-and-health/.

II. LONGEVITY HISTORY

6. Introduction to "A History of Life-Extensionism in the Twentieth Century"

Summary

The book *A History of Life-Extensionism in the Twentieth Century*[1] focuses on the history of the pursuit of life extension, even radical life extension, in the 20th century, with a primary focus on the first half of the century. Yet it also briefly explores the historical backgrounds of this pursuit in earlier periods as well as recent developments up to the present time. The term life-extensionism is meant to describe an ideological system professing that radical life extension (far beyond the present life expectancy) is desirable on ethical grounds and is possible to achieve through conscious scientific efforts. This work examines major lines of life-extensionist thought, in chronological order, over the course of the 20th century, while focusing on central seminal works representative of each trend and period, by such authors as Elie Metchnikoff, Bernard Shaw, Alexis Carrel, Alexander Bogomolets and others. Their works are considered in their social and intellectual context, as parts of a larger contemporary social and ideological discourse, associated with major political upheavals and social and economic patterns. The following national contexts are considered: France (Chapter One), Germany, Austria, Romania and Switzerland (Chapter Two), Russia (Chapter Three), the US and UK (Chapter Four).

This work pursues three major aims. The first is to attempt to identify and trace throughout the century several generic biomedical methods whose development or applications were associated with radical hopes for life-extension. Beyond mere hopefulness, this work argues, the desire to radically prolong human life often constituted a formidable, though hardly ever acknowledged, motivation for biomedical research and discovery. This work shows that novel fields of biomedical science often had their origin in far-reaching pursuits of radical life extension. The dynamic dichotomy between reductionist and holistic methods is emphasized.

The second goal is to investigate the ideological and socio-economic backgrounds of the proponents of radical life extension, in order to determine how ideology and economic conditions motivated the life-extensionists and how it affected the science they pursued. For that purpose, the biographies and key writings of several prominent longevity advocates are studied. Their specific ideological premises (attitudes toward religion and progress, pessimism or optimism regarding human perfectibility, and ethical imperatives) as well as their socioeconomic conditions (the ability to conduct and disseminate research in a specific social or economic milieu) are examined in an attempt to find out what conditions have encouraged or discouraged life-extensionist thought. This research argues for the inherent adjustability of life-extensionism, as a particular form of scientific enterprise, to particular prevalent state ideologies.

The third, more general, aim is to collect a broad register of life-extensionist works, and, based on that register, to establish common traits and goals definitive of life-extensionism, such as valuation of life and constancy, despite all the diversity of methods and ideologies professed. This work aims to contribute to the understanding of extreme expectations associated with biomedical progress that have been scarcely investigated by biomedical history.

Aims

Life-extensionism can be defined by a strong belief in the possibility and desirability of radical prolongation of human life. Champions of the life-extensionist intellectual movement extrapolated on contemporary scientific and technological achievements and perceived human progress to be unlimited, capable of radically extending the human life-span. For example, seminal biological developments of the late 19th-early 20th century – such as Jacques and Leo Loeb's and Alexis Carrel's concepts of potential cell immortality, Elie Metchnikoff's theory of phagocytosis or Charles-Édouard Brown-Séquard and Eugen Steinach's hormone replacement therapies – inspired far reaching popular expectations of radical longevity, even of a salvation by biomedical science. In fact, the desire to radically prolong human life often constituted a formidable, though hardly ever acknowledged, motivation for biomedical research and discovery. Novel fields of biomedical science often had their origin in far-reaching pursuits of radical life extension.[2] Thus, the development of endocrinology owed much to Eugen Steinach's "endocrine rejuvenation" operations (c. 1910s-1920s). Probiotic diets originated in Elie Metchnikoff's conception of radically prolonged "orthobiosis" (c. 1900). The world's first institute for blood transfusion was established by Alexander Bogdanov to find rejuvenating means (1926). Systemic immunotherapy derived from Alexander Bogomolets' "life-extending anti-reticular cytotoxic serum" (1930s). And cell therapy (and particularly human embryonic cell therapy) was conducted by Paul Niehans for the purposes of rejuvenation as early as the 1930s. Thus the pursuit of life extension has constituted an inseparable and crucial element in the history of biomedicine.

And yet despite this broad significance for the history of biomedicine, the subject has until now been marginalized and there have been relatively few attempts to research the history of life-extensionism and its underlying ideological and social motives.[3] The present research aims to redress this historiographic gap and to examine the major lines of life-extensionist scientific and philosophical thought, in chronological order, over the course of the 20th century. Seminal works in the field are considered in their social and intellectual context, as parts of a larger contemporary social discourse, associated with political upheavals and social and economic events, with state ideologies and cultural fashions.

   This work pursues three major aims. The first is to attempt to identify and trace throughout the century several generic biomedical methods whose development or application, were associated with hopes for life extension. In other words, this work inquires what kinds of biomedical interventions (actual or potential) raised the expectations of radical life extension enthusiasts over the years. There exists an extensive number of sources containing suggestions for possible methods of life prolongation, written by leading scientists and science popularizers, which when studied carefully reveal a taxonomy: idealistic/holistic/hygienic approaches emphasized the importance of psychological environment and hygienic regulation of behavior, whereas, on the other hand, materialistic/reductionist/therapeutic methodologies sought ways to eliminate damaging agents, to introduce biological replacements, to maintain homeostasis, and to bring about man-machine synergy. The apparent relative weight of each method in public discourse (in terms of notoriety and prestige, funding, amount and dissemination of relevant publications) has changed with time, reflecting the initial hopes, disappointments and reactions to those disappointments in a variety of scientific programs.

   The second goal is to investigate the ideological and socio-economic backgrounds of the proponents of radical life extension, in order to determine how ideology and social conditions motivated the life-extensionists and how this affected the science they pursued. Their specific ideological premises (attitudes toward religion and progress, pessimism or optimism regarding human perfectibility, ethical imperatives, adjustments to prevalent state ideologies) as well as their socioeconomic conditions (the ability to conduct and disseminate research in a specific social or economic milieu[4]) are examined in an attempt to find out what conditions have encouraged or discouraged life-extensionist thought.

   The third goal is to attempt to find common defining characteristics of life-extensionism in spite of all the diversity of the professed methods and socio-ideological backgrounds. This work endeavors to do this partly through examining shared traits among the varied forms of life-extensionism and partly through examining the relation of life-extensionism to general biomedical research and practice. Despite the wide variety, what seems to unify the diverse life extension advocates is an assertion of the unconditional value of human life, unmitigated optimism and belief in progress, perceived as reaching a long-lasting social and biological equilibrium, and a striving toward the absolute goal of maximal life prolongation for as many people as possible, or at least for the proponents themselves or for the groups to which they felt belonging. This desire was neither trivial nor self-explanatory, and was commonly frustrated. Its very expression required a certain daring on the part of life-extensionist writers. In the present work, the open expression of this desire is what defines adherence to "life-extensionism" or the "life-extensionist movement."

The precise definition of "life-extensionism" or "the life-extensionist movement" is difficult to articulate. The term "life-extensionism" is relatively recent (its precise origins are uncertain).[5] But of course the terms "life extension" (or "prolongation of life" in early texts), "longevity" or "rejuvenation" are very old.[6] The prolongation of life and rejuvenation were pursued by alchemy[7] and gerocomia[8] in the Middle Ages, and by experimental gerontology[9] and anti-aging medicine[10] in our time. Obviously they are not the same. In the second half of the 20th century, the advocates of life extension were alternatively called prolongevitists,[11] life-extensionists, immortalists[12] or transhumanists,[13] and did not seem to have an agreed title before that. How then can "life-extensionism" or the "life-extensionist movement" be defined in a way which is not "Whig-historical" – imposing contemporary terms on earlier phenomena? The current study proposes to use the term "life-extensionist" generally to designate "proponents of life extension" and then to seek various and often conflicting ways in which this common and definitive aspiration was expressed in particular historical contexts.

Well into the late 1930s there appeared to be no common organizational affiliation of the seekers of life extension whatsoever. In that early period, a wide variety of thinkers joined the quest: materialists and idealists, scientists and men of letters, socialists and conservatives. The research was multi-focal and multi-lingual. The proponents of life extension constituted a congeries rather than a synthetic entity. And even now, the advocates of life extension are very loosely and disparately affiliated, if they are affiliated at all. Still, I would suggest that they constituted a movement, that is to say an *intellectual* movement defined by a common aspiration. The model is that of other intellectual movements, such as the "Romantic Movement," the "Enlightenment Movement," or the "Feminist movement," having no clear organizational affiliations, but expressing similar aims. As in the latter cases, the writings of the proponents of the life-extensionist *intellectual* movement show an intricate dialogue and inter-textual influence, cross-fertilization and mutual encouragement. Moreover, the authors expressed an almost universal yearning for a broader cooperation and massive public support. No such broad cooperation and support seem to have occurred until the late 1930s in any of the countries under consideration, yet the striving for their establishment constituted a common ground which may have eventually led to the actual institutional cooperation.

Still, essentially, in the first half of the century, the model of this intellectual movement was "top down": After the publication of works by elite scientists and philosophers, some of their suggestions became adopted or propagandized by the public, or left at the top level – a subject of a learned and restricted discourse. A laboratory here, a club there, the movement could hardly claim any massive affiliated membership. The proponents had very clear and similar objectives and moral imperatives, yet they enjoined an almost endless variety of methods: theories of aging counting by the dozens and rejuvenating nostrums by the hundreds. As the book exemplifies, the proponents also diverged dramatically in their political philosophies, each in line with the native dominant socio-political paradigm in which the proponents were most closely integrated. Several central figures and general trends can be delineated. Yet, despite all this diversity, the expressed common aspiration allows one to see its proponents as belonging to a "movement."

The very notion of a "pursuit of life extension" also requires qualifications. It might be safe to assume that few people in the world would oppose healthy life extension *per se* (though some authors have expressed such opposing statements). The universal drive of medicine to prolong human life for some periods of time is also generally implied. How then can "life-extensionism" be distinguished as an intellectual movement apart from the aspirations of the whole of medicine or the whole of humanity? The difference may just consist in the extent of hopes, the openness with which such hopes were expressed, and the amount of effort directed toward their fulfillment. When the hopes are high and openly expressed, and the effort toward their implementation is great, the protagonist may be described as a "life-extensionist." In this sense, aspirations for life extension for very limited periods of time, as for example in terminal cases, would not be subsumed under the heading of "life-extensionism" (though these are highly compatible with life-extensionist goals, representing, so to say, a "first step"). As a rule of thumb, when the earnestly expressed aspirations amount to 100-120 years, the life-span attained by humanity's longest-lived,[14] the person who expresses them might be characterized as a "moderate life-extensionist" or simply a "life-extensionist." Beyond that period, the aspirant may be termed a "radical life-extensionist." And those who envision virtually no potential limit to the human life-span may be categorized as "immortalists." Yet, even without mentioning any specific time periods, life-extensionists can be identified by such expressions as "defeating/reversing aging,"

98

"fighting/overcoming death" or even by a prevalent emphasis on the "prolongation of life" or "longevity" generally. These emphases are prominent in the writings of life-extensionists, but almost conspicuously absent in those who might not be categorized as such. The desire to prolong human life may be generally implied in medicine, but it is not always *expressed*. And certainly, speaking of "radical life extension" is often considered bad taste among physicians and biomedical researchers.[15] Furthermore, biology textbooks often do not include aging and dying, not to mention longevity, among the processes of life.[16] For the life-extensionists, these topics are central.

A further distinction may be expected to be found in the specific methods proposed. Yet, it appears that the distinction may consist not so much in the specifics of the methods, but rather in their specific purposes. As the book exemplifies, several biomedical methodologies were developed for the explicit purpose of life extension and rejuvenation, rather than for the treatment of particular diseases, even though these methods also drew on and were applied to other fields of medicine. The non-identity of the pursuit of health/eradication of diseases and the prolongation of life was first expressed by Christoph Wilhelm Hufeland (1762-1836), the renowned German hygienist, physician to the King of Prussia, Friedrich Wilhelm III, and to Goethe and Schiller. Hufeland coined his own term for life extension – "macrobiotics." (The word "macrobiotes," designating the extremely long-lived, appears as early as Pliny the Elder (23-79 CE) who also notices the interest in this subject in Herodotus, c. 484-425 BCE, and Hesiod, c. 750-650 BCE.[17]) The term "macrobiotics" has survived to the present. In *Macrobiotics or the Art of Prolonging Human Life* (1796), Hufeland thus distinguished the art of life extension from the general medical art:[18]

"This art [of prolonging life], however, must not be confounded with the common art of medicine or medical regimen; its object, means, and boundaries, are different. The object of medical art is health; that of the macrobiotic, long life. The means employed in the medical art are regulated according to the present state of the body and its variations; those of the macrobiotic, by general principles. In the first it is sufficient if one is able to restore that health which has been lost; but no person thinks of inquiring whether, by the means used for that purpose, life, upon the whole, will be lengthened or shortened; and the latter is often the case in many methods employed in medicine. The medical art must consider every disease as an evil, which cannot be too soon expelled; the macrobiotic, on the other hand, shows that many diseases may be the means of prolonging life. The medical art endeavors, by corroborative and other remedies, to elevate mankind to the highest degree of strength and physical perfection; while the macrobiotic proves that here even there is a maximum, and that strengthening, carried too far, may tend to accelerate life, and consequently, to shorten its duration. The practical part of medicine, therefore, in regard to the macrobiotic art, is to be considered only as an auxiliary science which teaches us how to know diseases, the enemies of life, and how to prevent and expel them; but which, however, must itself be subordinate to the highest laws of the latter."

Indeed, the emphasis on the treatment of particular diseases may distinguish general medical practice from life-extensionism. The cure of a disease might be more readily and immediately perceived, while the ascertainment of human life extension may be a more lengthy and confounded process. Moreover, the possibility of "radical life extension" is not yet subject to empirical confirmation. These might be some of the reasons why "life extension" and even "longevity" are not often mentioned in biological or medical discourse.

Yet, it would be a great mistake to think that life-extensionism is somehow watertight and separated from general biology or medicine and that it can be defined by some particular and exclusive "method." Life-extensionism is not a method – it is an aspiration and a motivation. Or more precisely, it is a reason to develop and apply a method, primarily for the purpose of life extension, which however may also involve treatment of particular diseases. Hence, life-extensionists can be distinguished by their goals, rather than by their methods. Proponents of the very same methods can be perceived as life-extensionists or not, based on the expressed motivations. Moreover, most authors under consideration were not exclusively involved in life extension research, but also in other fields of biomedicine, often achieving high prominence in these fields. The research of aging, or "gerontology," was a primary field of study, but in no way the only one. Prominent and often world famous scholars and scientists from different fields who sympathized with the life-extensionist goals are the focus of the current study.[19] The interest of these authors in radical life extension has received little attention in biomedical history. The current work addresses these omissions. The scientific contributions of the protagonists were extensive, as was their public appeal, and their life-extensionist views and motivations need to be considered to create a more rich and balanced biomedical history. Insofar as the authors extrapolated on and created contemporary biological and medical advances, the history of life-extensionism represents an integral, though until now under-appreciated, part of the general history of biology and medicine.

When referring to the general difficulty of defining "holism" in twentieth-century medicine, the American medical historian Charles Ernest Rosenberg pointed out that "twentieth-century medical holism has to be understood primarily in terms of what it was not."[20] In a similar fashion, life-extensionism might be understood by "what it was not." That is to say, life-extensionist programs may be better appreciated by analyzing the reactions and criticisms raised against them and by their counter-reactions. I would like to suggest three general types of reactions to life-extensionist programs. The first (and very common) type is simply ignoring the topic of life extension, the kind of reaction which omits aging and longevity from processes of biological development. (Such a reaction might be due to the simple reluctance to think about dying or about struggle with the apparently inevitable end.) In this sense, life-extensionism stands out simply by emphasizing the topics which other authors do not.

The second type is the principal opposition to the task of life extension, seeing life extension far beyond the present life expectancy as ethically undesirable and theoretically impossible. The American historian Gerald Joseph Gruman, the author of the best available history of early life-extensionism (or "prolongevitism" to use the term coined by Gruman) – *A History of Ideas about the Prolongation of Life. The Evolution of Prolongevity Hypotheses to 1800* (1966)[21] – termed such principal opposition "apologism," an attitude rationalizing and even apologizing for our mortality. Earlier, the British philosopher Herbert Spencer defined the opposition as the "pessimistic" as contrasted to the "optimistic view" of increased longevity (1879). "Legislation conducive to increased longevity," Spencer wrote, "would, on the pessimistic view, remain blameable; while it would be praiseworthy on the optimistic view."[22] Several principal ethical and political objections are commonly raised, such as "overpopulation," "boredom," "injustice" and a few others. Such objections were reviewed and countered by the bioethicists Robert Veatch, John Harris and others.[23] The historical tradition of these ethical objections questioning the very desirability of life extension is considered in greater detail in this book, in Chapter 4, in the section "British Allies – Literary and philosophical life-extensionism: The optimistic vs. the pessimistic view. The reductionist vs. the holistic approach" and mentioned *passim* throughout the text.

Another branch of the principal opposition asserts the theoretical impossibility of radical life-extension. The most common argument has been that there is a "limit" to the human life-span which cannot be overcome. The various perceptions of this limit are focused on and referenced in Chapter 4, in the sections "Theories of Aging" and "Rectifying 'Discord' and conserving 'Vital Capital'" and *passim* throughout. Yet, it should be noted from the outset, that even when proposing a "limit" to the life-span, it was often realized by the proponents that this "limit" is quite flexible and theoretically not very limiting. As stated by the Nobel Prize winning physicist Richard Phillips Feynman, "there is nothing in biology yet found that indicates the inevitability of death."[24] Yet, *practical* limits, the constraints in our ability to greatly increase the human life-span with the current technological means, have been realized even by the most ardent life-extensionists. Their only distinctive feature appears to be the desire and the striving to overcome those limits.

The third type of reaction was the specific response (critical or accepting) to particular theories or methods proposed for life extension, or to particular research programs and therapeutic modalities directed toward this purpose. The discussions of this type occupy the bulk of the present history. It appears that the main responders to the specific life extension programs were life-extensionists themselves (for whom this was indeed a major topic of concern). Their responses to particular programs were often severely critical and fiercely controversial. Among the enthusiasts of life extension, the disagreements have been wide. A battle has been waged throughout the century between "reductionist" and "holistic" approaches, with alternate success. "Spiritualists" scorned what they perceived as the ineptitude of modern medicine and science; while "materialists" despised what they saw as unscientific quackery. Even within the "materialistic" branch, there has been much controversy: The more academic life-extensionists argued between themselves on theories, "limits" and funds, and all together attacked unproved remedies which were in turn defended by their providers. Yet, despite all these controversies, life-extensionism may still be seen as a significant intellectual movement, defined by the common goal. Beside the shared goals, other common denominators of life-extensionism are sought in this study, such as a pursuit of constancy, stability and adaptation.

In summary, the three aims of this survey are, first, to fill an important lacuna in biomedical history by looking at the understudied history of life-extensionist research and its diverse methodologies; second, to examine the motivating factors for life-extensionist research by looking at the people behind the work, their biographies, psychologies, philosophies, and social and political contexts; and the third, overarching aim is to collect a broad register of life-extensionist authors, and, based on that register, to find common and definitive characteristics of the life-extensionist intellectual movement and its role in science and society.

Argument

With specific reference to the scientific projects initiated by life-extensionists (the first aim), the current study examines an interrelation between holistic/hygienic approaches and reductionist/therapeutic approaches. The primary focus of the current research is on the formative first half of the twentieth century, with an extension to a later period. I argue that the failure of reductionist "endocrine rejuvenation" attempts,

102

that began at *fin-de-siècle* and culminated in the 1920s, impacted profoundly on the development of longevity research. The reactions to the failures of earlier reductionist rejuvenation were characteristic. A large number of researchers made a transition to a more holistic approach (such a reaction was particularly pronounced among life-extensionists in France and Germany of the 1930s-1940s). Others conceived of the failures as building blocks and signposts for a continued pursuit on the same path, viewing the human body as a machine in need of repair, and searching for new reductionist methods for its prolonged maintenance by surgery or pharmacological supplements (this type of reaction was prominent among many life-extensionist researchers in the US and the USSR of the 1930s-1940s). Thus, the disillusionment with reductionist endocrine rejuvenation exemplifies varied responses to a scientific failure and modifying research approaches in response to that failure. The conflict between reductionist and holistic approaches is shown to continue throughout the 20th century. Though, it should be noted that several researchers succeeded in combining reductionist and holistic methods. Moreover, several lines of biomedical research are shown to owe their beginnings and changing forms to particular life-extensionist enterprises.

With reference to the ideological and social determinants (the second aim), I argue that the hopes for life extension have been coupled to a wide variety of nationalities and ideologies. Insofar as the conditions at home had the most effect, the data are organized according to national contexts. The following contexts are considered: France (Chapter One), Germany, Austria, Romania and Switzerland (Chapter Two), Russia (Chapter Three), the US and UK (Chapter Four). (Unless otherwise specified, all the excerpts are in my translation.) No ideological system or nation seems to have had a monopoly, however strongly it asserted that it constituted the rock-solid foundation for the pursuit of longevity. It may even be that, rather than providing such a foundation, political ideologies enlisted the hope for life extension to increase their appeal. It therefore appears that radical life extension is a cross-cultural value, with a common humanistic appeal above and beyond any particular ideology. Nevertheless, life-extensionism was a strongly ideologically and socially constructed enterprise: In different national contexts, different, and often conflicting, ideological schemes – secular humanism or religion, socialism or capitalism, materialism or idealism, elitism or egalitarianism – yielded different justifications for the necessity of life prolongation and longevity research and impacted profoundly on the way such goals were conceived and pursued. This work investigates such ideological, socio-economic and national backgrounds, and exemplifies the integral adjustment of the specific scientific pursuits to prevalent state ideologies.

In attempting to establish common defining characteristics of life extensionism (the third aim), I argue that the persistent striving for adjustment indeed constituted such a defining trait. The term "adjustment" is used here as a general heading in its common dictionary sense. Thus, for example, the Merriam-Webster dictionary defines "adjustment" (synonymous with "adaptation") as achieving "balance" within a given environment. And "balance" (synonymous with "equilibrium") entails "stability," "steadiness" and "constancy."[25] All these terms have been key in life-extensionist writings, and they have been often used interchangeably. The emphasis on these notions could be expected. If adaptation is a defining feature of life, and if a harmonious, balanced state of equilibrium entails durability and constancy, it is hardly surprising that the proponents of the extension of life were determined to adapt and maintain equilibrium and stability without limits, for their own bodies, for their research projects, and for the societies in which they lived. Yet the task of defining specific local adaptations and equilibria is daunting, either for the body or the society. This work attempts to examine some of the more general forms of adaptation characteristic of particular national contexts and instantiates these general forms by more nuanced examples of adaptation of particular life-extensionist projects.

In relation to the society, I examine the adaptation of life-extensionist programs to what might be termed "dominant" or "hegemonic" socio-ideological orders. Such "dominants" can be most clearly perceived in the 1930s (a major focus of this work): Socialism in Russia, National Socialism in Germany, Capitalism in the US. In France, the "dominant" was more difficult to see, yet the strong rise of political "traditionalism" in the 1930s-early 1940s may be significant. I suggest three common types of adjustment of the life-extensionist thought, which are exemplified in particular contexts. The first is the rhetorical support of the ruling socio-ideological order (if only to ensure the continuation of the research). This is a kind of mimicry, "when in Rome, doing as the Romans." Sometimes it was difficult to distinguish whether such support was purely opportunistic or honestly believed in. (Often this distinction did not seem to have any implications for the authors' words or deeds; when a person was compelled to believe in something to survive, he would seem to believe in it with all his heart, if only to avoid cognitive dissonance.) The second form of adjustment was the positing of metaphorical socio-biological parallels between the workings of the body and of the society in which the authors lived. The society provided the frame of reference for scientific metaphor ("as above, so below") and when the perceptions of the "above" changed, so did those of the "below." And thirdly, and perhaps most importantly, specific research projects were often favored as compatible with the ruling socio-ideological order. As will be exemplified, under particular national ruling regimes,

104

certain lines of research were simply not allowed to flourish or were discouraged. In all these senses, life-extensionism was "adjusted" to the ruling national orders or to more local orders. Yet, the striving for adaptation, that is, maintaining stability within a particular environment, appears to be universal for the life-extensionists. Moreover, the support of the existing ruling regime, whatever it may be, may derive from the nature of life-extensionism that seeks stability and perpetuation. In this regard, a question may be raised regarding the forms of society that would indeed merit such a perpetuation.

In relation to the body, the striving for stabilization and equilibration has been equally persistent. Insofar as the stability and equilibrium of the body have been perceived to be under continuous threat of disruption and destruction, means for preserving the constancy of the body (or the constancy of the "internal environment") have been relentlessly sought through a variety of methods. And if some particular methods – "holistic" or "reductionist," "hygienic" or "therapeutic" – failed to maintain this constancy, new methods for stabilization would be sought, either by embracing a scientific or therapeutic paradigm opposed to the one that failed, or by continuing in the earlier paradigm hoping for its gradual perfection. Still, the desire for constancy appears to be universal and only sought by varied and often novel means. Thus, the underlying conservative (or conservationist) proclivity of prominent life-extensionist scientists in many countries, seeking stability and perpetuation, may have been a source for their diverse and often unorthodox scientific and medical developments.

References and notes

1. Ilia Stambler, *A History of Life-Extensionism in the Twentieth Century*, Longevity History, 2014, http://www.longevityhistory.com/.
2. Ilia Stambler, "The unexpected outcomes of anti-aging, rejuvenation, and life extension studies: an origin of modern therapies," *Rejuvenation Research*, 17(3), 297-305, 2014.
3. Valuable sources on the early history of aging research and care for the elderly (though for the most part omitting the authors' aspirations to radical life prolongation) include:
Joseph T Freeman, "The History of Geriatrics," *Annals of Medical History*, 10, 324-335, 1938; Frederic D. Zeman, "Life's Later Years: Studies in the Medical History of Old Age," *Journal of Mount Sinai Hospital*, 16, 308-322; 17, 53-68, 1950; Sona Rosa Burstein, "Gerontology: a Modern Science with a Long History," *Post Graduate Medical Journal* (London), 22, 185-190, 1946; Sona Rosa Burstein, "The foundations of geriatrics," *Geriatrics*, 12, 494-499, 1957; Sona Rosa Burstein, "The historical background of Gerontology," *Geriatrics*, 189-193, 328-332, 536-540, 1955; Gerald J. Gruman, "An

Introduction to Literature on the History of Gerontology," *Bulletin of the History of Medicine*, 31, 78-83, 1957; Mirko D. Grmek, *On Ageing and Old Age, Basic Problems and Historic Aspects of Gerontology and Geriatrics*, Monographiae Biologicae, 5, 2, Den Haag, 1958; Johannes Steudel, "Zur Geschichte der Lehre von den Greisenkrankheiten" (The history of the study of the diseases of old age), *Sudhoffs Archiv für Geschichte der Medizin und der Naturwissenschaften*, 35, 1-27, 1942; Paul Lüth, *Geschichte der geriatrie: Dreitausend Jahre Physiologie, Pathologie und Therapie des alten Menschen* (The history of geriatrics, three thousand years of physiology, pathology and therapy of the aged), Enke, Stuttgart, 1965; Pat Thane, "Geriatrics," pp. 1092-1115, in *Companion Encyclopedia of the History of Medicine*, Edited by W.F. Bynum and R.S. Porter, Routledge, London and NY, 2001; V.N. Anisimov, M.V. Soloviev, *Evoluzia Concepcy v Gerontologii* (The Evolution of Concepts in Gerontology), Aesculap, Saint Petersburg, 1999; David Boyd Haycock, *Mortal Coil. A Short History of Living Longer*, Yale University Press, New Haven and London, 2008; Lucian Boia, *Forever Young: A Cultural History of Longevity from Antiquity to the Present*, translated from French by Trista Selous, Reaktion Books, London, 2004. The latter two works do consider the aspirations to radical life extension, yet emphasize the time frame and national contexts other than the present work, i.e. give relatively little space to the first half of the 20th century (about 40 pages each); in the modern period they focus on the US/UK, and do not consider many authors and socio-ideological and scientific aspects examined in the current study.

4. The difficulties in funding, research and dissemination appear to be as old as life-extensionism itself, going back to the origins of Chinese Taoist immortalism. Thus, one of the earliest Chinese alchemists, Ko Hung (Ge Hong, 283-343 CE), wrote:

"I suffer from poverty and lack of resources and strength; I have met with much misfortune. There is nobody at all to whom I can turn for help. The lanes of travel being cut, the ingredients of the medicines are unobtainable. The result is that I have never been able to compound these medicines I am recommending. When I tell people today that I know how to make gold and silver, while I personally remain cold and hungry, how do I differ from the seller of medicine for lameness who is himself unable to walk? It is simply impossible to get people to believe you. Nevertheless, even though the situation may contain some unsatisfactory elements, it is not to be rejected in its entirety. Accordingly, I am carefully committing these things to writing because I wish to enable future lovers of the extraordinary and esteemers of truth, through reading my writings, to consummate their desires to investigate God [the Immortal Tao]."

(*Alchemy, Medicine, Religion in the China of A.D. 320: The Nei P'ien of Ko Hung (Pao-p'u tzu)*, translated by James R. Ware, Massachusetts Institute of

Technology Press, Cambridge, Massachusetts, 1966, Ch. 16 "The Yellow and the White," p. 262.)

And the very first known author of Chinese alchemy, the man reputed for the invention of gun-powder, Wei Boyang (Wei Po-Yang), said c. 142 CE:

"I have abandoned the worldly route and forsaken my home to come here. I should be ashamed to return if I could not attain the *hsien* [immortality]."

(*Lieh Hsien Ch'üan chuan, Complete Biographies of the Immortals*, Tenney L. Davis, 1932, p. 214.)

"O, the sages of old!" Wei Boyang said "They held in their bosoms the elements of profundity and truth. ... Their sympathy for those of posterity, who might have a liking for the attainment of the Tao (Way), led them to explain the writings of old with words and illustrations. They couched their ideas in the names of stones and in vague language so that only some branches, as it were, were in view and the roots were securely hidden. Those who had access to the discourses wasted their own lives over them. The same path of misery was followed by one generation after another with the same failure. If an official, his career was cut short; if a farmer, his farm was cluttered with weeds; if a merchant, his trade was abandoned; if an ambitious scholar, his family became destitute – in the vain attempt. These grieve me and have prompted the present writing. Although concise and simple, yet it embraces the essential points. The appropriate quantities [and processes] are put down for instruction together with confusing statements. However, the wise man will be able to profit by it by using his own judgement."

(Wei Po-Yang, "Ts'an T'ung Ch'i" ["The akinness of the three", i.e. of the alchemical processes, the Book of Changes, and the Taoist doctrines], Chapter LXII, pp. 257-258, in *An ancient Chinese treatise on alchemy entitled Ts'an T'ung C'hi, Written by Wei Po-Yang about 142 A.D., Now Translated from the Chinese into English by Lu-Ch'iang Wu, With an Introduction and Notes by Tenney L. Davis*, Massachusetts Institute of Technology, Cambridge, Massachusetts, *Isis*, Vol. 18, No. 2, Oct. 1932, pp. 210-289.)

5. The term "life-extensionism" has been increasingly used in on-line health forums and books about longevity since about 2000, though it was also used in the 1980s and 1990s. There were other kinds of "extensionism" in the US as early as the 19th century, such as "slavery extensionism," "church extensionism" and "university extensionism."

But the earliest reference to "Life-extensionism" that I could find was in 1929, in the journal *Eugenics: A Journal of Race Betterment.* The reference was by Dr. Clarence Gordon Campbell (1868-1956), president of the American Eugenics Research Association, addressing and criticizing the largely "euthenic"/"environmentalist" views of Dr. Eugene Lyman Fisk (1867-1931), director of the American Life Extension Institute (established in 1913). It is likely, though, that the term is even older. As Campbell's article

stated: "the life extensionists … might adopt the Irish toast: 'May you live to be a hundred, and then be hanged for rape.'"
(C.G. Campbell, "Eugenics and euthenics," *Eugenics: A Journal of Race Betterment*, 2(9), 21-25, September 1929.)

6. Ilia Stambler, "Longevity and the Indian Tradition," India Future Society, June 13, 2013, http://indiafuturesociety.org/longevity-and-the-indian-tradition/, republished at http://www.longevityhistory.com/articles/indian.php and https://ieet.org/index.php/IEET2/more/stambler20160316;
Ilia Stambler, "Longevity in the Ancient Middle East and the Islamic Tradition," Institute for Ethics and Emerging Technologies (IEET), January 13, 2015, http://ieet.org/index.php/IEET/more/stambler20150113;
Ilia Stambler, "Longevity and the Jewish Tradition," IEET, October 21, 2015, http://ieet.org/index.php/IEET/more/stambler20151021;
Ilia Stambler, "Longevity and the Christian Tradition," IEET, January 24, 2017, http://ieet.org/index.php/IEET/more/Stambler20170124.

7. The word "alchemy" apparently took root in Europe in the 12th century. The first alchemical text translated from Arabic into Latin was presumably done by Robert of Chester in 1144 and was entitled *Liber de compositione alchimiae* (The book of alchemical composition). This was allegedly a translation from Arabic into Latin of an epistle of the Egyptian-Greek-Christian alchemist Marianos to the Arab alchemical adept, the Umayyad prince Khalid ibn Yazid (665-704 CE).
(*Alchemy Academy Archive*, January 2002, "Maryanos," http://www.levity.com/alchemy/a-archive_jan02.html.)
The world "al-kimia" is of Arabic origin (originating with Khalid ibn Yazid?), "al" being the Arabic definite article, and the etymology of "kimia" being very uncertain, with hypotheses ranging from the Greek "Khemeioa" (appearing c. 296 CE in the decree of the Roman Emperor Diocletian banning the "old writings" of Egyptian "makers" (counterfeiters) of gold and silver; "Khemia" ("the land of black earth," the old name of Egypt); "khymatos" (pouring/infusing in Greek); "khymos (the Greek word for juice), etc.
(Douglas Harper, *Online Etymology Dictionary*, 2012, http://www.etymonline.com/index.php?search=alchemy;
Alchemy Academy Archive, June 2006, "Diocletian's Edict against alchemy," http://www.levity.com/alchemy/a-archive_jun06.html.)
See also: Gerald Joseph Gruman, *A History of Ideas about the Prolongation of Life. The Evolution of Prolongevity Hypotheses to 1800*, Transactions of the American Philosophical Society, Volume 56(9), Philadelphia, 1966, "Arabic Alchemy: The Missing Link?")

8. The term "gerocomia" ("gerocomica" or "gerontocomia" from the Greek "care for the aged") was used since the time of Galen (Aelius/Claudius Galenus, c. 129-217 AD, Galen, 5th Book, *De tuenda Sanitate. Gerontocomia* (5th book *On the Preservation of Health. Gerontocomia*), quoted in Sir John Floyer [1649-1734], *Medicina gerocomica, or, The Galenic art of preserving old men's healths*, J. Isted, London, 1725, p. 107).

Another influential work on gerocomia was Gabriele Zerbi [1445-1505], *Gerontocomia, scilicet de senium cura atque victu* (1489, "Gerontocomia, or, care and nutrition for old age," written in Rome upon request of Pope Innocent VIII, 1432-1492).

9. The term "gerontology" (the study of aging) was coined in Elie Metchnikoff, *Études sur la Nature Humaine* (Etudes on the Nature of Man), Masson, Paris, 1903. The Russian edition used here is I.I. Metchnikoff, *Etudy o Prirode Cheloveka* (Etudes On the Nature of Man), Izdatelstvo Academii Nauk SSSR (The USSR Academy of Sciences Press), Moscow, 1961 (1915, first published in 1903), Ch. 12 "Obshy Obzor I Vyvody" (General review and conclusions), p. 242.

10. The term "anti-aging" was first widely used in the 1920s-1930s, but mainly in chemical engineering, particularly with regard to the protection of rubber, using "anti-agers, age resisters, or anti-oxidants" (George Oenslager, Ch. 13. "Chemical and Engineering Advances in the Rubber Industry," in Sidney D. Kirkpatrick (Ed.), *Twenty-Five Years of Chemical Engineering Progress*, American Institute of Chemical Engineers, New York, 1933, p. 181).

A Canadian patent "for a process of treating rubber or similar material ... in the presence of anti-ageing material" was issued in 1917 (*The Canadian Patent Office Record*, September 1917, p. 2778).

The term was then very seldom used in the field of medicine, as for example in the cursory mention of "anti-aging treatment" in "The Cry for Youthfulness," *The Urologic and Cutaneous Review*, vol. 32, 1928, p. 40.

The term "anti-aging" seems to have become noticeable in medical discourse only in the late 1940s, with the appearance of such expressions as "anti-aging program" (Charles Ward Crampton, *Live Long and Like It*, 1948, p. 16); "anti-aging work" (*Science Digest*, vol. 21, 1947, p. 30), "anti-aging science" (*Nation's Business*, vol. 37, 1949, p. 76), "anti-aging factors" (*Conference on Problems of Aging, Transactions of the Tenth and Eleventh Conferences, 1948-1949*, Josiah Macy Jr. Foundation, NY, 1950, p. 168).

One of the earliest scientific reports on "anti-aging" substances as well as "gerontotherapeutics" that I could find, was made in 1948 by Thomas Samuel Gardner (1908-1963) from Rutherford, New Jersey, the original home base of the Becton-Dickinson medical technology company. (Thomas Samuel Gardner, "The design of experiments for the cumulative effects of vitamins as anti-aging factors," *Journal of the Tennessee Academy of Sciences*, 23(4), 291-306, 1948.)

As Gardner stated, "In conclusion it would not be an exaggeration to suggest that longevity research work may be the most profitable field of human well-being, as well as from the commercial returns, of all of the present fields of medical investigations" (p. 302).

Interestingly enough, T.S. Gardner's work inspired the philanthropist Paul Glenn to establish in 1965 the "Glenn Foundation," one of the earliest American sponsors of basic research into the molecular biology of aging and age-related diseases ("The Mysteries of Aging: Paul F. Glenn," MIT School of Science, http://web.archive.org/web/20130724035802/http://web.mit.edu/science /alumniandfriends/profiles/glenn.html).

11. The term "prolongevity" or "prolongevitism" was coined by the medical historian Gerald Joseph Gruman (1926-2007, University of Massachusetts), in *A History of Ideas about the Prolongation of Life. The Evolution of Prolongevity Hypotheses to 1800*, Transactions of the American Philosophical Society, Volume 56(9), Philadelphia, 1966, reprinted as Gerald J. Gruman, *A History of Ideas About the Prolongation of Life (Classics in Longevity and Aging)*, Springer Publishing Company, New York, 2003.

12. It seems, the term "Immortalism," referring to the advocacy of radical life extension, took hold in the late 1960s, after the inauguration of the journal *The Immortalist* in 1967 by the Immortalist Society, led by the American founder of cryonics Robert Ettinger. The term gained in popularity after the publication of Alan Harrington philosophical-apologetic book, *The Immortalist*, in 1969.

But the term appeared in English as early as the 18th century (though since then until the 1960s it mainly referred to the belief in the immortality of the soul). Thus in 1774, the book-seller, historian and philosopher William Creech (1745-1815) of Edinburgh, Scotland, wrote:

"The Immortalist, therefore, is the only philosopher, who can render the parts of Christianity consistent and homogeneous. For, if the essence of man be not evanescent and fluctuating, but immaterial and permanent; if the body be no more than a mere instrument of action and vehicle of perception, then is essential identity ascertained; then the idea of accountability remains; and the man is as much punishable in a new body for crimes committed in the old one, as a robber is amenable in a new suit of cloaths, for a theft committed in those he formerly wore."

(William Creech, "Review of New Publications. Institutes of Natural and Revealed Religion, vol. III. Containing a view of the Doctrines of Revelation. By Joseph Priestley LL.D. F.R.S," *The Edinburgh Magazine and Review by a Society of Gentlemen*, Volumes 1-2, November 1774, p. 714.)

13. The term "Transhumanism" appeared in varying contexts since the second half of the 20th century. Sources mentioning this term include:

Pierre Teilhard de Chardin, "From the Pre-Human to the Ultra-Human: The Phases of a Living Planet" (written in 1950 and first published in 1951) and "The Essence of the Democratic Idea: A Biological Approach" (written in 1949, but at the time unpublished), in Teilhard de Chardin, *The Future of Mankind*, translated by Norman Denny, Harper & Row, New York, 1959;

Julian Huxley, "Transhumanism," in *New Bottles for New Wine*, Chatto & Windus, London, 1957, pp. 13-17;

Fereydun M. Esfandiary (a.k.a. FM-2030), *Are You a Transhuman?* Warner Books, New York, 1989, and in FM-2030, "New Concepts of the Human," 1966, quoted in Nick Bostrom, "The Transhumanist FAQ. What is a transhumanism and the transhuman?" 1999, 2003;

Max More, "Transhumanism: Toward a Futurist Philosophy," 1990, 1996.

14. Jean-Marie Robine and Michel Allard, "The oldest human," *Science*, 279(5358), 1834-1835, 1998.

15. As of 2011, the PubMed database search on "life extension" yielded about 2,000 results, and only about 20 (~1%) contained "life-extension" or "life-span extension" in the title of the article. Apparently, in the vast majority of cases, "life" and "extension" are considered separately. As of 2014, the total number of such articles increased to about 3,400.

16. For example, Max Fogiel (Ed.), *The Biology Problem Solver. A Complete Solution Guide to Any Textbook* (Research and Education Association, Piscataway, New Jersey, US, 1990, republished in 2001) contains about 800 problems ("for undergraduate and graduate studies") relating to all areas of biology and physiology. Yet the single problem even remotely related to aging is that on the menopause. The term "death" is scarcely ever mentioned and is not indexed. And many more such examples can be cited.

17. *Natural History of Pliny* (translated by John Bostock and H.T. Riley), Henry G. Bohn, London, 1855, vol. 2, Book 7, Ch. 2 "The wonderful forms of different nations," p. 134, Ch. 49 "The greatest length of life," p. 200.

Herodotus (c. 484-425 BCE) spoke of the extremely long-lived "macrobii" and "Hyperboreans" in Herodotus, *The Histories* (edited by A.D. Godley, 1920), sections 3.17-25, 4.13.1, reprinted at the Perseus Project, Tufts University, Boston MA, http://www.perseus.tufts.edu/.

The extremely long-lived Hyperboreans are also mentioned in the *Pythian Odes* of Pindar (c. 518 - 438 BC) (Pindar, *Odes*, "Pythian Ode 10," edited by Diane Svarlien, 1990, Perseus Project, http://www.perseus.tufts.edu).

Hesiod spoke of the Hyperboreans in the "Catalogues of Women" (*Hesiod, The Homeric Hymns, and Homerica, by Homer and Hesiod*, Project Gutenberg, http://www.gutenberg.org/files/348/348-h/348-h.htm#2H_4_0024).

18. *Hufeland's Art of Prolonging Life,* Edited by Erasmus Wilson, Lindsay & Blakiston, Philadelphia, 1867, pp. IX-X, originally Christoph Wilhelm Hufeland, *Makrobiotik; oder, Die Kunst das menschliche Leben zu verlängern,* first published in Jena in 1796.

19. The scientists considered in this work, include (in rough chronological order):

In the period 1890-1930 – the Russian/French immunologist Elie Metchnikoff, the French physiologist Charles-Édouard Brown-Séquard, the Russian/French surgeon Serge Voronoff, the French philosopher Jean Finot, the Austrian physician Eugen Steinach, the French/American biologist Alexis Carrel, the Russian physician and politician Alexander Bogdanov, the German/American biologist Jacques Loeb, the American biologists Charles Stephens and Raymond Pearl, and the British playwright Bernard Shaw.

In the period 1930-1950 – the French biologist and inventor Auguste Lumière, the German physicians Ludwig Roemheld, Gerhard Venzmer and Max Bürger, the Romanian gerontologists Dimu Kotsovsky, Ana Aslan and Constantin Ion Parhon, the Swiss physicians Paul Niehans and Fritz Verzár, the Russian physiologists Alexander Bogomolets and Alexander Nagorny, the American physiologists Edmund Cowdry, Clive McCay and Walter Cannon, and the Russian/British physician Vladimir Korenchevsky.

In the period 1950-1980 – the Russian scientists Vasily Kuprevich, Lev Komarov and Nikolay Amosov, and the American scientists Linus Pauling, Robert Ettinger, Denham Harman, Johan Bjorksten and Bernard Strehler.

And in 1980-2017 – the British Aubrey de Grey, the Russian Vladimir Skulachev, the Americans Ray Kurzweil and Michael West, and many others.

20. Charles E. Rosenberg, "Holism in twentieth-century medicine," in Christopher Lawrence, George Weisz (Eds.), *Greater Than the Parts: Holism in Biomedicine, 1920-1950,* Oxford University Press, Oxford, 1998, p. 335.

21. Gerald Joseph Gruman, *A History of Ideas about the Prolongation of Life. The Evolution of Prolongevity Hypotheses to 1800,* Transactions of the American Philosophical Society, Volume 56(9), Philadelphia, 1966, reprinted as Gerald J. Gruman, *A History of Ideas About the Prolongation of Life (Classics in Longevity and Aging),* Springer Publishing Company, New York, 2003.

22. Herbert Spencer, *The Data of Ethics,* Ch. 3 "Good and Bad Conduct," § 9, Williams and Norgate, London, 1879, reprinted in the Online Library of Liberty, http://oll.libertyfund.org.

23. Robert Veatch, *Death, Dying, and the Biological Revolution. Our Last Quest for Responsibility,* Yale University Press, New Haven CT, 1977, Ch. 8 "Natural death and public policy," pp. 293-305;

John Harris, "Immortal Ethics," presented at the International Association of Biogerontologists (IABG) 10th Annual Conference "Strategies for

Engineered Negligible Senescence," Queens College, Cambridge, UK, September 17-24, 2003, reprinted in *Strategies for Engineered Negligible Senescence: Why Genuine Control of Aging May Be Foreseeable* (Aubrey de Grey, Ed.), *Annals of the New York Academy of Sciences*, 1019, 527-534, June 2004.

Further on the ethics of radical life extension, see: Christine Overall, *Aging, Death, and Human Longevity: A Philosophical Inquiry*, University of California Press, Berkeley, CA, 2003. The book finds "the usual arguments against seeking immortality" unconvincing (p. 153).

See also: Frida Fuchs-Simonstein, *Self-evolution: The Ethics of Redesigning Eden*, Yozmot, Tel Aviv, 2004. The book argues that "It seems improbable to find ethical objections to increasing life spans, or even immortality, when it means saving someone's life" (p. 181).

24. Richard P. Feynman, "What Is and What Should be the Role of Scientific Culture in Modern Society," presented at the Galileo Symposium in Florence, Italy, in 1964, in Richard P. Feynman, *The Pleasure of Finding Things Out: The Best Short Works of Richard P. Feynman*, Perseus Books, NY, 1999, p. 100.

25. *Merriam-Webster Dictionary*, in *Encyclopedia Britannica*, Deluxe Edition CD, London, 2000. Similar definitions of adjustment, adaptation, balance and equilibrium, are given in the Free Online Dictionary, http://www.thefreedictionary.com/.

7. Reductionism and Holism in the History of Aging and Longevity Research: Does the Whole have Parts?

Summary

The research of aging and life extension has been notoriously characterized by a multitude of often contradictory approaches, both in terms of theoretical concepts as well as possible practical interventions. This work will explore a general taxonomy of these approaches that seems to be ubiquitous in the history of aging and longevity research. The taxonomy will juxtapose between reductionist/therapeutic and holistic/hygienic approaches to potential life-extending interventions. Both approaches sought to achieve biological equilibrium and constancy of internal environment, yet emphasized diverging means and diverging perceptions of what constitutes equilibrium and constancy. The reductionist approach saw the human body as a machine in need of repair and internal adjustment and equilibration, seeking to achieve material homeostasis by eliminating damaging agents and introducing biological replacements, in other words, working by subtraction and addition toward balance. The holistic approach, in contrast, focused on the equilibration of the organism as a unit within the environment, strongly emphasizing the direct sustaining and revitalizing power of the mind and hygienic regulation of behavior. In the holistic approach, internal equilibrium was sought not so much through calibrating intrusions, but through resistance to intrusions. The apparent relative weight of each approach in public discourse will be shown to change with time, in several western countries, with a special focus on France in the first half of the twentieth century, reflecting the initial hopes, disappointments and reactions to those disappointments in a variety of scientific programs. The potential benefits and drawbacks of both the reductionist and holistic approaches to the problems of aging and longevity will be thus exemplified.

Introduction: Reductionism vs. Holism – a major dichotomy among potential life extension methods

The history of biomedical research of aging and longevity has been an integral part of general medical history, though this relationship is not always acknowledged. Yet, in fact, studies, explicitly aiming to ameliorate the degenerative aging process and prolong human life, often constituted a formidable motivation for biomedical research and discovery. Arguably, at

114

least several modern biomedical fields have originated directly from aging and life extension research. Some examples include hormone replacement therapy born in Charles-Edouard Brown-Séquard's rejuvenation experiments with animal gland extracts (1889), probiotic diets originating in Elie Metchnikoff's conception of radically prolonged "orthobiosis" (c. 1900), the cell therapy and tissue replacement therapy methods now currently referred to as "regenerative medicine" owing a lot to the experiments on cell and tissue culture and replacement by Eugen Steinach, Serge Voronoff, Alexis Carrel, Paul Niehans and others.[1,2] Yet, the field has also been notoriously controversial and diverse concerning the prospective actual or potential methods that should be pursued for the amelioration of aging and achievement of life extension, their scientific, methodological and practical merits. Historically, the research of aging and life extension has been teeming with a multitude of often contradictory approaches, both in terms of theoretical concepts as well as possible practical interventions. The present work will attempt to provide an over-arching categorical dichotomic framework for those diverse approaches.

I argue that, despite the great diversity of suggestions for possible methods and research directions toward life prolongation, a major basic dichotomy transpires: between what can be termed the "holistic/hygienic approaches" that emphasized the importance of psychological environment and hygienic regulation of behavior to maintain the harmony of the whole vs. the "reductionist/therapeutic approaches" which sought ways to eliminate damaging agents and to introduce biological replacements to maintain the human machine in good working order. Apparently, these approaches have always coexisted side by side, though it may be possible to observe that the ostensible relative weight of each approach in public discourse (in terms of notoriety and prestige, funding, amount and dissemination of relevant publications) changed with time, reflecting the initial hopes, disappointments and reactions to those disappointments in a variety of scientific programs in particular local contexts. The distinction between holistic and reductionist approaches has been definitive for the history of modern medicine,[3] and the history of longevity research illustrates and foregrounds this distinction.

France – a seedbed of modern aging and longevity research. The reductionist roots of this research

France represents probably one of the best examples of this distinction. France was a fertile, perhaps even a primary ground for the research of aging and longevity since the Enlightenment and even earlier. In mid-19th century, profound contributions to the practical treatment of the elderly were made by the founders of *Médecine de Vieillards* (medicine of the aged), in particular Charles-Louis-Maxime Durand-Fardel, Jean-Martin Charcot and others. Pioneering contributions were made to the theory of aging by Marie-Jean-Pierre Flourens (1794-1867) and Édouard Robin (c. 1859).[1] In the late 19th – early 20th century, the pursuit of human life extension was encouraged by peaceful and prosperous social conditions, and by the philosophical traditions of positivism, liberalism and progressivism. In this period, France produced some of the world's ground-breaking advancements in the theory of aging, methods of rejuvenation and life-extensionist philosophy. This is epitomized by the works of Elie Metchnikoff (1845-1916), a vice director of the Pasteur Institute in Paris, the Nobel Laureate in Physiology/Medicine of 1908 and the author of the concept of "gerontology."[4] Another crucial figure was Charles-Édouard Brown-Séquard (1817-1894), the President of the French Biological Society, Chair of Medicine at Collège de France in Paris and the founder of therapeutic endocrinology that emerged from a "rejuvenation" experiment. Other prominent figures included Serge Voronoff (1866-1951) – one of the pioneers of xeno-transplantation born of rejuvenation attempts, Jean Finot (1856-1922) – the author of the "philosophy of long life" and more. In this formative period of the French school of aging and longevity research, reductionist and mechanistic proclivities were unmistakable.

Notably, since the mid-19th through the early 20th century, reductionism and materialism, essentially viewing the human body as a machine in need of repair, underscored most of the ground-laying works of French researchers of aging and longevity. Thus, the primary methodology of the French founders of "medicine of the aged" and aging-ameliorating interventions in the mid-19th century – Charles-Louis-Maxime Durand-Fardel, Jean-Martin Charcot and others – was dissection. Through the autopsy dissection, they established the age-related pathological changes in separate organs and tissues, in fact, reducing the entire process of aging to these specific organ changes. Though Durand-Fardel spoke of the life-span being determined by a holistic "vital principle of limited duration"[5] – finding tissue-specific degeneration was for him by far more determinative. One of the most prominent French researchers of longevity of the mid-19th century, Marie-Jean-Pierre Flourens (1794-1867), asserted that "Just as the duration of growth, multiplied a certain number of times, say five times, gives the ordinary duration of life, so does this ordinary duration, multiplied a certain number of times, say twice, give the extreme duration. A first century of ordinary life, and almost a second century, half a century (at least) of extraordinary life, is then the prospect science holds out to man" (1854).[6] He thus determined that human longevity is preset by a mechanical body buildup, as if by winding of a clock-work. And the main line of Flourens' research on the localization of brain functions (the field he in fact founded) was an epitome of reductionism. Furthermore, one of the first

116

modern scientific theories of aging, proposed by Édouard Robin of the French Academy of Sciences in 1858, posited that aging is due to body "mineralization" or accumulation of "alkaline residues," "calcification" or "ossification." Robin's theory considered lactic acid and "vegetable acids" as possible means to dissolve the "mineral matters" and thus prolong life.[7,8] Thus, the body was essentially viewed as a rusting and clogging machine subject to a cleanup. (Unlike otherwise specified, hereafter all the excerpts are in my translation.)

The teachings of the most authoritative figures in aging and longevity research of the late 19th-early 20th century – the founder of therapeutic endocrinology Charles-Edouard Brown-Séquard and the founder of modern gerontology Elie Metchnikoff – were profoundly materialistic and reductionist. Brown-Séquard suggested that through the supplementation of deficient hormones, bodily equilibrium can be restored, youth returned, and life prolonged. In Brown-Séquard's seminal experiment of 1889 with self-injections with animal (dogs' and guinea pigs') sex gland extracts for rejuvenation (which laid down the foundation for modern therapeutic endocrinology), a chief concern was to rule out any psychosomatic influences and to reduce medical intervention to a subtraction or addition of matter.[9] Metchnikoff, in turn, in his foundational theory of aging (perhaps the first truly scientific theory of aging based on histological observations) divided the body into "noble" or "functional" elements (mainly the parenchymal tissues, such as the heart and the brain) and "primitive" or "harmful" elements (such as the "devouring phagocytes" and intoxicating putrefactive microflora). The former needed to be strengthened or replenished, the latter destroyed or attenuated. Thus the body was seen as a sort of a mechanical balance, with weights added or subtracted as needed to keep the balance steady. According to Metchnikoff, the direct effects of the mind on the body were limited to "some nervous disorders."[10]

Materialism and reductionism underwrote the work of yet another prominent fin-de-siècle French proponent of healthy longevity, the social scholar Jean Finot. In *The Philosophy of Long Life* (1900), Finot did speak of "Will as a means of prolonging life," yet for him reductionism held the key for understanding, manipulating and extending life. In Finot's philosophy, biology is reducible to chemistry and physics, and the complexity of a living organism is reducible to an interrelation of its components. Such a reduction, according to Finot, opens the possibility for engineering life, and eventually for life's prolonged maintenance:[11]

"What is the life of a man? The result of the lives of millions of plastides. For each plastide lives its own life, and there are even cases in which the man dies whilst the plastides composing him continue to live. Now,

117

biology proves to us that among the phenomena observable at a given moment in a living plastide there is none which has no affinity to physics and to the chemistry of inert bodies. Nothing in them permits us to separate them from the body of elements already studied and possible of reproduction."

Equally in favor of materialism and reductionism were Metchnikoff's French followers, the physiologists Albert Dastre and Sergey Metalnikov. According to Albert Dastre (1844-1917), Claude Bernard's pupil and Chair of the Department of General Physiology at the Sorbonne, reductionism opens the possibility to profoundly manipulate life's components, since biology "is a particular chemistry, but chemistry none the less. ... The vital action is not distinct in basis from physicochemical action, but only in form." Subjected to physicochemical manipulation, human beings may "remain forever in full health and guarded from disease."[12] And according to Metchnikoff's pupil at Institut Pasteur, Sergey Metalnikov (1870-1946), senescence and death arise from a disharmony of differentiated body components. (This fundamental tenet was shared by the majority of *fin-de-siècle* theorists of aging, from August Weismann to Metchnikoff.) The basic unit of life, the cell, however was seen as potentially immortal. Therefore, according to Metalnikov, the body, composed of such potentially immortal units, can be made potentially immortal, if only learning to bring the components into harmony.[13]

Essentially, reductionism formed the theoretical basis for the rejuvenation experiments in humans at that period. The "father" of rejuvenative hormone replacement therapy, Brown-Séquard, vigorously defended the specificity of sex hormone injections and countered critics (such as Dr. Amédée Dumontpallier, 1826-1899) who argued that their effects are due to auto-suggestion or non-specific stimulation (i.e. that any injection would produce the same stimulating effect on the body). Brown-Séquard's follower, the Russian-born Parisian surgeon Serge Voronoff, famous for the transplantation ("grafting") into humans of animal (mainly male ape) sex gland tissues for "rejuvenation," continued in his master's footsteps. Voronoff recapitulated the basic theoretical premise that the deterioration of aging is due to an imbalance of the components comprising the body machinery, and that the balance can be restored through supplementing or replacing failing components.[14-16] Voronoff's methodology of "rejuvenation" by sex gland "grafting" was reductionist almost by definition: by substituting (grafting) a single crucial element in the body mechanism (the sex gland tissue), the machine's 'run-time' could be increased. The grafting did affect the whole body, but the effect was believed to be analogous to replacing an energy carrier (a principal component or a "battery") to sustain the operation of the entire machine.

Voronoff's reductionist and mechanistic views were explicit. He spoke of the "essential mechanism of our body" where "each organ performs its part," the thyroid gland provides "the brain-motor's ignition spark," all the endocrine glands are "wonderful little factories" that "regulate the action of each organ" and, when some of these controls fail, the body is "put out of gear" and disintegrates. The sex glands, the main object of rejuvenating interventions, are akin to a battery, supplying the body with "vital energy." The removal of particular parts brings about disarray and death, while their replacement provides new "sources of energy," reestablishes the "controls" and restores the body's "equilibrium of functions." Hence, a major task of rejuvenative medicine is to establish "a stock of spare parts for the human machine." A central place in Voronoff's writings was reserved for anatomical and histological examinations, for detailing the surgical technique intended to rearrange the parts of the mechanism.[14-16] Indeed, Voronoff attributed great importance to the "psychic" effects of the grafting operation, but only to demonstrate how a material, "mechanistic" interference positively affects the mental sphere: improving intelligence, productivity, interest in life. But the opposite influence, from the mind onto the body, was thoroughly depreciated. Such mind-over-body effects would obscure the results of treatment and had to be ruled out.

The grafting appeared to be a novel, unorthodox intervention, but Voronoff's central claim was that the operation restored the natural equilibrium of the body. The ultimate aim of rejuvenation techniques was, in accordance to Claude Bernard's dictum, to achieve "the fixity of the internal environment" which is "the condition for free life."[17] And the means to attain this fixity were through supplementing or replacing those components whose deteriorative change would otherwise threaten the overall body stability. Reductionism might thus be pivotal for the rejuvenation enterprises of the early 20th century: the supplementation or replacement of an isolated component appeared to the rejuvenators a feasible task, perhaps more feasible than attempting to comprehend and/or manipulate the whole of the human reaction to the whole of the external environment. Beside Voronoff, the cohort of French pioneers of rejuvenation (mainly practicing sex gland tissue transplantations and various other means of endocrine rejuvenation) included Placide Mauclaire, Lois Dartigues, Raymond Petit, Léopold Lévi, Henri de Rothschild, and others, forming a "school."

In later assessments, however, reductionist rejuvenation techniques did not appear to live up to their promise.[18] With regard to Voronoff's method, the problem of graft rejection by the host organism appeared almost insurmountable. Replacing or supplementing a single gland did not appear to durably forestall the deterioration of the entire organism, and no conclusive evidence for extending the life-span by such means was offered.

Consequently, a recoil from immediate rejuvenation attempts occurred, accompanied by a recoil from their underlying mechanism and reductionism.

The research of aging and longevity in France in 1930-1950. The strengthening of the holistic approach

In the 1930s-1940s, an increasing number of French researchers of aging and longevity began to espouse holistic perceptions of the unity of the mind and body, and the subordination of an individual to society, gradually replacing the earlier prevalent notions of reductionism, physicalism and individualism. The holistic tone in French research of aging of the 1930s-1940s was set by the leading French longevity researcher, one of the pioneers of tissue culture and regenerative medicine, Alexis Carrel (1873-1944).[2] Echoing Auguste Comte, who asserted that "No sound treatment of either body or mind is possible, now that the physician and the priest make an exclusive study, the one of the physical, the other of the moral nature of man,"[19] Carrel urged:[20]

> "Man is much more than a sum of analytical components. One has to embrace at the same time both the parts and the unity of man, because he reacts like a unit, and not like a multiplicity, to the cosmic, economic and psychological milieu. The solution of grand problems of civilization depends on the knowledge not only of different aspects of humanity, but of the human being as a whole: as an individual within a group, a nation and a race. This is the true science of man…. The conquest of health is not sufficient. It is the progress of a human person that is sought, because the quality of life is more important than life in and of itself."

Such a holistic vision moved away from the earlier materialistic and reductionist proclivities of French life-extensionists.

The recoil from reductionist rejuvenation took many forms. First and foremost, since immediate rejuvenation appeared at the time untenable, the scholarly focus seems to have shifted to basic research of aging, predicated on the assumption that only after a comprehensive, lengthy and costly investigation, the complexity of the aging processes can be gradually unraveled, and consequently, in some distant future, actual life-extending interventions may be found. The concepts of bodily "equilibrium" of the early rejuvenators were rather qualitative and vague, and it was necessary to establish precisely what components and quantities constitute "steady states" or deviations from them. The practical aims of aging research became more modest: rather than attempting to effect an immediate and thorough rejuvenation, it became more presentable to seek a thorough understanding of the aging process and perhaps some mitigation of age-related diseases. Such an emphasis on basic research and caution in goals have been expressed by many researchers of aging, in particular in France, since the late 1930s through the early 1950s.[1] Another form of withdrawal was a rejection of "surgical" means of rejuvenation, in favor of more "natural" improvements in the life style.

Yet perhaps one of the central forms of withdrawal from rejuvenation attempts appears to have been a movement away from their underlying reductionism, and toward a more holistic perspective. This trend seems to have been salient in the "post-Voronoff" French longevity research community, and was epitomized by the work of Auguste Lumière, the crusader for the revival of "humoralist" medicine, among many other contemporary French physicians and biologists.

Auguste Lumière (1862-1954) could be considered as one of the leading actors in the "holistic turn" in French research of aging and longevity of the 1930s-1940s. Auguste and Louis Lumière (1864-1948) are renowned for the creation of cinematography in 1895. Perhaps less known is their deep involvement in biomedical research, especially that of Auguste.[21] Thus, during WWI Louis constructed articulated arm prostheses for amputees, while Auguste developed a non-adherent anti-septic bandage (tulle gras) that dramatically reduced the time of wound healing, introduced oral anti-typhoid vaccination, anti-tetanus serum booster (sodium persulfate), and more. While Louis concentrated more on research and development of photographic technology, Auguste fully dedicated his efforts to biomedical research proper, with a notable emphasis on aging, rejuvenation and life-extension.[22]

Lumière's medical theory and practice were based on the most ancient and widespread holistic medical tradition of all – the "Humoralism." For thousands of years, the balance and stability of different body liquids (or "humors") was seen as the necessary condition for health and longevity. Auguste Lumière's most ambitious and pervasive project was "The Renaissance of the Humoral Medicine."[23] It was Lumière's task to revive the humoralist tradition, to create a new "scientific humoralism" that would focus on establishing the balance of all types of liquids throughout the body, especially intracellular and interstitial liquids. As for the earlier "humoralist" theories, for Lumière the key concepts were "balance," "equilibrium," "stability" and "fixity." He just introduced other constituents of "equilibrium," different from the equilibrium of "essential elements" in Roger Bacon, Paracelsus and other alchemists, or the equilibrium of "cell types" in Metchnikoff, Steinach, Voronoff and great many other life-extensionist physiologists in the first quarter of the century. Instead, Lumière's theory considered the equilibrium and stability of cell colloids – dispersed liquid suspensions of macro-molecules (particularly proteins), or micelloids (colloid droplets). And this is the gist of his theory: When the colloids are stable and balanced (maintained dispersed in suspension), this state is characteristic of health and vitality; but when the colloids become unstable or imbalanced, they precipitate and flocculate – and this is the state of pathology and aging.[24] For Lumière, at the infancy of molecular biology, the colloids were essentially blobs of matter that "congest" or "dissolve," with molecular composition and mechanisms unknown. Nonetheless, he was able to detect the colloids' "stability" or "perturbations" and incorporated that knowledge into a vast explanatory apparatus and therapeutic methodology, including anti-aging strategies aimed to "stabilize the cell colloids."

One of Lumière's favorite "stabilizing substances" (essentially emulsifiers) was Magnesium Hyposulfite ($Mg\text{-}S_2O_3$), an anti-shock substance, capable of "reestablishing humoral equilibrium" and "inhibiting the disorganization of colloids, with all the cortege of disorders this entails." It was also supposed to exert a general "desensitizing" (immunizing or tempering) effect on the entire body.[25] A wide variety of other "desensitizing" and "stabilizing" agents were tested and clinically applied by Lumière: "Anti-bacterial desensitization" (the regular immunization by specific antigens, e.g. Koch bacillus extracts), "Auto-hemotherapy" (injection of the patient's own blood, presumably exerting "desensitizing" effects), as well as a wide assortment of metal compounds: magnesium benzoate, copper glycocholate, sodium undecylate, etc. etc. A special place was reserved for compounds of gold, partly realizing the ancient dream of alchemists. Chrysotherapy, using salts of gold, such as Allochrisine, was employed to stabilize innumerable "humoral imbalances" (and gold particles are still used today in the treatment of rheumatoid arthritis and other diseases, even in "nanomedicine"[26]). "Granulotherapy" or "Anthrotherapy" employed small carbon or other particles, not just to absorb toxins, but to produce a "mild mechanical irritation" in order to achieve general desensitization and stimulate phagocytosis (also reminiscent of some more recent "nanomedicine" experiments[27]). Changing the blood volume was yet another mechanical means to influence the colloidal state. Changing fluid pressure would change the vasomotor sensitivity to the pressure of flocculates, and consequently affect the sensitivity or immunity to shock. Accordingly, the most ancient methods of "balancing the humors" – the blood-letting or water intake – remained in the arsenal and were given a new rationale. Yet another therapy dear to Lumière's heart was "negative ionization," using the "aero-ionization lamp" introduced by the Russian biophysicist Alexander Chizhevsky in 1919. In Lumière's view, negative ions presumably stabilize the colloids' electrical charge. Endocrine extracts too were employed for colloids' stabilization, for maintaining the "equilibrium of humors," continuing the studies of "endocrine rejuvenation" started by Voronoff and others.

Despite some similarities of methodology, Lumière in fact broke away from the "rejuvenators" of the 1920s, such as Voronoff. The dissent manifested in the criticism and skepticism of the actual effectiveness of their methods, and in the fact that hormone replacements played only a very minor part in Lumière's clinical practice. But perhaps the strongest point of departure was Lumière's withdrawal from the mechanistic reductionism that underscored the majority of rejuvenation techniques. Not only did he emphasize the importance of purely psychological motivation for longevity, but the body itself was seen as much more than a combination of its parts. In *Sénilité et Rajeunissement* (Aging and Rejuvenation, 1932, pp. 94-95), Lumière wrote:

> "The most important [characteristic of living beings] consists in the prodigious faculty of synthesis that only the living cells possess and that does not appear in any measure and in any degree in other molecular arrangements... Experience and observation, unaffected by all the reasoning of logicians, demonstrate that the properties of a substance essentially depend on the arrangement, the assemblage, the aggregation of atoms and molecules that compose it, and that these assemblages give birth, out of all the pieces, to novel properties that are present in no way and in no degree in the constituent parts."

Lumière's model of the body just could not be easily broken down into parts, because it was mainly composed of "balanced fluids."

The therapeutic implications of this "holistic" theory followed. As Lumière insisted, all therapy should be combined, multi-faceted or "polyvalent" (*Les Horizons de la Médecine*, 1937, p. 60):

> "One grand principle must dominate the methods of treatment of chronic functional afflictions: in pathological states, the disequilibrium and the instability of humors depend on accidents that have multiple causes; with rare exceptions, the stabilizing and curative therapy directed against them cannot achieve its goal except when it addresses simultaneously all the causes, that is to say, it must be "polyvalent" in order to be completely efficient.... [It is necessary] to remedy, in the same time, all the dysfunctions and eliminate all the factors that are involved in their production."

Furthermore, he strove to provide a unifying framework for the phenomena of therapeutic non-specificity that may explain many therapeutic and rejuvenative effects (*La Renaissance de la Médecine Humorale*, 1937, p. 267):

"This conception [of humoral destabilization through flocculation of colloids] allows us to understand medical mysteries that would remain impenetrable without it. This notion explains to us why a single agent can cause diverse afflictions; why a multiplicity of essentially different agents can generate the same disease; why a single remedy can cure multiple distinct afflictions; why many completely different medications can cure the same syndrome; and why the major symptoms of acute maladies present a remarkable similarity. This is because all these phenomena share one common factor – the flocculate."

Both Voronoff and Lumière sought "equilibrium" and "fixity." According to Lumière, "the great principle of life appears to be fixity" that must be maintained in all life forms, from individual cells to organisms, to species to societies (*La Vie, La Maladie et La Mort, Phénomènes Colloïdaux*, 1928, pp. 66-67). The task of therapy, for Lumière as well as for Voronoff, consisted in maintaining the fixity, safeguarding it against catastrophe or degenerative change. But, paradoxically, in the quest for "fixity," in the struggle against formidable change, both scientists became great medical innovators, introducing new "stabilizing" treatments that may appear unorthodox even by contemporary standards.

Yet, an important difference may be pointed out between Lumière and Voronoff. In Lumière, the "vital equilibrium" appears to be much more complex than Voronoff's "human machine." In Lumière's vision, the equilibrium must involve the responses of the body as a whole, including diverse environmental and psychological factors. Compared to Voronoff, Lumière was much more willing to admit to his almost complete ignorance of these intricacies. In *Sénilité et Rajeunissement* (p. 91), he stated:

"If, generally, we perceive the existence of a relation between matter and intelligence, we are completely ignorant of the mechanisms that govern this relation, and the cause for psychic equilibrium completely evades us. Not only in this order of phenomena has the vital equilibrium remained an enigma: the processes of the regulation of all organic functions, the thermal, the respiratory, the cardiac, etc.... remain entirely obscure. We are ignorant!"

It was perhaps this realization of the immense complexity of the "vital equilibrium," of integrating elements that could not be readily "removed" or "supplemented," that contributed to Lumière's withdrawal from the current rejuvenation methods, and caused him to seek solace in anticipating the results of "future research."

Intriguingly, despite the humility before the grandeur of the "organism as a whole," Lumière remained a "therapeutic activist" and "scientific optimist" to the end of his nonagenarian life. A similar coexistence of therapeutic and scientific optimism with the great "holistic" awe before the complexity and wholeness of the human being, in his/her infinite connectedness to the society and the universe, is salient in the work of other French contemporary longevity researchers and seekers of "equilibrium", members of the so-called "Neo-Hippocratic" holistic movement. After his return to France from the US in 1939, Carrel became one of the leaders of this movement. Yet many other prominent figures supported the movement. The supporters included prominent physicians, some of them members of the French Academy of Sciences and the Medical Academy, heads of medical departments. They were united against the "analytical," "materialistic," "mechanistic" and "dehumanizing" approaches in medicine, and unanimous in their advocacy of "synthesis," treating the human being as "a whole," with due consideration of his mental or "psychic" activities, "imponderable" factors in healing, the recognition of the patients' individuality, the integration of an individual with the grander social and physical environment. These emphases are now firmly associated with a "holistic" medical paradigm.

The proponents of the movement did not use the term "holism," but rather saw themselves as "Neo-Hippocratists." From the teachings of Hippocrates, they derived the basis for considering the human being as a "whole" in an unbreakable rapport with the environment, with season and place. Following Hippocrates, they sought to maintain a physiological and mental equilibrium, never considering a disease as an entity, but as a temporal imbalance of the equilibrium. The equilibrium, according to them, could be restored not so much by chemicals and operations, but rather by a more "natural" and "moderate" way of life. Depreciating heroic interventions, they strove to assist the "healing power of nature" through adjusting the life-style, and most of all, by cultivating the healing power of the mind. These principles were, according to them, neglected by the "official" or "materialistic" medicine and must be restored.

In the 1930s-early 1940s, France was at the forefront of the "Neo-Hippocratic" and "Naturist" movement, upheld by such prominent physicians as Jean Poucel, Claude Sigaud, Paul Carton, René Biot, Louis Corman, Pierre Winter and others.[28] In 1933, the world's first journal dedicated to natural and integrative medicine – *Hippocrate* – was inaugurated by Prof. Maxime Laignel-Lavastine of Paris. In the same year, on the initiative of Dr. Jérome Casabianca, there was organized in Marseille "La Société de Médecine Naturiste de Marseille – Médecine Préventive et Néohipppocratique" (the Marseille society for naturist, preventive and neo-Hippocratic medicine). The first International Congress on Neo-Hippocratism was held in July 1937 in Paris, under Laignel-Lavastine's presidency. Then, the first grand, national conference in the field took place in Marseille in November 1938, presided over by Prof. Lucien Cornil, dean of the Marseille medical faculty. In 1939, there was founded the "Union pour la defense de l'espèce" ("The union for the defense of the species") dedicated to developing agriculture "conforming to our physiological needs." At the time, these were pioneering institutions on the world scale, and they manifest a "holistic turn" in French medical science generally,[29] and in the approach to aging-related ill health in particular.

After the "holistic turn" France seems to have lost its leading position in the life-extensionist movement. The diminishing impact of French life-extensionists after the departure from reductionist rejuvenation endeavors is understandable, as it signified a departure from daring interventions toward a more protective and conservative attitude. Since the 1930s through the 1950s, the (predominantly critical and cautious) discussions of rejuvenation continued in France, notably by the founders of the French Society of Gerontology (formed in 1939) – Leon Binet (1891-1971) and Francois Bourlière (1913-1993). Leon Binet, who became president of the French Academy of Sciences in 1957, focused on clinical geriatrics and experimented with oxygen therapy and embryonic extracts. Francois Bourlière, who became the founding director of the Claude Bernard Center of Gerontology in Paris in 1956, conducted comparative studies of average longevity from various animal species and supported the use of hormones (mainly sex hormones) in geriatric therapy.[30] In the late 1940s, Michel Bardach of the Pasteur Institute in Paris advanced a "rejuvenative"/"orthobiotic"/"stimulating" cytotoxic serum.[31] In the 1950s and 1960s, the biologist and philosopher of science Jean Rostand (1894-1977) was an outspoken supporter of radical life extension and pioneer of cryo-preservation.[32] But none of these researchers seems to have had the notoriety and ambition of the French "founding fathers" of life-extensionism – Brown-Séquard, Metchnikoff and Voronoff. Was the therapeutic optimism "dissolved in the whole"?

A similar trend in the German-speaking aging research community

A very similar change of attitudes and approaches occurred in the German-speaking world, mainly in Austria and Germany (to a lesser extent in Switzerland). In the 1920s, "endocrine rejuvenation" became a world wide movement, spreading from the US to Russia and Japan. Yet, France and Austria emerged as the primary and competing rejuvenation superpowers. Beside the Parisian Voronoff and his "sex gland transplantations," a crucial figure in the rejuvenation movement was the Viennese physician Eugen Steinach (1861-1944), famous for the "Steinach operation," first performed in a human patient on November 1, 1918, which involved the ligation of seminal ducts ("vasoligation" or vasectomy). The theory behind the operation was quite reductionist and mechanistic. The vasoligation was supposed to suppress the sperm-producing activity and thereby to stimulate the hormone-producing activity of the "interstitial tissue" of the testis. Such enhanced sex hormone production was assumed to effect "rejuvenation," "revitalization" or "reinvigoration." The general rejuvenating effects were ascribed by Steinach to the whole-body increase in the blood flow (hyperemia) produced by the sex hormones (though Steinach recognized other methods of blood flow increase, such as diathermy, massage, exercise and baths). To avoid infertility, the operation was commonly performed only on one of the two spermatic ducts. Simply put, the operation was supposed to tweak and boost the energy supply mechanism.

Under Steinach's leadership, Austria (beside France) became a world leader in all matters of endocrine rejuvenation, renowned by the works of Erwin Last, August Bier, Karl Doppler, Emerich Ullmann, Paul Kammerer, Robert Lichtenstern, Otto Kauders, Gottlieb Haberlandt and others. Sigmund Freud (1856-1939) was enthusiastic enough about Steinach's rejuvenating operation to have it performed on himself in 1923 by the Viennese surgeon Victor Blum. In Germany too, in the first quarter of the century, the rejuvenation movement boomed, though perhaps to a lesser extent than in Austria. The German physiologist Jürgen Harms (1885-1956) performed the first testis transplantations in guinea pigs at about the same time as Steinach, in 1911, while Voronoff conducted the first testis transplantations in animals (he-goats and rams) only in 1917. In the 1920s, Harms was one of the most active proponents of sexual rejuvenation in humans, though Voronoff's work stirred a much greater sensation. One of the most energetic practitioners of Steinach's procedure in Germany was Peter Schmidt, having performed hundreds of operations in his clinic in Berlin. Other Berlin practitioners, such as Richard Mühsam and Ludwing Levy-Lenz, followed suit. Indeed, in the 1920s, Steinach's procedure was widely applied all across the world. In Germany, however, the application of Steinach's operation was among the widest. Beside operative interventions, by the late 1920s, hormonal preparations for rejuvenation became an object of keen interest in Germany. Sex gland extracts and stimulants became widely available for men and women: Testiglandol from Grenzach and Testifortan from Promonta, Novotestal from Merck and Plazentaopton from Kalle, Pituglandol and Neosex, Testogan and Yohimbin, Progynon and Menformon, Follikulin and Unden, dried ovaries, testis and erectile tissue powder. The majority of German founders of endocrinology (many of whom incidentally were Jewish) actively researched, developed and advertised the rejuvenating and eroticizing effects of such supplements. The proponents included Magnus Hirschfeld (the founder of the Institut für Sexualwissenschaft – the Institute for Sex Research in Berlin, and one of the first gay rights activists), Bernhard Schapiro (Hirschfeld's co-worker and co-developer of Testifortan), Max Hirsch (editor of the monumental *Handbuch der Inneren Sekretion* - Handbook of Inner Secretion, 1926-1933), Bernhard Zondek and Selmar Ascheim (developers of the first reliable pregnancy test), and Hermann Zondek (Bernhard's older brother, also a prominent endocrinologist) and others. In summary, in the 1920s the rejuvenation through "artificial" operative or pharmacological/organotherapeutic interventions flourished in Germany and Austria, and from this intertwined research into sex and rejuvenation a large part of modern endocrinology was born.[33]

Yet, similarly to the French-speaking scientific community, also for the German-speaking researchers of aging and longevity, by the early 1930s it was becoming increasingly clear that the "rejuvenation" methods did not quite live up to their promise. A corresponding recoil from the underlying reductionism occurred. A striking testimony to the disenchantment with "rejuvenation" and its underlying reductionism can be found in *Altern und Verjüngung. Eine Kritische Darstellung der Endokrinen "Verjüngungsmethoden," Ihrer Theoretischen Grundlagen und der Bisher Erzielten Erfolge* (Aging and Rejuvenation: A Critical Presentation of Endocrine "Rejuvenation Methods," Their Theoretical Foundations and Up-to-Date Successes), by Benno Romeis (1931).[34] Prof. Dr. Benno Romeis (1888-1971), at the time director of the Department of Experimental Biology of the Institute of Anatomy at the University of Munich, was an active member of the rejuvenation movement, having conducted in the 1920s extensive original studies on the effects of rejuvenating interventions (particularly Steinach's operations and hormonal supplements). *Altern und Verjüngung* (initially published as a part of Max Hirsch's *Handbuch der Inneren Sekretion*) was one of the most authoritative and thorough accounts of the worldwide rejuvenation research up-to-the-date, a watershed monograph, summarizing the rejuvenators' successes and failures and pointing out possible directions for future study. For most instances, Romeis's criticisms were devastating. Perhaps most importantly, the extensive anatomical and physiological data on age-related changes of various endocrine organs (thyroid, parathyroid, pituitary, adrenals, testes and ovaries) did not permit to ascribe to any of these organs the predominant or primary causative role in senescence, as many reductionist rejuvenators would have liked to believe. The whole appeared to be bigger than any particular component or the simple sum of them.

Generally, the rejuvenation methods were found thoroughly wanting methodologically. They did not fulfill the high popular expectations associated with them. Indeed, these methods demonstrated "some effects," such as increased appetite, improved libido and work power, in a large percentage of cases. Yet, these effects were mostly temporary and unpredictable, confounded by an immensity of other contributing factors and relativized by (mostly unknown) individual idiosyncrasies of each and every patient, under particular environmental circumstances and conditions. The evidence presented was often doctored or even falsified, and in any case contradictory and inconclusive. Neither operative nor supplementary rejuvenating methods provided any real evidence for a significant life extension or long-lasting health improvement. The effects of the "rejuvenation therapies" were shown to be usually of short duration, and stronger in younger patients (due to their generally better reactivity and reserves) rather than in the older patients for whom those therapies were presumably intended. The dominant reductionist theories of aging that underwrote those therapies, emphasizing the primary role of particular (mainly endocrine) organs in the aging process and in the reestablishment of organic equilibrium upon rejuvenation, were also found to be too rudimentary and restricted, requiring a profound elaboration.

Hence the strong disappointment with the therapeutic effectiveness of the rejuvenation methods was also accompanied by the disappointment with their underlying reductionist theories. And hence, similarly to France, the discussion of life extension in Germany in the 1930s showed a notable shift of emphasis from "materialistic-reductionist" or "artificial" rejuvenation toward more "natural" and "holistic" macrobiotic hygiene.[35] A good example of this shift of attitude can be seen in the book *Lang leben und jung bleiben!* (Live long and stay young!) (1937)[36] by Dr. Gerhard Venzmer (1893-1986) of Stuttgart, one the best known popularizers of life sciences in Germany, since the 1920s well into the 1950s, having written many books on diverse aspects of biomedicine, with a peak of acclaim during the Nazi period, with hundreds of thousands of copies in circulation. Venzmer's attitude to "rejuvenation" may be a prime example for the valorization of "natural" holistic hygiene over "artificial" and reductionist rejuvenative surgery and pharmacology. The very term "rejuvenation" was vilified: "The word 'rejuvenation'," Venzmer wrote, "was earlier severely abused. Overreaching reports, much more 'sensational' than factual, awakened false hopes, which were necessarily followed by bitter disappointments. All the endeavors to fight premature aging were thereby made 'unsavory'" (pp. 147-148).

In place of the "unsavory" (*anrüchig*) rejuvenation procedures, there comes the "natural" and holistic self-help, particularly emphasizing the health improvement systems practiced in Germany. Among the many

German life-extending projects promoted in the work, the anti-tobacco campaign was waged by Fritz Lickint. The life-prolonging breathing exercises or "gymnastics of the cardiovascular system" were recommended by Lothar Tirala and Ludwig Roemheld. The importance of physical exercise (particularly walking) against age-related cardiovascular diseases was emphasized by Julius Hermann Greeff. (Greeff was the author of apparently one of the world's first dedicated studies of centenarians, published in 1933.[37]) Relaxation techniques against cardiovascular and nervous diseases were suggested by Karl Fahrenkamp.[38] All these means were recommended by Venzmer as essential props to strengthen the vitality of the individual, and to maintain the entire "National Body" (*Volkskörper*). The emphasis on "natural" and holistic preventive measures was overwhelming. Several other examples of this trend of recoil from reductionist rejuvenation toward holistic life style improvement in Germany may be cited.[39-41] In Austria, the former seedbed of rejuvenation research, following its "Anschluss" (annexation) to Germany in 1938, the attitudes to rejuvenation became hardly distinguishable from those in Germany, as can be exemplified by the work on aging and longevity by the Austrian neurologist, president of the Austrian League for National Regeneration and Heredity, Julius Wagner-Jauregg (1857-1940).[42] This shift of attitudes to rejuvenation and life extension may have corresponded to the more general trend toward naturism and holism that was noted with reference to medicine in Nazi Germany in that period.[43]

With the "holistic" and "naturist" turn, it seems, the German-speaking aging and longevity research community also lost much of the pioneering drive that characterized the earlier "rejuvenators." It may be argued that the rise and fall of interest in rejuvenation attempts and their underlying reductionism was a global trend. After a surge of publications in the 1920s, in the 1930s the very term "rejuvenation" was rapidly disappearing from the scientific literature. According to Nathan Shock's *Classified Bibliography of Gerontology and Geriatrics* (1951, 1957, 1963), the number of publications on "rejuvenation" dropped from a maximum of 27 in 1928 to a minimum of 2 in 1940.[44] Yet, France alongside Austria and Germany represent perhaps the most salient examples of this trend. The scope of this work does not allow going into further details regarding other contexts.

Conclusion: Reductionism and Holism – which is "better"?

Admittedly the above examples are limited, and the scope of this work does not permit a more extensive further elaboration. For example, a thorough analysis of changes of attitudes in other national contexts or periods, especially after WWII until the present time, would go beyond the scope of this illustrative work. Yet, the examples above may serve well to illustrate the paradigmatic opposition and temporal succession between "reductionist" and "holistic" approaches in aging and longevity research. What philosophical or practical lessons can be learned from the examples of this opposition?

First of all, it is rather difficult to set in stone any definitive "oppositions" or temporal and local "trends" and "periods" in the pursuit of life extension. Just some apparent trends and predominant emphases can be observed. It should be noted, for example, that even at the peak of the "rejuvenation boom" in the 1920s, the reductionist endocrine rejuvenation was practiced by only a negligible proportion of the population (perhaps thousands operated and tens of thousands taking organotherapeutic supplements worldwide), leaving the rest of the world unaffected or even unfamiliar with these methods. In contrast, some forms of holistic physical culture and "healthy diet" could always be practiced by almost anybody. Thus "natural" and holistic means could have always predominated over the "artificial" and reductionist ones in popular practice. In the literature, however, the trends might be different. Indeed, in the scientific and popular-scientific literature, the "reductionist methods" may "leap to the eye" in the 1920s and disappear from view later on. Thus, the "reductionist" approach may be in a sense more "elitist," with a stronger appeal for the scientific community, perhaps even more fruitful for the development of science. After all, the reductionist understanding of the "mechanism" may require more intellectual rigor than the rather vague discussions of "wholeness." In contrast, holistic approaches may be more "populist," more easily accessible to lay audience and perhaps even more practical, following a set of rather simple and traditional recommendations for a healthy life style (such as cheerful attitude, rest and sleep, exercise, moderate and balanced nutrition). On the other hand, with all the valorization of holistic life style improvements, hormonal and other pharmacological supplements for rejuvenation and life extension have not vanished, but in fact formed the foundations for therapeutic endocrinology which became a part of massive healthcare practice. The balance and tradeoffs concerning the broadness of appeal and applicability of the different approaches should be kept in mind.

Another potential lesson is the suggestion of a strong relation between scientific perceptions and general social perceptions. It may not be an accident that many proponents and researchers of aging and life extension in Nazi Germany weighed heavily (though not exclusively) in favor of "natural" and holistic macrobiotic health regimens, despite many antagonistic undercurrents. The "natural" hygienic life style improvements were emphasized, as the German society was supposed to be reverting to a "natural" and therefore "healthy" state of the nation.[45] Moreover, the fear of reductionist intervention may have been a part of the general fear of any intervention into the "national body" from within or from without. In France, ideological parallels are more difficult to find. Nonetheless, it may not be accidental that the "holistic shift" occurred concomitantly with the strengthening of the so-called French political "traditionalism," reinforcing in the 1930s and culminating during the Vichy regime. The term "traditionalism" (*traditionalisme*) generally refers to an attempt to return to pre-Enlightenment values, for example, replacing the values of "Liberty, Equality, Fraternity" with "Labour, Family, Fatherland."[46] Yet, its extension into the field of longevity research is conceivable. It is difficult to speculate whether the attempts of rejuvenators to dissect and make far-reaching "progressive" intrusions into the "human nature" became increasingly suspicious within the political "traditionalist" paradigm; or whether the failure of the "rejuvenative" intrusions somehow contributed to the general rise of "traditionalism." In any case, the concomitance of the "holistic shift" with the rise of "traditionalism" may be significant. The same underlying psychological factors of populism and suspicion of "excessive" intellectualism, valorization of simplicity, alongside the fear of intrusion, and rejection of "modish" and presumably unsubstantiated novelty, may be implicated. Of course it would be a grave injustice to claim that all proponents of holism must necessarily also tend to nationalism and traditionalism, nonetheless, a significant correlation can be observed with reference to the specific historical examples.

The temporal succession of the trends may also be significant. The "strain" of reductionist analysis may be followed by a period of holistic "relaxation" (it may not be accidental that during relaxing meditation, unity and wholeness are commonly envisioned). The period of holistic relaxation may then again be followed by a period of reductionist effort. Though not elaborated here, a "comeback" of reductionist medical thinking may be observed after WWII in several national contexts, in particular with the development of "transplantation medicine."[1] The periodic change of attitudes may also point to a certain cyclicality in scientific thought, rather than unidirectional upward march of scientific progress. Such a cyclicality was noted earlier with reference to social structure and ideology, with analogies in human physiology. Thus, one of the prominent Russian longevity researchers of the early 20th century, Alexander Bogdanov (1873-1928, b. Alexander Malinovsky) – the creator of the science of "tectology" or the "universal science of organization" (1913-1928), a leader of the "Scientific Organization of Labor" movement in Russia, and the founding director of the State Institute for Blood Transfusion in Moscow, apparently the first such dedicated institute in the world – wrote in *Tectology*:[47]

"The increasing complexity of life's relations, the increase of their heterogeneity – decrease the harmonious order and stability of the entire

132

system… In all such cases, sooner or later, the accumulated instability leads to crisis. … Those crises that arise as a result of positive selection (and it must be remembered that this is not the only type of crisis) are usually accompanied by a change in the very direction of selection, which then becomes negative. … It manifests in destruction of those elements, connections or groups that are the least stable and vital, that in the largest measure disturb the internal organization of the whole. There takes place the simplification of the system, and increase of its harmonious order. Therefore, if the negative selection does not lead to a complete or profound destruction of the system, but is again followed by positive selection, then the subsequent growth and development of the system assume the characteristics of greater organization, the viability of the society increases, similar to how it happens under analogous cases concerning the viability of the organism."

The strengthening of reductionism may correspond to a period of "increasing complexity" or "heterogeneity", while holism may become more prevalent at the period of "simplification."

A question may arise: Which approach, the reductionist or the holistic, is conceptually "better"? Many clarifications are required to such a question. That is to say, "better" for which purposes? What is "better" – "the trees" (reductionism) or "the forest" (holism)? And can one see the forest for the trees, or the trees for the forest, or both at the same time? Presumably, at any given moment, one may either perceive "the whole" or "the parts," but not both at the same time. In this sense, what would be the meaning of "parts" within the "whole"? Perhaps some kind of "time-sharing" or "zooming" faculty is involved in shifting from reductionist analytical thinking to holistic synthetic thinking. These questions are rather speculative and hypothetical, yet hopefully they will encourage additional consideration. More rigorous definitions of medical "holism" and "reductionism" may be required to address these questions.

A more practical question may be: Which approach is "better" for therapy? Some authors argue against the predominance of "reductionism" in current medical thought, particularly in aging research, as being too limited, with its focus on selected mechanisms being too narrow and thus fraught with the danger of one-sided and partial, and therefore ineffectual and even potentially harmful treatment.[48] Yet, the impression that the reductionist method is completely without merit when attempting to understand and intervene into the aging process, in fact elevating the aging process above reductionism, may also be one-sided and ineffectual. The relative merits and shortcomings of reductionist vs. holistic thinking may be considered in a more balanced way. Thus, even when valorizing the wholeness, the unity of the mind and the body, highlighting "synthesis," and criticizing the limited mechanistic, materialistic, deterministic or reductionist views, we perhaps should not discard the reductionist, "analytical" approach altogether. The anti-reductionist, anti-mechanistic views often mask lacunas in the understanding of physiological processes, and sometimes amount to vagueness and superstition. On the other hand, with all its drawbacks, the conquests of "materialist," "quantitative" and "analytical" medicine, include veritable life-saving and life-prolonging means (for example, consider transplantation as a reductionist "engineering" approach[49]). Arguably, reductionism should not be discarded simply because we do not yet understand completely the mechanisms of aging. But the mechanisms of aging should not be the exclusive focus either, when devising therapy for the aging individual, at the risk of discarding a vast array of emerging, environmental and social properties and factors. Rather, analysis must be complemented by synthesis, or some "time sharing" may be employed. Reductionism and holism may have their specific indications and uses for particular therapeutic circumstances and purposes. Hopefully, the search for such indications and uses will continue.

Perhaps an even more pressing question is how the choice of either reductionist or holistic perception affects the actual choice of therapy in each particular case. As this work has argued and exemplified, both approaches sought to achieve biological equilibrium and constancy of internal environment. Yet, their implied perceptions of what constitutes equilibrium and constancy were diverging. The reductionist approach saw the human body as a machine in need of repair and internal adjustment and equilibration, seeking to achieve material homeostasis by eliminating damaging agents and introducing biological replacements, in other words, working by subtraction and addition toward balance. The holistic approach, in contrast, focused on the equilibration of the organism as a unit within the environment, strongly emphasizing the direct sustaining and revitalizing power of the mind and hygienic regulation of behavior. In the holistic approach, internal equilibrium was sought not so much through calibrating intrusions, but through resistance to intrusions. These approaches may in fact entail conflicting therapeutic strategies – the valorization vs. prevention of intrusions! How can these be reconciled, or how can the physicians and patients be empowered to make an informed and most therapeutically beneficial choice? And what are the biological equilibrium, balance or stability that are being sought in the first place?! Instead of "equilibrium" or "balance," sometimes the terms "homeostasis" or "homeodynamics" are used, with reference to the stability of particular tissues or the entire organism, at particular moments or during the entire life course. But how can these concepts be quantitatively and formally defined, and how would these definitions apply for particular clinical cases? How much is "too much" that needs to be removed, and how much is "too little" that needs to be supplemented to maintain "balance"? Or when does the equilibrium need to be preserved by avoiding disturbances, or when does it have to be rescued by interventions? Without a formal and mathematical definition of stable biological balance or equilibrium it may be difficult to answer these questions.[50] Hopefully, such agreed definitions and practicable suggestions could be elaborated in time.

References and notes

1. Ilia Stambler, *A History of Life-Extensionism in the Twentieth Century*, Longevity History, 2014, http://www.longevityhistory.com/.
2. Ilia Stambler, "The unexpected outcomes of anti-aging, rejuvenation, and life extension studies: an origin of modern therapies," *Rejuvenation Research*, 17(3), 297-305, 2014.
3. Charles E. Rosenberg, "Holism in twentieth-century medicine," in Christopher Lawrence, George Weisz (Eds.), *Greater Than the Parts: Holism in Biomedicine, 1920-1950*, Oxford University Press, Oxford, 1998, pp. 335-356.
4. Ilia Stambler, "Elie Metchnikoff – the founder of longevity science and a founder of modern medicine: In honor of the 170th anniversary," *Advances in Gerontology*, 28(2), 207-217, 2015.
5. Charles-Louis-Maxime Durand-Fardel, *Traité clinique et pratique des maladies des vieillards* (Clinical and practical treatise on the diseases of the aged), 1854, quoted in Joseph T. Freeman, "The History of Geriatrics," *Annals of Medical History*, 10, 324-335, 1938, and in Ignatz Leo Nascher, *Geriatrics, the Diseases of Old Age and their Treatment. Including Physiological Old Age, Home and Institutional Care, and Medicolegal Relations*, P. Blakiston's Son & Co, Philadelphia, 1914, p. 41.
6. Marie Jean Pierre Flourens, *On Human Longevity and the Amount of Life upon the Globe translated from the French by Charles Martel*, Bailliere, London, 1855 (first published in French in 1854), pp. 54, 75.
7. Chaillé SE, "Longevity," *New Orleans Medical and Surgical Journal*, 16, 417-424, 1859, reprinted in Geraldine M. Emerson (Ed.), *Benchmark Papers in Human Physiology*, *Vol. 11, Aging*, Dowden, Hutchinson and Ross, Stroudsburg PA, 1977, pp. 28-47.
8. Legrand M, "Peut-On Reculer le Bornes de la Vie Humaine?" (Can we reverse the limitations of human life?), *L'Union Médicale*, 13(5), 65-71, 1859, reprinted in Geraldine M. Emerson (Ed.), *Benchmark Papers in Human Physiology*, *Vol. 11, Aging*, Dowden, Hutchinson and Ross, Stroudsburg PA, 1977, pp. 28-47.
9. Brown-Séquard CE, "Des effets produits chez l'homme par des injections sous-cutanées d'un liquide retiré des testicules frais de cobaye et de chien" (Effects in man of subcutaneous injections of freshly prepared liquid from guinea pig and dog testes), *Comptes Rendus des Séances de la Société de Biologie*,

Série 9, 1, 415-419, 1889, reprinted and translated in Geraldine M. Emerson (Ed.), *Benchmark Papers in Human Physiology, Vol. 11, Aging,* Dowden, Hutchinson and Ross, Stroudsburg PA, 1977, pp. 68-76.

10. Elie Metchnikoff, *Etudy o Prirode Cheloveka* (Etudes On the Nature of Man), The USSR Academy of Sciences Press, Moscow, 1961 (1915, first published in 1903), p. 178.

11. Jean Finot, *The Philosophy of Long Life* (translated by Harry Roberts), John Lane Company, London and New York, 1909, p. 273, first published in French as *La Philosophie de la Longévité,* Schleicher Freres, Paris, 1900.

12. Albert Dastre, *La Vie et la Mort* (Life and Death), Flammarion, Paris 1907 (first published in 1903), pp. 1-51, 337, 348-349.

13. Sergey Metalnikov, *Problema Bessmertia i Omolozhenia v Sovremennoy Biologii* (The Problem of Immortality and Rejuvenation in Modern Biology), Slovo, Berlin, 1924 (1917).

14. Serge Voronoff, *The Sources of Life,* Bruce Humphries, Boston, 1943.

15. Serge Voronoff, *The Conquest of Life,* translated by G. Gibier Rambaud, Brentano's Ltd, London, 1928.

16. Serge Voronoff, *Rejuvenation by Grafting,* translated by Fred F. Imianitoff, George Allen and Unwin Ltd, London, 1925.

17. Claude Bernard, *Leçons sur les Phénomènes de la Vie Communs aux Animaux et aux Végétaux* (Lectures on the phenomena of communal life in animals and plants), J.-B. Baillière, Paris, 1878, edited by Albert Dastre, vol. 1, p. 113, subsection "La vie constante" (the constant life).

18. David Hamilton, *The Monkey Gland Affair,* Chatto and Windus, London, 1986.

19. Auguste Comte, *The Catechism of Positive Religion* (translated by Richard Congreve), John Chapman, London, 1858 (first published in French as *Catéchisme positiviste ou Sommaire exposition de la religion universelle,* Paris, 1852 – The Positivist Catechism or Summary Exposition of the Universal Religion), pp. 498-450.

20. Alexis Carrel, "Le Rôle Futur de la Médecine" (The future role of medicine), in *Médecine Officielle et Médecines Hérétiques* (Official Medicine and Heretical Medicines), Plon, Paris, 1945, pp. 1-9.

21. Bruno Salazard, Christophe Desouches, Guy Magalon, "Auguste and Louis Lumière, inventors at the service of the suffering," *European Journal of Plastic Surgery,* 28(7), 441-447, 2006.

22. Auguste Lumière, *Sénilité et Rajeunissement* (Aging and Rejuvenation), Librairie J.-B. Baillière et Fils, Paris, 1932.

23. Auguste Lumière, *La Renaissance de la Médecine Humorale,* Deuxie edition (The Renaissance of Humoral Medicine), Imprimerie Léon Sézanne, Lyon, 1937.

24. Auguste Lumière, *La Vie, La Maladie et La Mort, Phénomènes Colloïdaux* (Life, Disease and Death as Colloidal Phenomena), Masson & Cie, Libraires de L'Académie de Médecine, Paris, 1928.

25. Auguste Lumière, *Les Horizons de la Médecine* (The horizons of medicine), Albin Michel, Paris, 1937, pp. 42-47.

26. Yamada M, Foote M, Prow TW, "Therapeutic gold, silver, and platinum nanoparticles," *Wiley Interdisciplinary Reviews: Nanomedicine and Nanobiotechnology*, 7(3), 428-445, 2015.

27. Baati T, Bourasset F, Gharbi N, Njim L, Abderrabba M, Kerkeni A, Szwarc H, Moussa F, "The prolongation of the lifespan of rats by repeated oral administration of [60] fullerene," *Biomaterials*, 33(19), 4936-4946, 2012.

28. Jean Poucel, "La Médecine Naturiste" (The Naturist Medicine), in *Médecine Officielle et Médecines Hérétiques* (Official Medicine and Heretical Medicines), Plon, Paris, 1945, pp. 159-182.

29. George Weisz, "A moment of synthesis: medical holism in France between the wars," in Christopher Lawrence, George Weisz (Eds.), *Greater Than the Parts: Holism in Biomedicine, 1920-1950*, Oxford University Press, Oxford, 1998, pp. 68-93.

30. Léon Binet & François Bourlière (Eds.), *Précis de Gérontologie* (Precis of Gerontology), Masson e Cie., Paris, 1955.

31. Bardach M, Sobieski EJ, Tosquelles M, "Premièrs Résultats obtenus avec le sérum orthobiotique en médecine humaine" (The first results obtained with the orthobiotic serum in human medicine), *Archives Hospitalières*, 9, 269-275, 1949.

32. Jean Rostand, *La biologie et l'avenir humain* (Biology and the human future), Albin Michel, Paris, 1950, pp. 15-23.

33. Eugene Steinach and John Loebel, *Sex and Life; Forty Years of Biological and Medical Experiments*, Faber, London, 1940.

34. Benno Romeis, *Altern und Verjüngung. Eine Kritische Darstellung der Endokrinen "Verjüngungsmethoden", Ihrer Theoretischen Grundlagen und der Bisher Erzielten Erfolge*, Verlag von Curt Kabitzsch, Leipzig, 1931 (Aging and Rejuvenation. A Critical Presentation of Endocrine "Rejuvenation Methods", Their Theoretical Foundations and Up-to-Date Successes).

35. Heiko Stoff, *Ewige Jugend. Konzepte der Verjüngung vom späten 19. Jahrhundert bis ins Dritte Reich* (Eternal Youth. Concepts of Rejuvenation from the late 19th century until the Third Reich), Böhlau Verlag, Köln, 2004.

36. Gerhard Venzmer, *Lang leben und jung bleiben!* (Live long and stay young), Franckhsche Verlag, Stuttgart, 1937, republished in 1941.

37. Julius Hermann Greeff, "Hundertjahrige" (Centenarians), *Archiv für Rassen- und Gesellschafts-Biologie* (Archive for Racial and Social Biology), 27 (3), 241-270, 1933.

38. Karl Fahrenkamp, *Kreislauffürsorge und gesundheitsführung* (Care of the circulation system and healthy life-style), Hippokrates-Verlag, Stuttgart, 1941.

39. Ludwig Roemheld, *Wie verlängere ich mein Leben?* (How do I prolong my life?) Ferdinand Enke Verlag, Stuttgart, 1941, first presented in 1933.

40. Johannes Steudel, "Zur Geschichte der Lehre von den Greisenkrankheiten" (On the history of the study of the diseases of old age), *Sudhoffs Archiv für Geschichte der Medizin und der Naturwissenschaften*, 35, 1-27, 1942.

41. Wladislaw Klimaszewski, *Gründliche Gesundung. Vollkraft, Erfolg, Verjüngung*, 7. Auflage, München, 1937 (Fundamental health improvement: Full power, Success, Rejuvenation, 7th edition, first published in 1925).

42. Julius Wagner-Jauregg, *Über die menschliche Lebensdauer. Eine populär-wissenschaftliche Darstellung* (On the duration of human life. A popular scientific presentation), Deutscher Alpenverlag, Innsbruck, 1941 (published posthumously).

43. Robert N. Proctor, *The Nazi War on Cancer*, Princeton University Press, Princeton, 1999.

44. Nathan W. Shock (Ed.), *A Classified Bibliography of Gerontology and Geriatrics*, Stanford University Press, Stanford CA, 1951; *Supplement One 1949-1955*, 1957; *Supplement Two 1956-1961*, 1963 (reprinted in 1980 by Stanford University Press), Subcategory: "Rejuvenation."

45. Adolf Hitler, *Mein Kampf*, 1923, translated into English by James Murphy, Hurst and Blackett, NY, 1939, reprinted in Project Gutenberg of Australia, esp. Vol. 2, Ch. 1 "Weltanschauung and Party", Vol. 2, The National Socialist Movement, Ch. 2 "The State", Vol. 1, A Retrospect, Ch. 4 "Munich", Vol. 1, Ch. 11 "Race and People", http://gutenberg.net.au/ebooks02/0200601.txt.

46. René Rémond, *Les Droites en France* (The right-wingers in France), Aubier, Paris, 1982, pp. 473, 493.

47. Alexander Bogdanov, *Tektologia: Vseobshaya Organizatsionnaya Nauka* (1913-1928), "4. Ustoychivost i organizovannost form, 1. Kolichestvennaya i strukturnaya ustoychivost" (*Tectology: the universal science of organization* (1913-1928), Ch. 4. Stability and organization of forms, Section 1. Quantitative and structural stability), Economica, Moscow, 1989.

48. Marios Kyriazis, "Third phase science: defining a novel model of research into human ageing," *Frontiers in Bioscience*, 22, 982-990, 2017.

49. Ilia Stambler, *A History of Life-Extensionism in the Twentieth Century*, Longevity History, 2014, Ch. 4, Section 16, "The 1950s-1960s. The evolution of rejuvenation methods: From organotherapy to replacement medicine. The cycle of hopefulness," pp. 215-217, http://www.longevityhistory.com/.

The issue was partly raised at the presentation: Ilia Stambler, "On the history of life-extension research: Does the whole have parts?" *Sixth SENS Conference (SENS6). Reimagine Aging.* Queens' College – Cambridge UK, September 3-7, 2013, proceedings at *Rejuvenation Research*, 16, S41, 2013, http://www.sens.org/videos/history-life-extension-research-does-whole-have-parts-ilia-stambler;

https://www.youtube.com/watch?v=EoBkf8rEGOo.

50. David Blokh and Ilia Stambler, "The application of information theory for the research of aging and aging-related diseases," *Progress in Neurobiology*, S0301-0082(15)30059-9, 2016,

http://dx.doi.org/10.1016/j.pneurobio.2016.03.005.

8. Life-extensionism as a Pursuit of Constancy

When speaking of the extension of life, or radical extension of life, the question that should immediately arise – what is it exactly that we desire to extend or preserve during life extension? What is that thing that we would wish to preserve in continuity or even in perpetuity? I would argue that the goal of life extension has been associated with a striving for stability and equilibrium, desiring to stabilize and thus perpetuate the current state of the body or personality, and the present social system.[1] In this sense, life-extensionism may be a fundamentally conservative (or conservationist) enterprise. Therefore, the impression that life-extensionism represents a form of utopianism, a fringe or revolutionary movement, or an advocacy of a radical change of human nature – should be rejected or accepted only with profound reservations. Historically, the proponents of radical life extension may have envisioned no greater change to human nature than the extent to which maintenance of an ancient edifice changes the nature of that edifice, or the extent to which the (often high-tech) restoration and conservation of an old work of art make it a forgery. The life-extensionists may indeed have strived for a perfected society, which one might call a "utopia," but that "utopian" society, they hoped, would uncannily resemble the one they lived in, with all or most of its institutions intact and all the near and dear ones alive and around.[2] The life-extensionist movement may have been profoundly anti-revolutionary, if only for the simple reason that opposing the existing social system would nullify public support for longevity research. After a revolution has won, the life-extensionists may side with the winner (either opportunistically or in a firm belief, or both).

The adaptability of life-extensionists to the changing social patterns may be rapid, but paradoxically, once an adaptation had been established, it would appear that the new pattern would continue indefinitely, or only with very minor modifications. Hence, rather than speaking of life extension generally, it may be necessary to speak of the extension of particular "life-forms" or "life patterns" – personal or social – the forms that are being perpetuated or fixated upon. We may perhaps want to select or at least discuss the patterns that we indeed wish to perpetuate. In other words, we may consider what social practices, ethical precepts or power structures may be involved in the pursuit of life extension, or what would be the form of society in which we would wish to live long. An undesirable yet unchangeable pattern may be a dystopian prospect indeed. The question may still be raised regarding the form of society that is most conducive to longevity research or to actually increasing human longevity.

The desire to preserve constancy is difficult to fulfill, as changes in general and deteriorative changes in particular are difficult to resist. This might be one of the reasons why radical life-extensionism has not become entrenched in the public mind. The task of maintaining constancy, equilibrium or homeostasis, is daunting and goes against too many odds. Yet, the human desire to maintain constancy, in spite of all change, has been persistent as well, and in this regard life-extensionism is nothing exceptional. The inevitability of change has been acknowledged in many conceptions of social organization. But the desire for constancy and stability has been acknowledged as well. Thus according to Hegel's classical conception of the "Zeitgeist," or the "Spirit of the Age," prolonged periods of stability are not tolerated, but subverted by internal oppositions. "Periods of happiness," Hegel wrote in *The Philosophy of History* (1837) "are blank pages in [the History of the World], for they are periods of harmony – periods when the antithesis is in abeyance." Civilizations are always changing, manifesting the development and realization of Spirit. But Spirit itself does not change. "Spirit is immortal; with it there is no past, no future, but an essential now ... the present form of Spirit comprehends within it all earlier steps. ... what Spirit is it has always been essentially; distinctions are only the development of this essential nature."[3] Moreover, according to Hegel, as far as human capacity for reasoning goes, constancy is always sought for. As Hegel stated in the *Encyclopedia of the Philosophical Sciences* (1830), "reflection is always seeking for something fixed and permanent, definite in itself and governing the particulars."[4] Also in Marxism, owing a great deal to Hegelianism, change and constancy are pervasive concerns. In Marxism, "social formations" constantly change, being subverted by economic developments and class struggle; that is, until the "social formation" of communism will be reached, where there will be no class struggle and which will presumably continue indefinitely.[5] Even much earlier, transformative change has been a fundamental concept of Taoism, the "Book of Changes" being one of the most venerated texts of Chinese philosophy. Yet, Taoism also envisions the attainment by the society of the state of "Taiping" – the state of Great Peace – that will enjoy stability and harmony for eternity.[6] (Ironically, the historical Kingdom of Taiping (1850-1864) was one of the most turbulent and violent in Chinese history.)

The recognition of the inevitability of change and the desire for perpetuation are also present in many works of cultural history, particularly the works on the history and sociology of science. Thus, in Thomas Kuhn, paradigms constantly shift, being subverted by anomalies. Yet Kuhn also points out the resilience of established paradigms. "And at least part of that achievement always proves to be permanent" (1962).[7] (Or else, logically, the paradigmatic belief in paradigm shifts may itself pass.) Bruno Latour speaks of "reference" as "our way of keeping something constant through a series of transformations"(1999).[8] Steven Shapin speaks of "broad European changes in attitudes to knowledge in general and to the relations between

141

knowledge and social order." Yet, immediately afterwards, he notices "a state of permanent crisis affecting European politics, society and culture" (1996).[9] Michel Foucault, in *The Order of Things* (1966), speaks of "fixism" and "evolutionism" as "two simultaneous requirements," and "these two requirements are complementary, and therefore irreducible."[10] Stability and fixity are intrinsically related to order. And the striving for stable equilibrium has been related to rationalism.[11]

Further confirming the inexorable presence of both the concepts of change and of constancy, the American social historian Peter Burke (2005) defines "modernity" as "the assumption of fixity" and "post-modernity" as "the assumption of fluidity," "the collapse of the traditional idea of structure," "destabilization and decentering." In a "modern" or "modernizing" discourse, the rhetoric of progressive change is persistent, but it may conceal a deep-seated desire for fixity and stability. And in a "post-modern" discourse, "change" is a commendation in and of itself, and "constancy" or "stability" are commonly either ignored or vilified. Yet the desire to preserve constancy cannot be easily rejected. Burke points out numerous attempts "to freeze the social structure," to "resist change." "Such activities," Burke suggests, "surely deserve a place in any general theory of social change."[12]

On a continuum between the desire for absolute change and the desire for absolute constancy, the life-extensionists would seem to stand closer to the pole of constancy. Indeed, without some notion of constancy, the concept of life extension, even of survival, would be meaningless. Consider such cases as the atoms of a decomposing human body merging with the Universe, or human life being transformed into the life of grave worms, as discussed by Jean Finot in *The Philosophy of Long Life* (1900).[13] Many boundaries are "transcended" in such "transformations," but one can hardly speak of "life-extension." If extinction is determined by "a critical rate of long-term environmental change beyond which extinction is certain"[14] (notice, any change), then life-extensionists would wish to be as far from this rate of change as possible.[15] Or else, they would wish to design the technological armor that would make us impervious to such changes. Without work invested in maintaining constancy, spontaneous deteriorative change may be expected. Thus, in the sense of Burke's definition, life-extensionism is a very "modern" endeavor. The rhetoric of progressive change is emphasized, but not just any change for the change's sake, but only such change that would serve to perpetuate some existing structure. In the words of the protagonist of Giuseppe di Lampedusa's *The Leopard* (1960) "If we want things to stay as they are, things will have to change."[16] And in the words of Lewis Carroll, "it takes all the running you can do, to keep in the same place" (1871).[17]

The question may again arise: what is it exactly that the life-extensionists would endeavor to fix? For a religious person, the answer might be easier. The things that require preservation might be the eternal, imperishable soul maintained in a robust temple of the body, and a God-decreed social order and way of life. But for a materialist, believing in the contingent and temporal construction of physical objects, the answer may be much more difficult. Should the preservation efforts be directed to some arbitrary structure, archetype, memory, connections, the Zeitgeist? Hegel's classical notion of the "zeitgeist" has now been generally discarded. As succinctly stated by the Austrian-British art historian Ernst Gombrich in his book *In Search of Cultural History* (1969), in place of the Hegelian search for expressions of the universal spirit of the age, there comes the search for connections within the surrounding culture, since "any event and any creation of a period is connected by a thousand threads with the culture in which it is embedded."[18] And thus, an historian may observe distinctions between specific social and ideological environments or "embedding cultures" (for example, French liberalism followed by conservatism, German fascism, Russian communism or American capitalism), even without providing exact definitions, and may detect specific adaptations.[1]

With reference to life-extensionism, the adaptations can be clearly perceived. Even the very terms for life-extensionism have varied according to period and context – internal alchemy, gerocomia, macrobiotics, rejuvenation, experimental gerontology, anti-aging, prolongevity, life-extensionism, immortalism, transhumanism – as befits the circumstance of political correctness. And the terms for progress, within which life-extensionism has been commonly embedded, have changed as well: in place of the somewhat archaic "meliorism" and the somewhat ominously sounding "progressivism," now the more popular terms are "making the world a better place," "sustained human development" or "continuous evolution." An apparent persistent opposition in life-extensionist methodologies, between what may be termed here "reductionist" vs. "holistic" approaches to life extension, emphasizing, respectively, targeted repairs of the human machine vs. psychosomatic effects, also seems to have undergone shifts of terminological fashions. These were manifested in the dichotomies of "mechanism" vs. "vitalism," "materialism" vs. "idealism," "invasive/artificial therapeutics" vs. "non-invasive/natural hygiene."[1] The respective terms are not entirely synonymous. Moreover, "reductionist" and "holistic" methods for life extension were often combined by the proponents. Yet, similarities and continuities between the respective terms can nonetheless be observed.

But perhaps the most salient adaptations were to what might be termed the "dominant socio-ideological order" – "liberalism" or "conservatism," "fascism," "communism" or "capitalism" – whose prevalence in the specific countries and periods under consideration is apparent. Though these "dominants" may seem similar to Hegelian manifestations of the "Spirit of the Age," they are rather expressions of the "interconnected embedding culture," not something "essential" but rather categorical and contingent. The adaptations of life-extensionism to particular contexts took various forms. These included the rhetorical support of the ruling socio-ideological order (if only to ensure that the research is not shut down by the authorities), and the positing of metaphorical socio-biological parallels between the workings of the body and the society in which the authors lived. Moreover, specific research projects were favored as compatible with the ruling socio-ideological order.[1] But variation was only a part of the adaptation process; another was conservation. The life-extensionists did not simply "adapt" to the changing socio-ideological conditions, but sought to conserve the adaptation, sought to make their relations to the environment or "embedding culture" stable. I argue that the support of the existing ruling regime, whatever it may be, may derive from the nature of life-extensionism that seeks stability and constancy.

The life-extensionists' inherent desire for constancy has stood in stark contrast to "apocalyptic" beliefs. Such beliefs have been present throughout the century, and they had been recently intensifying. There has existed an extensive literature expecting (and accepting) "the world as we know it" to end anytime soon.[19] In morbid excitement, the prophets of the apocalypse have often stressed the great corruption of humanity, expressing what the novelist John Updike termed "a smug conviction that the world was doomed" (1972).[20] Insofar as humanity was seen as inherently corrupt and self-destructive, a thorough "cleansing" appeared to be in order, through an all-out war between "the sons of light" and "the sons of darkness," separating the bad "weeds" from the good "wheat." Often the apocalyptists, both secular and religious, have had some very strong convictions about who the "sons of darkness" and the "weeds" are.

Historically, the life-extensionists have exhibited none of this attitude. They might find it difficult to distinguish and separate between the "weeds" and the "wheat" and would request a longer life-span to figure it out. Until then, the entire societal and personal 'bundle' may need to be conserved. Alternatively, many life-extensionists appear to have realized the existence of corruption and exploitation in the current society, whose perpetuation would be highly undesirable. But at the same time they also extrapolated on the manifestations of creativity, benevolence and justice, as well found in the current society, and considered them to be worth preserving indefinitely. Thus they would follow the ancient Talmudic command that "the sins will cease" but not "the sinners."[21] While the "apocalyptic" view largely assumed that human attempts to resist catastrophic changes are

144

destined to failure, the life-extensionists, even though recognizing existential threats (and the threat of senescent death in the first place), valorized our ability to defend ourselves.[22] Whatever the explanation or underlying motives, life-extensionism appears to be a profoundly anti-revolutionary, anti-catastrophic, anti-apocalyptic ideology. As the American author William Bailey emphasized in his bibliography on *Human Longevity from Antiquity to the Modern Lab* (1987), "Death be not proud, this heartening literature opposes Armageddon and the perniciousness of nature to say that we can extend life and enjoy many another springtime."[23]

The questions still remain considering what exactly the life-extensionists would desire to maintain constant, and whether anything at all can be maintained constant. An answer may be again suggested by Taoism. As the great teacher of Taoist immortalists, Lao Tse said of the Tao (the Way or Course): "How still it was and formless, standing alone, and undergoing no change. ... Great, it passes on in constant flow." Moreover, human beings should "possess the attributes of the Tao."[24] No wonder then that in Taoism, radical life extension and conservation of order have always been all-pervasive aspirations. If Heraclites could not "step twice into the same river; for other waters are continually flowing in"; Lao Tse could, for the course of the flow may remain constant. It seems as if Walter Cannon's concept of homeostasis, described in *The Wisdom of the Body* (1932), follows directly Lao Tse's notion of the Tao. In Cannon, some constancy is provided by what he terms "the interesting fact that we are separated from the air which surrounds us by a layer of dead or inert material." Yet, for Cannon, the organism is not entirely separated from the environment, but related to it through a constant flow of materials and energy: "the internal, proximate environment of the cells is made favorable by keeping the fluids on the move and constantly fresh and uniform."[25] A modern textbook definition of homeostasis would say the same. The materials may be exchanged, but the course and the form of their flow remain constant: "life is characterized by a continuing flow of material and energy, and a steady state is reached if all possible disturbing factors remain constant."[26]

A ramification of this idea can be found in the philosophy of Arthur Schopenhauer (1788-1860) who postulated that "the dead body is a mere excrement of a constant human form."[27] That is to say, all materials in the human body are being incessantly replaced, and only their form or arrangement is constant. Schopenhauer's "pessimistic philosophy," calling for reconciliation with death, was hardly compatible with life-extensionism. The life-extensionist founder of gerontology, Elie Metchnikoff took great pains to refute it, among other reasons, because he did not believe that the "form" or "ideal," either of an individual or of a species, can exist without a material substrate (1903).[28] Yet, the particular idea of Schopenhauer's

145

regarding the constancy of the human form, despite the material replacements, was approvingly cited by the German gerontologist Max Bürger, the proponent of "biorhesis" or stable biological flow (1947).[29] Indeed, various "replacement therapies" – ranging from hormones through vitamins and minerals to stem cells, artificially grown organs and bionic prostheses, while maintaining the constancy of the human form – have constituted the core of proposed methodologies of life-extensionism throughout the century, mainly in its "reductionist" and "materialistic" branches. In the "holistic" and "idealistic" branches, some essential core of human personality was believed to be able to directly control the body and resist bodily changes.

The idea of maintaining the constancy of structure and function through a continuous replacement of material components can be traced even further back to the "Paradox of the Ship of Theseus" first mentioned by Plutarch (c. 46-120 CE).[30] The great quandary was whether a ship, all of whose parts are replaced, will retain its identity. For the life-extensionists this has been a vital issue and their implicit (and often explicit) answer has been that it would indeed remain essentially the same, since its structure and function would be preserved. And if some new components were to be added to the "Theseus' Ship" to improve and prolong its performance, it would be essentially the same as well, since a major part of its structure and function would remain constant. However, if it were to break down into components, even though the materials would remain, the constancy of form would be lost.[31]

Science fiction related to life extension had a field-day with this paradox. Among many examples, in Stanislaw Lem's "Do you exist, Mr. Johns?" (1955),[32] the protagonist has all his biological components replaced by artificial ones, and the company that produced them claims ownership over him. The cybernetic human vehemently defends his right to an identity (that is, being identical to the former biological human), since his personal memories are uniquely his own and are only preserved in a different substrate. Even as a biological entity, all of the materials in his body were being replaced in a very short time. By analogy, he is now no more the property of the company than he was the property of the grocer who formerly supplied him with food.

Beyond science fiction, for practicing life-extensionist scientists, the "Theseus' Ship Paradox" has been a practical concern, as it informed the search for replacement therapies. And the paradox has been resolved in a similar, positive manner. Thus Aubrey de Grey wrote in *Ending Aging* (2007):[33]

"I emphasized ... that the body is a machine, and that that's both why it ages and why it can in principle be maintained. I made a comparison with vintage cars, which are kept fully functional even 100 years after they were built, using the same maintenance technologies that kept them going 50 years ago when they were already far older than they were ever designed to be."

The main point is that for the life-extensionists, the possibility of maintaining the constancy of form has been certain.

The same valorization of the constancy of form recurs in Ray Kurzweil's *The Singularity Is Near: When Humans Transcend Biology* (2005).[34] Yet, instead of the classical notion of the "form," Kurzweil uses the term "pattern." Kurzweil is a world-renowned expert in pattern recognition, having pioneered several ground-breaking developments in optical character recognition, speech recognition, stock-market pattern recognition and more. The entire world, according to Kurzweil, consists of "patterns of information": patterns of matter and energy, biological and social patterns. And there are precise procedures in information theory to determine the extent to which various patterns, material, biological or social, are similar or different (for example through the use of entropy and mutual information).[35] Hence, for Kurzweil, the maintenance of specific patterns is a very tangible and practical task. Insofar as orderly information patterns are constantly maintained by biological systems, such patterns can be similarly (perhaps even better) maintained by machines. A dedicated life-extensionist, Kurzweil suggests the constancy of an information pattern, comprising the human body and mind, as an underlying concept for indefinite survival (*The Singularity Is Near*, 2005, pp. 371-372):

"My body is temporary. Its particles turn over almost completely every month. Only the pattern of my body and brain have continuity. ... Knowledge is precious in all its forms: music, art, science, and technology, as well as the embedded knowledge in our bodies and brains. Any loss of this knowledge is tragic. ... Death is a tragedy. It is not demeaning to regard a person as a profound pattern (a form of knowledge), which is lost when he or she dies. That, at least, is the case today, since we do not yet have the means to access and back up this knowledge."

By perfecting the means of preserving our "information patterns" and eventually "backing them up," human life can be preserved indefinitely: "We are now approaching a paradigm shift in the means we will have available to preserve the patterns underlying our existence." And further down the line, "As we move toward a nonbiological existence, we will gain the means of 'backing ourselves up' (storing the key patterns underlying our knowledge, skills, and personality), thereby eliminating most causes of death as we know it" (p. 323). Thus the conservation of the existing patterns is an explicit goal. Kurzweil admits that he cherishes all his memories and never discards any memorabilia, since they constitute the unique pattern of his personality. Furthermore, one might suggest, Kurzweil's valorization of "democracy and capitalism" (p. 406) is a part of the overall program to conserve the "pattern" in which he exists.

It should be noted, however, that, in Kurzweil, the conserved pattern is not perceived as entirely stagnant. Rather, the underlying metaphor is that of a continuous growth, building new structures on the existing foundation or "core" and including the already existing building blocks. Kurzweil uses the analogy of an old computer file that may be preserved in a new computer, yet with many new files added to it. Similarly, our general "mind file" will be conserved, yet augmented with new extensions. The "core pattern" is not entirely unchangeable either, but it changes slowly and gradually. Still, the continuity of the pattern is maintained: "You change your pattern – your memory, skills, experiences, even personality over time – but there is a continuity, a core that changes only gradually." Technological enhancement will not radically modify this "core": "that's just a surface manifestation. My true core changes only gradually" (p. 258). Kurzweil uses as an epigraph to his discussion of longevity the statement by the American computer scientist Vernor Vinge (1993) that the technologically enhanced human "would be everything the original was, but vastly more."[36] Still, it would be "everything the original was." Thus, the underlying desire for constancy is affirmed once again.

The assumption of constancy may also answer the frequently raised question: 'Why would we want to prolong life?' If human life is an absolute value now, and its value will remain the same tomorrow or in a hundred years, then all the efforts to preserve human life at any moment and for any period of time are justified. It is important to bear those philosophical considerations in mind when researching the historical motivations for life-extensionism.

Finally, and paradoxically, out of the desire for constancy, novelty arises. It is easy to dismiss the pursuit of life extension as a "pipe dream." Yet, many examples show that the scientific contributions of life-extensionist researchers have been considerable, and often pioneering: the first attempts at therapeutic endocrinology, blood transfusion, transplantation, cell and tissue therapy, probiotic diets, cryobiology, general hygiene, and more.[37] These developments may have been not just due to 'aiming high' and in the process bound to achieve at least some results, even though most often falling short of the original aspirations. Rather, the scientific advances made by the life-extensionists may be the product of their underlying conservative bent on stability and perpetuation. As the stability of the internal milieu could not be achieved by contemporary medical technology, innovative interventions were sought. Consider, for example, such late 19th-early 20th century developments as Nikolay Pirogov's plaster casts to fixate the bone (c. 1870), Porfiry Bakhmetiev's preservation of animals by freezing (c. 1900), or Auguste Lumière's introduction into biomedicine of film and auto-chrome plates to safeguard images of the body (c. 1900). All these can be viewed as technological novelties employed in the service of maintaining constancy. And if some methods of maintaining constancy failed, such as the reductionist "endocrine" rejuvenation – new methods of maintaining homeostasis would emerge, such as improved (and still reductionist) replacement techniques or more systemic, holistic or hygienic approaches.

Many life-extensionist scientists spoke explicitly about their desire to maintain constancy through novel technological means. Thus, the British pioneer of X-ray crystallography, John Desmond Bernal, asserted that new technological extensions of existing human capabilities will lead to an indefinite extension of life and a greater "fixity" of human personality (1929): "This capacity for indefinite extension might in the end lead to the relative fixity of the different brains; and this would, in itself, be an advantage from the point of view of security and uniformity of conditions." At any rate, the technologically modified man may have a better chance for self-preservation than an unmodified one, even at an early and imperfect stage of the modifying technology: "But though it is possible that in the early stages a surgically transformed man would be at a disadvantage in capacity of performance to a normal, healthy man, he would still be better off than a dead man."[38] The Russian pioneer of neurophysiology, Ivan Pavlov, spoke about the fundamental drive of science toward equilibration of living systems (1923): "There will be a time, even though a remote one, when mathematical analysis, based on natural science, will encompass, by magnificent mathematical equations, all existing equilibria."[39] And as one of the foremost twentieth century life-extensionists, the French-American pioneer of organ transplantation and tissue engineering, Alexis Carrel contended (1935): "Science has supplied us with means for keeping our intraorganic equilibrium, which are more agreeable and less laborious than the natural processes. ... the physical conditions of our daily life are prevented from varying."[40] Thus the desire for fixity and equilibration may have been a pervasive motive in life-extensionism and often a source of new developments in biomedical science and technology. As the "philosopher of long life," Jean Finot asserted (1900), the primary purpose of biomedical advances is not to change, but to "preserve and greatly strengthen existing life."[13]

References and notes

1. Ilia Stambler, *A History of Life-Extensionism in the Twentieth Century*, Longevity History, 2014, http://www.longevityhistory.com/.
The present article is the conclusion of that book.
2. Historically, there have been life-extensionist utopias, such as Tommaso Campanella's *The City of the Sun* (1602), where "The length of their lives is generally 100 years, but often they reach 200" (http://www.gutenberg.org/files/2816/2816-h/2816-h.htm).
And there have also been anti-life-extensionist utopias, such as Thomas More's *Utopia* (1516), where "when any is taken with a torturing and lingering pain," they "choose rather to die since they cannot live but in much misery" (http://www.gutenberg.org/files/2130/2130-h/2130-h.htm).
But in both cases, the utopian society is preserved in a perpetual equilibrium, and the authors' values are hoped to triumph for all posterity.
3. Georg Wilhelm Friedrich Hegel [1770-1831], *The Philosophy of History*, Translated by J. Sibree, Colonial Press, New York, 1900 (first published in 1837), pp. 26-27, 77.
4. G.W.F. Hegel, *Encyclopaedia of the Philosophical Sciences*, Third and Final Edition, 1830, translated by William Wallace, first published 1873, Part II. Preliminary, "Universals apprehended in Reflection" §21n, reprinted at http://www.marxists.org/reference/archive/hegel/index.htm.
5. Karl Marx and Frederick Engels, *Manifesto of the Communist Party*, London, 1848, http://www.anu.edu.au/polsci/marx/classics/manifesto.html.
6. Livia Kohn, "Told you so: Extreme Longevity and Daoist Realization," in *Religion and the Implications of Radical Life Extension*, Edited by Calvin Mercer and Derek F. Maher, Macmillan Palgrave, New York, 2009, pp. 85-96;
The Book of Changes - The I Ching, translated by James Legge, *Sacred Books of the East, vol. 16*, 1899, http://www.sacred-texts.com/ich/index.htm.
7. Thomas S. Kuhn, *The Structure of Scientific Revolutions*, Third Edition, The University of Chicago Press, Chicago, 1996 (first published in 1962), p. 25.
8. Bruno Latour, *Pandora's Hope. Essays on the Reality of Science Studies*, Harvard University Press, Cambridge MA, 1999, p. 58.
9. Steven Shapin, *The Scientific Revolution*, The University of Chicago Press, Chicago, 1996, p. 123.
10. Michel Foucault, *The Order of Things*, Pantheon Books, New York, 1971, reprinted by Random House / Vintage Books, New York, 1994, p. 150 (first published in 1966).
11. M. Norton Wise, "Mediations: Enlightenment Balancing Acts, or the Technologies of Rationalism," in Paul Horwich (Ed.), *World Changes. Thomas Kuhn and the Nature of Science*, The MIT Press, Cambridge MA, 1993, pp. 207-256.

12. Peter Burke, *History and Social Theory* (Second Edition), Cornell University Press, Ithaca, New York, 2005, pp. 166-167, 173.

13. Jean Finot, *The Philosophy of Long Life* (translated by Harry Roberts), John Lane Company, London and New York, 1909, pp. 122-145, 278, first published in French as *La Philosophie De La Longévité*, Schleicher Freres, Paris, 1900, https://archive.org/details/philosophyoflong00finouoft.

14. Reinhard Burger, Michael Lynch, "Evolution and Extinction in a Changing Environment: A Quantitative-Genetic Analysis," *Evolution*, 49(1), 151-163, 1995.

15. In a recent evolutionary model, André C. R. Martins argued almost precisely to that effect: "when the system is completely stable, no mutation going on and no changing conditions for worse, ... it is to be expected that a population that shows senescence will be driven to extinction." However, "When conditions change, a senescent species can drive immortal competitors to extinction." The author concludes: "We age because the world changes."

(André C. R. Martins, "Change and Aging: Senescence as an Adaptation," *PLoS One*, 6(9):e24328, 2011, https://www.ncbi.nlm.nih.gov/pmc/articles/PMC3174959/.)

Several other contemporary researchers, such as Joshua Mitteldorf, Theodore Goldsmith and Vladimir Skulachev, have pondered a return to August Weismann's theory (originated in 1882-1884) proposing a direct evolutionary selection for senescence. A major suggested reason for such a selection, in these new interpretations, is that an absence of senescence would diminish the species' variability and diversity, hence impair its adaptability and evolvability.

(August Weismann, *Über die Dauer des Lebens* (On the duration of life), G. Fischer, Jena, 1882; August Weismann, *Über Leben und Tod* (On Life and Death), G. Fischer, Jena, 1884; Theodore C. Goldsmith, "Aging as an Evolved Characteristic – Weismann's Theory Reconsidered," *Medical Hypotheses*, 62(2), 304-308, 2004; Joshua Mitteldorf, "Ageing selected for its own sake," *Evolutionary Ecology Research*, 6, 937-953, 2004; Vladimir Skulachev, "Aging is a Specific Biological Function Rather than the Result of a Disorder in Complex Living Systems: Biochemical Evidence in Support of Weismann's Hypothesis," *Biochemistry* (Moscow), 62(11), 1191-1195, 1997.)

Furthermore, a link has been suggested between increasing longevity and the level of inbreeding (keeping the genome stable), even for humans. (A. Montesanto, G. Passarino, A. Senatore, L. Carotenuto, G. De Benedictus, "Spatial Analysis and Surname Analysis: Complementary Tools for Shedding Light on Human Longevity Patterns," *Annals of Human Genetics*, 72(2), 253-260, 2008.)

Notably, all these authors seem to be in favor of finding effective anti-aging means for humans, suggesting that through a better understanding of the evolutionary mechanism, factors affecting longevity can be identified and manipulated.

16. Giuseppe Tomasi di Lampedusa, *The Leopard*, translated by Archibald Colquhoun, Pantheon Books, NY, 1960, p. 40.

17. Lewis Carroll, *Through the Looking-Glass*, 1871, reprinted at Project Gutenberg, http://www.gutenberg.org/files/12/12-h/12-h.htm.

18. Ernst Hans Josef Gombrich, *In Search of Cultural History*, Clarendon Press, Oxford, 1969, p. 30.

19. To cite just a few recent examples of the preoccupation with the Apocalypse:

"List of dates predicted for apocalyptic events"

https://en.wikipedia.org/wiki/List_of_dates_predicted_for_apocalyptic_ev ents;

A large register of millennial and apocalyptic organizations, both religious and secular, active around 2000, is provided by the Boston University Center for Millennial Studies, http://www.bu.edu/mille/links.html.

See also Daniel Wojcik, *End of the World as We Know It: Faith, Fatalism, and Apocalypse in America*, New York University Press, NY, 1997.

20. John Updike, "When Everyone was pregnant" (1972), *Museums & Women And Other Stories*, Alfred A. Knopf, NY, 1972, p. 93, quoted in Donald J. Greiner, "Updike, Rabbit, and the myth of American exceptionalism," p. 153, in Stacey Michele Olster, Stacey Olster (Eds.), *The Cambridge Companion to John Updike*, Cambridge University Press, Cambridge, 2006.

21. *Talmud [Gemara] – Masechet Berachoth [Tractate on Blessings]*, 10a, in *English Babylonian Talmud*, Rabbi Dr. J. H. Hertz, Rabbi Dr. I Epstein, et al. (Eds.), Talmudic Books, 2012, at http://halakhah.com/.

22. It should be emphasized that many transhumanists and life-extensionists are well aware of a wide variety of global existential risks – either natural threats, such as increasing solar activity, or technogenic threats, such as uncontrolled industrial pollution, or combined natural and man-made threats, such as global warming – yet they seek ways to mitigate and endure potential disasters.

(See, for example, the stated missions of the Lifeboat Foundation, http://lifeboat.com/ex/boards.)

23. William G. Bailey, *Human Longevity from Antiquity to the Modern Lab: A Selected, Annotated Bibliography*, Greenwood Press, Westport CN, 1987, p. ix.

24. *Lao-Tse. The Tao Teh King. The Tao and Its Characteristics*, Translated by James Legge, 1880, reprinted at Project Gutenberg, Ch. 1. 25. 1-3, http://www.gutenberg.org/files/216/216-h/216-h.htm.

25. Walter Cannon, *The Wisdom of the Body*, Norton, NY, 1932, pp. 27-28.

26. Richard W. Jones, *Principles of Biological Regulation. An Introduction to Feedback Systems*, Academic Press, NY, 1973, Ch. 2 "Flow Processes in the Steady State," p. 7.

27. Schopenhauer's exact words were: "Die Leiche ist ein blosses Exkrement der stets bestehenden menschlichen Form."
(*Arthur Schopenhauers Sämtliche werke*, hrsg. von Dr. Paul Deussen, R. Piper & Co., München, 1913, Bd. 10. Arthur Schopenhauers handschriftlicher Nachlaß. Philosophische Vorlesungen: Hälfte 2, Metaphysik der Natur, des Schönen und der Sitten, S. 374 – The Complete Works of Arthur Schopenhauer, edited by Dr. Paul Deussen, R. Piper & Co., Munich, 1913, Vol. 10, Arthur Schopenhauer's hand-written papers, Philosophical Lectures, Half 2, The metaphysics of nature, of beauty and of manners, p. 374.)
This passage is quoted in Max Bürger, *Altern und Krankheit* (Aging and Disease), Zweite Auflage, Georg Thieme, Leipzig, 1954 (1947), p. 41.

28. Elie Metchnikoff, *Etudy o Prirode Cheloveka* (Etudes on the Nature of Man), Izdatelstvo Academii Nauk SSSR (The USSR Academy of Sciences Press), Moscow, 1961 (1903), Ch. 8 "Popytki filosofskich system borotsia s disharmoniami chelovecheskoy prirody" (Attempts of philosophical systems to combat the disharmonies of human nature), pp. 151-153.

29. Max Bürger, *Altern und Krankheit* (Aging and Disease), Zweite Auflage, Georg Thieme, Leipzig, 1954 (1947), p. 41.

30. Plutarch, *Theseus*, c. 75 CE, translated by John Dryden (1683), reprinted in The Internet Classics Archive, http://classics.mit.edu/Plutarch/theseus.html.

31. In contrast, two identically constructed "Theseus' Ships" or "copies" would not be the same, following Aristotle's principle that the same body cannot occupy separate places at the same time. According to Aristotle's *On the Soul*, the existence of "two bodies in the same place" is impossible. And one can also infer that one body in separate places simultaneously is equally impossible. Aristotle, who equates the Soul with Vitality, establishes the immateriality of the soul precisely on this principle, since "there must be two bodies in the same place, if the soul is a body." Rather, according to Aristotle, the soul (or vitality) is a particular faculty or form of matter.
(Aristotle [384 BCE - 322 BCE], *On the Soul*, translated with notes by Walter Stanley Hett, in *Aristotle in Twenty-Three Volumes*, William Heinemann Ltd., London, 1975 (1936), Vol. 8, Book 1, Part 5, 409b1-5, p. 53.)
The preservation of each human "copy" separately would of course be necessary unless someone embraces the notion of a "quantum mechanical body," spoken of in some life-extensionist circles, which would allow a person to be in several places simultaneously or alternatively.
(E.g. Frank J. Tipler, *The Physics of Immortality: Modern Cosmology, God, and the Resurrection of the Dead*, Doubleday, NY, 1994, pp. 173, 234; Ben Goertzel

and Stephan Vladimir Bugaj, *The Path to Posthumanity: 21st Century Technology and Its Radical Implications for Mind, Society and Reality*, Academica Press, Bethesda MD, 2006, "Physics and Immortality," pp. 342-348; Tel Peters, Robert John Russell, and Michael Welker (Eds.), *Resurrection: Theological and Scientific Assessments*, William B. Eerdmans, Grand Rapids, Michigan, 2002; Deepak Chopra, *Ageless Body, Timeless Mind. The Quantum Alternative to Growing Old*, Harmony Books, New York, 1993, p. 288.)
The ideas about "quantum immortality" and transcending spatial confines, may be too unorthodox for a "traditional" life-extensionist wishing to defend his/her body from decay and disintegration.

32. Stanislaw Lem, "Czy pan istnieje, Mr Johns?" Przekroj, Krakow, Poland, 1955, № 553 ("Do you exist, Mr. Johns?" Translated from Polish into Russian by A. Yakushev, "Sushestvuete li vy, Mister Johns?" 1960, http://samlib.ru/w/wladimir_pro/mister_djons.shtml).

33. Aubrey de Grey and Michael Rae, *Ending Aging. The Rejuvenation Breakthroughs That Could Reverse Human Aging in Our Lifetime*, St. Martin's Press, NY, 2007, p. 326.

34. Ray Kurzweil, *The Singularity Is Near: When Humans Transcend Biology*, Penguin Books, New York, 2005.

35. As stated by one of the pioneers in the application of Information Theory to biology, Henry Quastler (1908-1963): "The basic concepts of information theory – measures of information, of noise, of constraint, of redundancy – establish the possibility of associating precise (although relative) measures with things like form, specificity, lawfulness, structure, degree of organization. ... Closely related is the problem of destruction of orderliness. In biology, this is the problem of aging and decay."
(Henry Quastler, "The Domain of Information Theory in Biology," *Symposium on Information Theory in Biology, Gatlinburg, Tennessee, October 29-31, 1956*, Edited by Hubert P. Yockey, with the assistance of Robert L. Platzman and Henry Quastler, Pergamon Press, NY, 1958, pp. 187-196.)
See also: David Blokh and Ilia Stambler, "The application of information theory for the research of aging and aging-related diseases," *Progress in Neurobiology*, S0301-0082(15)30059-9, 2016, http://dx.doi.org/10.1016/j.pneurobio.2016.03.005.

36. Vernor Vinge, "Technological Singularity," *Whole Earth Review*, 81, 89-95, 1993, reprinted at http://mindstalk.net/vinge/vinge-sing.html.

37. Ilia Stambler, "The unexpected outcomes of anti-aging, rejuvenation and life extension studies: an origin of modern therapies," *Rejuvenation Research*, 17, 297-305, 2014 http://online.liebertpub.com/doi/abs/10.1089/rej.2013.1527.

38. John Desmond Bernal, *The World, the Flesh & the Devil. An Enquiry into the Future of the Three Enemies of the Rational Soul*, 1929, III "The Flesh,"

Reprinted at the Marxists Internet Archive Library, http://www.marxists.org/archive/bernal/works/1920s/soul/.

39. Ivan Pavlov, *Dvadzatiletniy opyt objektivnogo izuchenia vyshey nervnoy deyatelnosti povedenia zhivotnikh. Uslovnie reflexy* (Twenty years of objective study of the high nervous activity of animal behavior. Conditioned reflexes), Gosudarstvennoe Izdatelstvo, Moscow, 1923, p. 77.

Quoted in Alexander Chizhevsky, *Physicheskie Factory Istoricheskogo Processa* (Physical Factors of the Historical Process), Kaluga, 1924, IV. "Vlianie geofizicheskikh i kosmicheskikh faktorov na povedenie individov i kollektivov" (The influence of geophysical and cosmic factors on the behavior of individuals and collectives, http://www.astrologic.ru/library/chizhevsky/index.htm).

40. Alexis Carrel, *Man, The Unknown*, Burns & Oates, London, 1961 (1935), p. 180.

9. The Legacy of Elie Metchnikoff

The years 2015-2016 mark a double anniversary of the founder of gerontology, a foundational figure of modern immunology, aging and longevity science, and of modern medicine generally – Elie Metchnikoff (May 15, 1845 – July 15, 1916). On May 15, 2015, we celebrated the 170th anniversary of his birth, and on July 15, 2016, we marked 100 years since his death. For the proponents of healthy longevity and advocates of aging research, Metchnikoff has a special significance. Metchnikoff is of course known as a pioneering immunologist and microbiologist, a vice director of the Pasteur Institute in Paris, and the Nobel Laureate in Physiology or Medicine of 1908 for the discovery of phagocytosis (a major contribution to the cellular theory of immunity). Yet, he may also be well credited as "the father" of gerontology – the disciplinary term he coined. Both the terms "gerontology" ("the study of aging") and "thanatology" ("the study of death") were coined by him in the *Etudes On the Nature of Man*, published in 1903, which may mark the beginning of these scientific fields.[1] To the present day, his scientific reputation has remained high around the world. In fact, Metchnikoff can be considered a unifying cultural symbol for many nations.

Metchnikoff was either a direct originator or one of the primary researchers for a variety of key aging-ameliorating and life-extending methods, experiments and research programs that are still being followed today.[2] They include in fact the first truly scientific theory of aging and longevity, based on meticulous histological observations and on a model of dynamic behavior of living tissues, in particular showing the critical role of the immune system (phagocytes) and intoxication of intestinal microflora (microbiome) in degenerative aging processes. Metchnikoff also made a foundational contribution to the discussions of the evolutionary theory of aging, in particular regarding the possibility of "programmed aging." Thanks to him, there began the development of many practical geroprotective means, including probiotic diets, systemic and adjuvant immunotherapy (serum therapy, in particular the use of cytotoxic sera for tissue stimulation), the study of replacement therapy and regenerative therapy.[3]

In view of the immense significance of degenerative aging processes for the emergence of virtually all diseases, both communicable and non-communicable, and in view of the accelerating development of potential means to intervene into and ameliorate these processes for the sake of achieving healthy longevity, Metchnikoff's pioneering contribution to this field assumes an ever greater global significance. The world is rapidly aging, threatening grave consequences for the global society and economy, while the rapidly developing biomedical science and technology stand in the first line of defense against the potential threat. These two ever increasing forces bring gerontology, describing the challenges of aging while at the same time seeking means to address those challenges, to the central stage of the global scientific, technological and political discourse. At this time, it is necessary to honor Metchnikoff, who stood at the origin of gerontological discourse, not just as a scientific field, but as a social and intellectual movement.

There is a tradition to celebrate the anniversaries of great persons (scientists, artists, writers, politicians, generals) to promote the area of their activity and popularize their ideology. It may be hoped that honoring the anniversary of Metchnikoff can serve to promote and popularize the science and ideology of healthy life extension, including the state level. The "Metchnikoff Day" (held on the day of his birth) can provide an impulse for organizing topical meetings and conferences, a stimulus for research, and publications in the media, dedicated to Metchnikoff's legacy and continuation of his life's work – the study of aging and longevity. This may play a positive role not only for the advancement and popularization of research of aging and healthy longevity, but also for the promotion of optimism, peace and cooperation.

Indeed, in 2015, events in honor of the Metchnikoff Day were held in Ukraine, Russia, UK, Israel, Cyprus.[4] It may be hoped that, following these examples, more events and publications will be held around the world in honor of this day in the future. It is possible to dedicate additional special days to organize internationally coordinated actions and educational campaigns in support of longevity science. Thus, in 2013 through 2016, such actions were organized on October 1 ("The International Day of Older Persons" or "The International Longevity Day"), March 1 ("The Future Day"), February 21 ("Jeanne Calment's day" in honor of the longest lived human, with a certified 122.5 years lifespan, February 21, 1875 - August 4, 1997).[5] Yet, "Metchnikoff's day" on May 15, can be one of the most unifying, uplifting and educational.

Thus thanks to Metchnikoff's continuing inspiration and authority, the interest in aging and longevity research can be increased in all the walks and segments of society. And thanks to the increased interest and education, the research itself may intensify, producing an improved capacity to contribute to the achievement of healthy longevity for all.

Consider, for example, several statements by Metchnikoff that can inspire thought and action even now. As he stated in *Etudes on the Nature of Man* (1903, p. 201):[1]

"It has been long noted that aging is very similar to disease. Therefore it is not surprising that human beings feel a strong aversion to aging. ... Undoubtedly, it is a mistake to consider aging as a physiological phenomenon. It makes as much sense to accept aging as a normal phenomenon, because everybody ages, as it makes sense to accept childbirth pain as normal, because only very few women are spared it. In both cases, we deal, of course, with pathological and not with purely physiological phenomena. Inasmuch as people endeavor to mitigate or eliminate the pains of a woman in labor, it is as natural to endeavor to eliminate the evils brought by aging. However, while during childbirth pains, it is enough to apply an anesthetic, aging is a chronic evil against which it is much more difficult to find a cure."

And as he asserted in *Forty Years in Search of a Rational Worldview* (1914):[6]

"The second of Bergson's questions "What are we doing in this world?" should be formulated differently: "What *should* we do in this world?" Our answer to this, presented in this work and elsewhere, can be stated as follows: "We should, by all means, strive that people, ourselves included, live their full life cycle in harmony of feeling and of mind, until reaching, in the ripest old age, a sense of saturation with life. The main misfortune on earth is that people do not live to that limit and die prematurely." This statement is the basis of all moral actions… It is difficult to imagine that, in some more or less distant future, science will not accomplish this goal and will not solve the problem of the prolongation of human life to a desired limit, as well as rectify other disharmonies of the human nature."

Can there be a stronger call to thought and to action for the combat of degenerative aging and for the prolongation of healthy human life? Let us hope this call will continue to be heard and acted upon.

References and notes

1. I.I. [Ilya Ilyich] Metchnikoff, *Etudy o Prirode Cheloveka* (Etudes On the Nature of Man), Izdatelstvo Academii Nauk SSSR (The USSR Academy of Sciences Press), Moscow, 1961 (1903). The first French edition, Elie Metchnikoff, *Études sur la Nature Humaine,* was published in Paris (Masson) in 1903. The Russian translation used here was done by Elie Metchnikoff and his wife Olga. The book is also available in English (*The Nature of Man: Studies in Optimistic Philosophy,* translated by P.C. Mitchell, Putnam, NY, 1908 (1903), https://archive.org/details/prolongationofli00metciala). Unless otherwise specified, all the excerpts quoted in the present work are in my translation.
2. Ilia Stambler, "Elie Metchnikoff – the founder of longevity science and a founder of modern medicine: In honor of the 170th anniversary," *Advances in Gerontology*, 28(2), 207-217, 2015 (Russian), 5(4), 201-208, 2015 (English).

3. Ilia Stambler, *A History of Life-Extensionism in the Twentieth Century*, Longevity History, 2014, http://www.longevityhistory.com/.

4. Ilia Stambler, "The 170th anniversary of Elie Metchnikoff – the founder of gerontology, May 15, 2015," Longevity for All, http://www.longevityforall.org/170th-anniversary-of-elie-metchnikoff-the-founder-of-gerontology-may-15-2015/;
http://hplusmagazine.com/2015/05/06/may-15-2015-170th-anniversary-of-elie-metchnikoff-the-founder-of-gerontology-an-opportunity-to-promote-aging-and-longevity-research/.

5. Ilia Stambler, "International Longevity Day - October 1" (2013, 2014, 2015, 2016),
http://ieet.org/index.php/IEET/more/stambler20131029;
http://ieet.org/index.php/IEET/more/stambler20140110;
http://www.longecity.org/forum/topic/72013-promoting-longevity-research-on-october-1-%E2%80%93-the-international-day-of-older-persons/;
http://www.longevityforall.org/international-longevity-day-october-1-2015/;
http://www.longevityforall.org/longevity-day-and-longevity-month-october-2016/;
Ilia Stambler, "For the Future of Longevity – Celebrating longevity on the international "Future Day" March 1, 2013" http://longevityalliance.org/?q=future-longevity;
http://www.longevityforall.org/future-day-march-1-2013-theme-longevity/;
Victor Björk, "A Celebration Of The Oldest Person On Record: Calment's Day – February 21, 2016," February 1, 2016 http://longevityreporter.org/blog/2016/1/31/a-celebration-of-the-longest-lived-person-on-record-calments-day;
http://www.longevityreporter.org/blog/2016/1/31/a-celebration-of-the-longest-lived-person-on-record-calments-day;

6. Elie Metchnikoff, *Sorok Let Iskania Razionalnogo Mirovozzrenia* (Forty Years in Search of a Rational Worldview), 1914, in I.I. Metchnikoff, *Academicheskoe Sobranie Sochineniy* (Elie Metchnikoff. Academic Collected Works, Ed. G.S. Vasezky), Academia Medizinskikh Nauk SSSR (The USSR Academy of Medical Sciences), Moscow, 1954, vol. 13, pp. 9-22.

10. The Historical Evolution of Evolutionary Theories of Aging

How have aging and natural death emerged in the course of evolution? According to the very definition of fitness, i.e. survival and reproductive ability, aging and natural death (that is death inherent in a living organism and not brought about by external factors) are obviously detrimental, while an increased healthy life span would seem an obvious evolutionary advantage. Why then haven't the organisms evolved into immortal, super-long-lived or non-aging life-forms? On the contrary, the phenomena of biological immortality and absence of aging are present only among unicellular organisms and somewhat higher forms like the hydra, but not in more complex evolved forms, such as mammals. These are not just theoretically intriguing questions. Many gerontologists have believed that the understanding of the evolutionary mechanisms of aging and natural death may help pinpoint specific ways of intervention into human life span to achieve life extension.

The idea that death is an integral part of life, moreover that it is a necessary condition for life, has been long present. Its proponents included founding figures of modern biology. Thus, according to Xavier Bichat (1771-1802), life has developed in response to the threat of death from the environment: "life is the totality of functions which resist death." According to Carl Linnaeus (1707-1778) and Georges-Louis Buffon (1707-1788), death plays a crucial role in the "balance of nature" by regulating the population size of each species and thus maintaining harmony. According to Georges Cuvier (1769-1832), the threat of death defines not only population numbers, but the very structure and function of every given organism.[1] In Charles Darwin's *On the Origin of Species by Means of Natural Selection* (1859), this idea is further reinforced. Without death, the mechanism of natural selection would be inoperative.

At the end of the 19th century, the German biologist August Weismann (1834-1914) posited the first evolutionary theory specifically regarding aging and natural death.[2] According to Weismann, death is not an integral part of all life, as he affirmed that unicellular organisms are immortal. However, in higher organisms, there exists a distinction between immortal germ cells and mortal body cells (the "soma"). According to Weismann, the increasing complexity of the soma and tissue differentiation in higher organisms brought about the phenomena of aging and natural death. Highly differentiated tissues have a diminished ability to replicate and restore themselves, thus aging and death are the price paid for the complexity. Another crucial aspect of Weismann's theory is that aging and natural death are necessary conditions for evolution. Without them, aged organisms would fill the earth, exhausting all the resources, and stifling the emergence of new generations and new life forms.

Weismann's ideas seem very cogent, even intuitive. However this is largely teleological thinking: 'death is needed for something' (generations shift, innovation, diversity, availability of resources, etc.). But what can be the actual causal mechanisms of such a selection for aging deterioration (remembering that prolonged life and vigor are clear advantages for an individual organism)? Already in the beginning of the 20th century, the Russian immunologist Elie Metchnikoff (1845-1916) raised several important arguments against Weismann's theory.[3] Metchnikoff agreed with Weismann in that death is not a necessary prerequisite of all life: unicellular organisms are immortal, and even if they show signs of degeneration, they can be completely rejuvenated by conjugation. However, Metchnikoff did not believe that natural death can be an evolutionary advantage. According to him, "normal aging" and "natural death" almost never occur in nature. According to Metchnikoff, a relative weakening of an organism is enough to remove it from competition. There is just no chance (and no need) for it to 'age gracefully' or 'die a natural death' to assist evolution. Weakened organisms are eliminated by external causes – predation, disease, accidents, scramble or contest competition. And if aging and natural death almost never occur in nature, then natural selection cannot operate on them, let alone select for them. Regarding humans, Metchnikoff strongly asserted that we all die a "violent" and not a "natural death", and that if we are ever able to combat the pathogens that cause our premature death, human life can be greatly prolonged.

During the twentieth century, the possible evolutionary mechanisms of aging have continued to be hotly debated. The majority of researches reached the conclusion that aging (which is mainly observed in humans and animals held in captivity) is by no means an evolutionary advantage, but a result of "evolutionary neglect."[4] In the 1940s, the British geneticist John Haldane suggested a possible evolutionary mechanism for Huntington's progeria. The victims of this disease lead a relatively normal life and are capable of reproduction until about the age of 40. After that, they begin to show signs of rapidly accelerated aging and die within a short period. Why isn't this genetic defect eliminated from the population? According to Haldane, it is because of the fact that the victims are completely normal during their reproductive period and able to pass on the gene to the progeny. Thus, the genetic defect operating late in life is preserved.[5]

In 1952, the British immunologist Peter Medawar developed this idea into a general theory of *"Mutation Accumulation."*[6] According to this theory, only the genes expressed earlier in life, during the reproductive period, are selected for and important from the evolutionary perspective. What happens after the reproductive period is largely irrelevant for the evolutionary success. The late-acting mutations accumulate and cause the damage of aging. An important implication of this theory is that under conditions favorable for survival, the late acting genes have a better chance to be expressed and hence selected for or against. Much evidence confirms this prediction. For example, bats and mice are mammals of approximately the same size, yet bats can have a maximum life span of up to 30 years, while mice live only 2 or 3 years. The explanation for this is that bats are better protected and have fewer predators. The favorable conditions for survival allowed their late-acting genes to get expressed and selected. Under such favorable conditions, long-lived animals had an advantage over short-lived ones (bats generally were able to develop an effective anti-oxidant defense system and the ability to hibernate). In contrast, in mice, it did not matter whether they had a large or small longevity potential – they just needed enough time to reproduce before getting eaten by predators. This theory, however, has its drawbacks. It seems that evolution is not completely indifferent to events happening late in life, after the reproductive period is over: even a small degree of senescence damage affects survival rates and reproductive success. For example, a prolonged post-reproductive period can improve the success in raising the young. The Mutation Accumulation theory, thus, neglects intergenerational transfers and the "Grandmother effect."[7] Another problem is that genes that have been so far found to affect aging do not appear to be random mutations, but rather have orderly patterns.[8] This issue will be discussed later on.

In 1957, the American evolutionary biologist George Williams added an important specification.[9] (According to the British gerontologist Alex Comfort, writing in 1956, very similar principles were posited by the British marine biologist George Bidder in 1932.[10]) According to Williams, it is not just the mere accumulation of late-acting mutations that causes senescence. According to him, the very same genes that aid survival and reproduction in an early period of life history, can be damaging and cause senescence in a later period. This concept came to be known as the *"Antagonistic Pleiotropy"* theory. A large number of observations seem to support it. In Williams's reasoning, the rapid accumulation of calcium ("calcification") early in life can be beneficial for bone and muscle development, hence increased stamina. However, later in life, enhanced calcium deposition can contribute to atherosclerosis. Another hypothetical example Williams uses is that "a gene that favored erythrocyte longevity might be far from ideal for the maximization of oxygen-carrying capacity."[9] Other examples can be adduced along those lines. Thus, high levels of testosterone may give a good edge in sexual competition, yet later in life may contribute to prostate growth. Even at a more fundamental level, oxidative phosphorylation in the respiratory chain is what sustains life, yet the free radicals, formed in the process, cause aging damage. In another instance, the shortening of telomeres plays a part in cell differentiation and prevents cancer, but it also leads to cell replication limit and thus aging and death.

This is indeed a very cogent theory, but also not unproblematic. The concept of temporal antagonism is still largely hypothetical and its epigenetic timing mechanism remains unclear: Why would a gene that helps survival, until say age 40, suddenly become detrimental at the age of 41? Not all discovered genes that affect aging rate, also affect fertility early in life. In fact almost no such genes were found[8] – perhaps with just a few exceptions, such as the decay-accelerating factor (DAF) genes.[11] In the experiments of the British-American biogerontologist Michael Rose, some strains of extremely long-lived fruit flies were bred without any decrease in early fertility.[12] Perhaps even more persuasive, arguably, are the observations showing that people who have good athletic abilities early in life also often live longer and are more active later in life.[13]

The propositions of the above two theories were formalized in 1966 by the British evolutionary biologist William Hamilton. Using Fisher's reproductive value or the "Malthusian parameter," he showed that there is always a greater selective premium on early rather than late reproduction, since a probability to survive to a certain age, declines with age. The problem is that these equations apply both to the "Mutation Accumulation" and "Antagonistic Pleiotropy" theories. According to the British evolutionary biologist Brian Charlesworth, "it is at present hard to be sure which of the two most likely important mechanisms by which this property of selection influences senescence (accumulation of late-acting deleterious mutations or fixation of mutations with favorable early effects and deleterious late effects) plays the more important role."[14]

Later on, in 1977, the British gerontologist Thomas Kirkwood suggested the *"Disposable Soma"* theory.[15] This is in fact an extension of the "Antagonistic Pleiotropy" theory, but instead of genetic and phenotypic terms, Kirkwood mainly uses terminology of energy expenditure. According to this theory, the expenditure of energy on reproduction (early in life) is more important for evolutionary success than the energy expended on a prolonged body/soma maintenance (throughout the life history). In this view, the body is "disposable": most energy resources are spent on reproduction at the expense of individual longevity. The life histories of semelparous organisms (the organisms having a single reproductive episode before death) offer perhaps the best demonstration of this principle. Thus, organisms like may-flies or the marsupial antechinus, copulate so vigorously that after several hours of it, they burn out and die of exhaustion. This trade-off mechanism seems to operate also in non-semelparous animals. Thus, the British researchers Jens Rolff and Michael Siva-Jothy demonstrated that frequent mating of beetles shortens their life ("Copulation corrupts immunity" 2002).[16] Also, Michael Rose showed that delayed reproduction in drosophila flies drastically increases their life-span.[17] Related effects may also exist in humans. Thus, several studies of monks and nuns showed that monks have a greater than average longevity (according to a recent German study about 5 years above average men, however in earlier Polish and Dutch studies only 1 or 2 years higher).[18]

Still, there exists a wide array of data contradicting this theory. This concept has been challenged by studies professing that sexual activity may actually strengthen the immune system and prolong life, and that survival is not necessarily antagonistic to reproduction. This was suggested for ants by Schrempf et al. ("Sexual cooperation: mating increases longevity in ant queens" 2005, Germany)[19] and for humans by Davey Smith et al. ("Sex and Death: Are They Related?" 1997, UK).[20] This was also the conclusion of the US Duke Longitudinal Study which showed that more sexually active people live longer.[21] According to the Russian-American gerontologist Leonid Gavrilov, childless women do not live longer. On the contrary, greater longevity seems to correlate with greater fecundity. Gavrilov's findings agree with those made by the British statisticians Karl Pearson and George Yule over a hundred years ago, but seem to completely contradict both the Disposable Soma theory and Kirkwood's own demographic observations.[22]

There seems to be a large number of methodological problems on both sides of the dispute. It is generally difficult to project animal studies (e.g. of insects or marsupials) on humans. Human studies also seem to be indeterminate. Regarding, for example, the longevity of monks, the positive effect of their supposed abstinence on longevity may be confounded by many other factors, such as absence of alcoholism or smoking. On the other hand, Davey Smith's et al. "Caerphilly study" ("Sex and Death: Are They Related?")[20] has become famous for suggesting that high sexual activity reduces mortality rates. It appeared in 1997 and has been making the headlines since. However, it may be argued that the Caerphilly study's representation is rather uncertain. Its sample size is by an order of magnitude less than that of Marc Luy's "Cloister Monks/Nuns study"[18] (2006, Germany-Austria). The Caerphilly study examines 918 men aged 45-59, with a 10 year follow up. Thus, it disregards earlier sexual habits and activities that might be determinative for the life span. This may even be a case of "delayed reproduction." The effect on the actual life span is also unclear. It may well be that a short-term increase in well-being is followed by rapid deterioration (as in the famous case of the French physiologist Charles-Édouard Brown-Séquard's experiment of 1889 with self-injection of animal testicular extracts, where some transient "rejuvenation" effects were soon followed by deterioration.[23]) And most importantly, this may be a case of "reversed causality" – Do the more sexually active people become healthier, or are the healthier people more active? It is difficult to disentangle these issues.

The "disposable soma" theory also seems to be at odds with data on calorie restriction in animals. Since the 1930s, calorie restriction has been consistently shown to increase the life span in almost all animals tried. It is perhaps the only well substantiated experimental method of life prolongation known so far. In mice, it can increase the life span by 50%.[24] Yet, according to the disposable soma theory, well fed animals should live longer (because they will have enough energy for both reproduction and body maintenance). This, however, does not occur. Moreover, in many calorie restricted models, fertility does not diminish as predicted by the theory. Still, the "Disposable Soma" theory is now a most widely accepted evolutionary theory of aging.

It is interesting to observe how ideological agendas affect areas of scientific interest. The above mainstream theories (with the exception of Williams, by British evolutionists) figure prominently in almost every review of evolutionary theories of aging.[25] However, in several books by advocates of radical life extension (mostly Americans), such as Durk Pearson and Sandy Shaw's *Life Extension. A Practical Scientific Approach* (1982)[26] or Saul Kent's *The Life Extension Revolution* (1983)[27] – Peter Medawar, George Williams and Tom Kirkwood are hardly ever mentioned. In contrast, the theories by the American gerontologists Richard Cutler and George Sacher receive there the utmost notice and are cited as the primary authority. This might be an issue of possible British-American rivalry (according to the American gerontologist George Martin, Sacher was "singularly unimpressed" by Medawar's theory, and only thanks to the British born Michael Rose, it made its entrance in the US).[28] Another, perhaps even more plausible explanation that could be offered, is that the three mainstream theories by Medawar, Williams and Kirkwood sound somewhat pessimistic. According to them, aging has emerged as a result of evolutionary neglect, it is due to an enormous multitude of intractable random mutations, it is inevitable if species are to survive early in life and reproduce. The implied message is that there is not much we can do about it.

The theories by Sacher and Cutler, on the other hand, offer a glimpse of hope. Both authors show a consistent increase in longevity during the evolution of mammalian species, including man. Sacher[29] posited a general formula relating the weight of an animal and the weight of its brain to its maximum life span (MLS):[30]

$$MLS = (10.83) \times (Brain\ wt.,\ g)^{0.636} \times (Body\ wt.,\ g)^{-0.225}$$

This formula gives correct results with 25% accuracy for a large number of species. (Assuming 1400-1500 g weight of the human brain,[31] the maximal life span would be somewhere around 90-100 years.) Large animals have been long known to live longer[32] (this may be due to a lower surface/volume ratio, hence slower metabolism per unit weight, hence less toxic metabolites/free radicals). A larger brain, on the other hand, allows for a better internal regulation, and intelligence and social behavior reduce extrinsic mortality. Thus, an increase in brain size correlates with an increase in longevity. Sacher's formula weighs these two parameters. (Interestingly, according to it, in any given species, lower body weight is associated with greater longevity, and only the combination of the brain and body weight distinguishes between the life spans of different species.)

Using the above formula, as also the formula relating sexual maturation age and life span: *Sexual maturation age = (0.2) (MLS)*, carbon dating, and mutation rate estimates – Richard Cutler calculated a consistent increase in longevity during human evolution. During the past 100,000 years, it presumably increased by ~14 years, associated with changes in ~0.6% of the genome (~250 genes according to his calculations). The optimism implied here is, first of all, that even if conscious human life-extensionist efforts fail, the human race can still rely on evolution for increased longevity (of course, if still granted favorable environmental conditions). The second source of optimism is that the amount of genetic change associated with increased longevity is rather limited (compared to the immense complexity and randomness implied in the "Mutation Accumulation" theory). The limited number of genes associated with aging raises the hopes to pinpoint specific intervention targets.

A possible problem that may be raised in this regard is that Cutler's calculations are likely not very accurate. There are obviously huge blank spots in the hominid ancestral descendant sequence. Moreover, Cutler's calculations of genetic change are based on Haldane's estimation that "the maximum rate of adaptive gene substitution in mammalian evolution could not be more than one substitution per genome per 300 generations" and he assumes the adaptive nucleotides fixation rate of about 6×10^{-3} AA/gene per 10^4 generations and 4×10^4 genes per genome. However, Cutler himself admits that estimations of adaptive gene substitutions differ by orders of magnitude among different authors. And the estimate of 40,000 genes per human genome is now known to be about twice the actual value.[33]

Nevertheless, the suggested tendency of longevity increase is very uplifting. For example, the prominent Ukrainian gerontologist Vladimir Frolkis, in his *Aging and Life-Prolonging Processes* (1982)[34] was truly inspired by Cutler's findings and quoted them at least a dozen times. According to Frolkis, mainstream evolutionary theories of aging give too much emphasis on genes causing aging damage, forgetting that alongside them there evolved deliberate mechanisms prolonging life, what he called *"vitauct"* roughly equivalent to *"anti-aging."* These mechanisms include genes for anti-oxidant defense enzymes, enzymes for DNA repair (various types of ligases, polymerases and nucleases), mechanisms of membrane hyper-polarization (necessary for cell resting state, ATP replenishment and protein synthesis). These types of genes could be included in the 0.5% genetic change suggested by Cutler and can be reasonably manipulated.

Inconsistencies in the three mainstream evolutionary theories of aging made several contemporary researchers, such as the Americans Josh Mitteldorf and Theodore Goldsmith and the Russian Vladimir Skulachev, ponder a return to Weismann's theory.[35] According to Skulachev, there are several "deliberate" mechanisms which seem to have no other function than to cause aging and death. These mechanisms seem to be too well orchestrated and directional to be randomly accumulated mutations. In Skulachev's metaphor, "we will not accuse a person of kleptomania if he only steals money." Among these "deliberate" mechanisms, Skulachev lists: "1) telomere shortening due to suppression of telomerase at early stages of embryogenesis; 2) age-related deactivation of a mechanism that induces the synthesis of heat shock proteins in response to denaturing stimuli; and 3) incomplete suppression of generation and scavenging of reactive oxygen species (ROS)." By analogy to apoptosis or programmed cell death, Skulachev terms these evolved programmed mechanisms of aging and death of the entire organism "phenoptosis." In organisms like salmon fish, aging is strictly programmed (they die right after spawning), while in man it is more pliable, but programmed nonetheless. Hence, Skulachev concludes that "Aging is a specific biological function rather than the result of a disorder in complex living systems." But what biological function? The specter of teleology is raised again. Skulachev, Mitteldorf and Goldsmith offer explanations. First of all, according to these authors, an absence of aging would impair variation and thus reduce the species evolvability and adaptability. For example, an ideal DNA repair mechanism would make mutability impossible (all mutations would be immediately corrected). And without mutability, there would be no diversity and no evolution. Any new threat (e.g. a new infection) could then wipe out the entire stagnant population. (Still, improved immunity and DNA repair may be assumed to provide improved defense against a greater range of pathogens and environmental threats, such as radiation, temperature changes and toxins, including bio-toxins, hence it seems not entirely clear how this can be an unequivocal evolutionary disadvantage.) Secondly, there remains the threat of resources exhaustion. A population that cannot regulate its size through programmed "natural death" will be wiped out by resource scarcity and famine. (However, in this case, selection should rapidly operate on a group rather than on an individual, insofar as longevity is a clear advantage for the individual. Since George Williams, the possibility of "group selection" has been hotly debated. Metchnikoff's earlier observation that "natural death" almost never occurs in nature might be recalled as well. There is no evidence of extinction of non-aging animals, such as protozoa or the hydra.)

The belief in the "programmed," "designed" nature of aging does not hinder the life-extensionists' optimism – rather to the contrary. For example, academician Skulachev has been one of the leading Russian life-extensionists. He is a self-avowed "fighter for human longevity," developing super-antioxidants aimed to correct oxidative damage at its source within the mitochondria, and hoping that "man will live hundreds of years."[36] He strongly believes that human beings are now at the stage when they can rise above the blind Darwinian selection and create our own destiny. Moreover, he believes that because of the fact that the number of "programmed" mechanisms of aging is limited, a restricted number of specific interventions can be designed to target them. Even under the mainstream "evolutionary neglect" paradigm, there is still a hope of intervention, for example by eliminating accumulated damage before it becomes pathological and irreparably harms the organism's regulation,[37] or by environmental adjustments aimed to induce prolongevity epigenetic effects.[38]

Whatever theory prevails, a deep and practical understanding of evolutionary mechanisms of aging and longevity entails a hope for positive ameliorative interventions. Despite the intense controversies, this is the hope (even though a distant one) that most aging researchers share. It is believed that through evolutionary investigations, factors affecting longevity (including genetic factors, pathogens and environmental conditions, constitutional and metabolic properties) can be identified and then manipulated to improve human health and longevity.

References and notes

1. William Randall Albury, "Ideas of Life and Death," in *Companion Encyclopedia of the History of Medicine*, Edited by William F. Bynum and Roy Porter, Routledge, London and NY, 2001, pp. 253-254.
2. August Weismann, "Ueber die Dauer des Lebens" (On the duration of life), Jena, 1882; August Weismann, "Ueber Leben und Tod" (On life and death), Jena, 1884. These works appear in English translation in August Weismann, *On Heredity*, Claredon Press, Oxford, 1891.
3. Elie Metchnikoff, *Etudy o Prirode Cheloveka* (Etudes On the Nature of Man), The USSR Academy of Sciences Press, Moscow, 1961, First published in 1903, "An introduction to the scientific study of death," pp. 214-245.

4. Aubrey de Grey, "Do we have genes that exist to hasten aging? New data, new arguments, but the answer is still no." *Current Aging Science*, 8(1), 24-33, 2015.

5. John B.S. Haldane, *New Paths in Genetics*, George Allen and Unwin, London, 1941.

6. Peter Brian Medawar, *An Unsolved Problem of Biology*, H.K. Lewis, London, 1952.

7. Ronald D. Lee, "Rethinking the evolutionary theory of aging: transfers, not births, shape senescence in social species," *Proceedings of the National Academy of Sciences USA*, 100(16), 9637-9642, 2003.

8. Jeff Bowles, "Shattered: Medawar's test tubes and their enduring legacy of chaos," *Medical Hypotheses*, 54(2), 326–339, 2000.

9. George C. Williams, "Pleiotropy, natural selection and the evolution of senescence," *Evolution*, 11, 398-411, 1957.

10. George P. Bidder, "The mortality of plaice," *Nature*, 115, 495, 1925; George P. Bidder, "Senescence," *British Medical Journal*, 2, 5831, 1932, quoted in Alexander Comfort, *The Biology of Senescence*, Butler & Tanner, London, 1956, pp. 11-12.

11. Cynthia J. Kenyon, "The genetics of ageing," *Nature*, 464, 504-512, 2010; Jacob J.E. Koopman, Jeroen Pijpe, Stefan Böhringer, et al., "Genetic variants determining survival and fertility in an adverse African environment: a population-based large-scale candidate gene association study," *Aging* (Albany NY), 8(7), 1364-1374, 2016.

12. Michael R. Rose, *Evolutionary Biology of Aging*, Oxford University Press, New York, 1991.

13. Some studies indicating the enhanced longevity of athletes include: Louis Dublin, "Longevity of College Athletes," *Harper's Monthly Magazine*, 157, 229-238, July 1928; Marti Karvonen, "Endurance sports, Longevity and Health," *Annals of the New York Academy of Sciences*, 301, 653-655, 1977. However, contrary data exist as well pointing out life-shortening effects of strenuous physical activity, e.g.: Peter Kaprovich, "Longevity and Athletics," *Research Quarterly*, 12: 451-455, 1941; Henry Montoye et al., *The Longevity and Morbidity of College Athletes*, Indianapolis, Phi Epsilon Kappa, 1957; Anthony Polednak and Albert Damon, "College Athletics, Longevity and Cause of Death," *Human Biology*, 42, 28-46, 1970; Charles Rose and Michel Cohen, "Relative importance of physical activity for longevity," *Annals of the New York Academy of Sciences*, 301, 671-702, 1977. The results also vary widely depending on the type of sports, level of athleticism, period of practice, and many other factors. (Anthony P. Polednak (Ed.), *The Longevity of Athletes*, Charles C. Thomas, Springfield IL, 1979.)

14. Brian Charlesworth, "Fisher, Medawar, Hamilton and the Evolution of Aging," *Genetics*, 156, 927-931, 2000; William D. Hamilton, "The moulding

of senescence by natural selection," *Journal of Theoretical Biology*, 12(1), 12-45, 1966.

15. Thomas B.L. Kirkwood, "Evolution of aging," *Nature*, 270, 301-304, 1977; Fotios Drenos, Thomas B.L. Kirkwood, "Modelling the disposable soma theory of ageing," *Mechanisms of Ageing and Development*, 126(1), 99-103, 2005.

16. Jens Rolff, Michael Siva-Jothy, "Copulation corrupts immunity," *Proceedings of the National Academy of Sciences USA*, 99, 9916-9918, 2002.

17. Michael R. Rose and Theodore J. Nusbaum, "Prospects for postponing human aging," *The FASEB Journal*, 8, 925-928, 1994; Ricki L. Rusting, "Why Do We Age," *Scientific American*, 87-95, December 1992.

18. Marc Luy, "Leben Frauen länger oder sterben Männer früher?" (Do women live longer or do men die earlier?), *Public Health Forum*, 14(50), S.18-20, 2006, part of *Klosterstudie zur Lebenserwartung von Nonnen und Mönchen* (The "Closter" study of life-expectancy in nuns and monks) http://www.klosterstudie.de/; Bartosz Jenner, "Changes in average life span of monks and nuns in Poland in the years 1950-2000," *Przegl Lek*, 59(4-5), 225-229, 2002; de Gouw H.W., Westendorp R.G., Kunst A.E., Mackenbach J.P., Vandenboucke J.P., "Decreased mortality among contemplative monks in The Netherlands," *American Journal of Epidemiology*, 141(8), 771-775, 1995.

19. Alexandra Schrempf, Jürgen Heinze, Sylvia Cremer, "Sexual cooperation: mating increases longevity in ant queens," *Current Biology*, 15, 267-270, 2005.

20. George Davey Smith, Stephen Frankel, John Yarnell, "Sex and Death: Are They Related?" *British Medical Journal*, 315, 1641-1644, 1997.

21. Maxon P.J., Gold C.H., Berg S., "Characteristics of long-surviving men: results from a nine-year longitudinal study," *Aging* (Milano), 9(3), 214-220, 1997; Ostbye T., Krause K.M., Norton M.C., et al., "Ten dimensions of health and their relationships with overall self-reported health and survival in a predominately religiously active elderly population: the cache county memory study," *Journal of the American Geriatrics Society*, 54(2), 199-209, 2006; Linda George and Stephen Weiler, "Sexuality in Middle and Late Life" pp. 12-19, Erdman B. Palmore, "Predictors of the Longevity Difference" pp. 20-29, in *Normal Aging: Reports from the Duke Longitudinal Study By Duke University Center for the Study of Aging and Human Development*, Duke University Press, Durham NC, 1985.

22. Natalia S. Gavrilova, Leonid A. Gavrilov, "Human longevity and Reproduction. An evolutionary perspective," in *Grandmotherhood: The Evolutionary Significance of the Second Half of Female Life*, Rutgers University Press, New Brunswick, NJ, USA, 2005, pp. 59-80.

23. Ilia Stambler, *A History of Life-Extensionism in the Twentieth Century*, Longevity History, 2014, http://www.longevityhistory.com/.

24. Richard Weindruch, Rajindar S. Sohal, "Caloric intake and aging," *New England Journal of Medicine*, 337(14), 986–994, 1997.

25. Leonid Gavrilov, Natalia Gavrilova, *Biologia Prodolzhitelnosti Zhizni* (Biology of the Lifespan), Vladimir Skulachev (Ed.), Nauka, Moscow, 1991, Ch. 4.1; Vladimir Anisimov, *Molekuliarnie i Physiologicheskie Mechanismy Starenia* (Molecular and Physiological Mechanisms of Aging), Nauka, St. Petersburg, 2003, Ch. 1.3. Accessible at: http://gerontology.bio.msu.ru/notourpublications.htm, http://gerontology-explorer.narod.ru/.
See also: Wikipedia, "Senescence" http://en.wikipedia.org/wiki/Senescence, "Evolution of Aging," http://en.wikipedia.org/wiki/Evolution_of_ageing; João Pedro de Magalhães, "The Evolutionary Theory of Aging," http://www.senescence.info/evolution_of_aging.html.

26. Durk Pearson, Sandy Shaw, *Life Extension. A Practical Scientific Approach*, Warner Books, NY, 1982, Part 1, Ch. 1. "The Evolution of Aging," pp. 18-23.

27. Saul Kent, *The Life-Extension Revolution. The Source Book for Optimum Health and Maximum Life-span*, Quill, NY, 1983, Ch. 1, "Why do we grow old and die?" pp. 19-20.

28. George M. Martin, "How is the evolutionary biological theory of aging holding up against mounting attacks?" *American Aging Association Newsletter*, March 2005, http://web.archive.org/web/20160328164647/http://www.americanaging.org/news/mar05.html.

29. George A. Sacher, "Relationship of lifespan to brain weight and body weight in mammals," in *CIBA Foundation Colloquia on Aging*, Churchill, London, 1959, Vol. 5, pp. 115-133; George A. Sacher, "Longevity and Aging in Vertebrate Evolution," *BioScience*, 28(8), 497-501, 1978.

30. Richard Cutler, "Evolution of human longevity and the genetic complexity governing aging rate," *Proceedings of the National Academy of Sciences USA*, 72(11), 4664-4668, 1975, https://www.ncbi.nlm.nih.gov/pmc/articles/PMC388784/.

31. Miller A.K., Corsellis J.A., "Evidence for a secular increase in human brain weight during the past century," *Annals of Human Biology*, 4(3), 253-257, 1977.

32. William A. Calder, *Size, Function, and Life History*, Harvard University Press, Cambridge, 1984; Knut Schmidt-Nielsen, *Scaling: Why is Animal Size So Important?* Cambridge University Press, Cambridge, 1984; João Pedro de Magalhães, "Comparative Biology of Aging," Senescence Info, http://www.senescence.info/comparative_biology.html.

33. International Human Genome Sequencing Consortium, "Finishing the euchromatic sequence of the human genome," *Nature* 431(7011), 931-45,

2004,
http://www.nature.com/nature/journal/v431/n7011/full/nature03001.html.

34. Vladimir Frolkis, *Aging and Life-Prolonging Processes*, Springer-Verlag, Wien, 1982.

35. Theodore C. Goldsmith, "Aging as an Evolved Characteristic – Weismann's Theory Reconsidered," *Medical Hypotheses*, 62(2), 304-308, 2004; Joshua Mitteldorf, "Ageing selected for its own sake," *Evolutionary Ecology Research*, 6, 937-953, 2004; Vladimir Skulachev, "Aging is a Specific Biological Function Rather than the Result of a Disorder in Complex Living Systems: Biochemical Evidence in Support of Weismann's Hypothesis," *Biochemistry* (Moscow), 62(11), 1191-1195, 1997, http://humbio.ru/humbio/phenopt/00000934.htm.

36. Vladimir Skulachev, "Starenie – atavism, kotory sleduet preodolet" (Aging is an atavism which must be overcome), Moscow University Seminar, 21.02.2005, http://azfor.narod.ru/geront/Skulachev.htm; Vladimir Skulachev (interview by Sergey Leskov), "Chelovek budet zhit sotni let i umirat ot neschastnich sluchaev" (Man will live hundreds of years and die of accidents), *Izvestia*, 28.11.2003, http://www.ras.ru/digest/showdnews.aspx?id=78f6851b-2371-4e58-9ab5-818770417192&print=1.

37. Aubrey de Grey, Michael Rae, *Ending Aging: The Rejuvenation Breakthroughs That Could Reverse Human Aging in Our Lifetime*, St. Martin's Press, New York, 2007.

38. André C. R. Martins, "Change and Aging: Senescence as an adaptation," *PLoS One*, 6(9):e24328, 2011, https://www.ncbi.nlm.nih.gov/pmc/articles/PMC3174959/; Marios Kyriazis, "Third phase science: defining a novel model of research into human ageing," *Frontiers in Bioscience*, 22, 982-990, 2017; Thomas A. Rando, Howard Y. Chang, "Aging, rejuvenation, and epigenetic reprogramming: resetting the aging clock," *Cell*, 148, 46-57, 2012.

III. LONGEVITY PHILOSOPHY

11. Longevity and the Indian Tradition

Does the pursuit of longevity, or even radical longevity, have future in India? The following article will consider this question mainly in ideological, cultural and historical terms, rather than in terms of analyzing current technological and demographic trends. In demographic terms, as was also noted earlier, the life expectancy in India is still relatively low compared to other countries (about 68 years), yet it is clearly on the rise[1] and no limit can be set for this increase. Important innovative initiatives for research of aging and longevity are on the way, such as the International Longevity Center India,[2] whose purpose is "to work towards healthy, productive and participatory ageing" (or healthy longevity). Also the future of general biomedical research in India, including longevity research, looks bright. According to one analyst, "India is a promised land, offering much in the medical and scientific research."[3]

Yet, apparently, the biomedical research of aging and longevity, has not yet received a considerable attention in India, judging from the absence of dedicated research institutes or governmental, or even large private, programs to address this issue.[4] One suggestion why this negligence happens was that the research of aging and longevity is somehow incompatible with Indian traditional values. It is sometimes assumed that Indian cultural beliefs are opposed to preservation of the material body, due to the belief in the transience of the body and reincarnation. The belief in the supremacy of the spirit and mind over matter and body supposedly makes maintenance of the body unimportant.

As formulated by Prof. Kalluri Subba Rao, Hon. Coordinator for Center for Research and Education in Aging (CREA) University of Hyderabad:[5]

"The summary of [this] argument was simple and straightforward. In India we have the faith that this life is only a transitory phase of never ending cycle of birth and death. Every one who is born is certain to die. In fact, according the Indian ethos, every one should strive to attain *janmarahityam* or *moksha*, a state where one becomes free from the cycle of birth and death. Under these circumstances why to worry that we are aging which inevitable? Instead, one should adopt *vanaprastha* and indulge in such activities that might take one nearer to *moksha* or even to *moksha* itself. Therefore, it is silly for any nation to spend a good chunk of its resources on finding out how we become old and die."

Yet, apparently the above argument against longevity research presents a very incomplete and even distorted view of Indian cultural tradition. As a

174

matter of fact, in Indian tradition, particularly in the religious tradition of Hinduism (or rather in the variety of religions of India designated by this term), the pursuit of longevity and even radical life extension has been a persistent theme since a very early time.

Here are some examples:

The entire Book 9 of *The Rigveda* (c. 1700-1100 BCE) is dedicated to praises of the immortality-giving "Soma" plant.[6] (The plant is called "Haoma" in ancient Iranian (Aryan) religious sources, such as *Avesta*, c. 1200-200 BCE.[7])

In India, the immortal Rishis, Arhats, and the Ciranjivas (the "extremely long-lived persons") are revered to the present. Their extreme longevity is often attributed to "Amrit" – अमृत – or the "nectar of immortality" – a revered and desired substance.

The traditional Indian medicine of Ayurveda, or "the science of (long) life," includes a special field of Rasayana, mainly dedicated to rejuvenation.

According to one of the earliest Ayurvedic texts, *The Sushruta Samhita* (Sushruta's Compilation of Knowledge, c. 800-300 BCE):[8]

"Bramha was the first to inculcate the principles of the holy Ayurveda. Prajapati learned the science from him. The Ashvins learned it from Prajapati and imparted the knowledge to Indra, who has favoured me [Dhanvantari, an incarnation of Lord Vishnu, the protector of life and the giver of Ayurveda on earth] with an entire knowledge thereof." This knowledge was in turn "disclosed by the holy Dhanvantari to his disciple Sushruta."

(Notably, within the Trimurti – Hindu Trinity: Brahma the creator, Vishnu the preserver and Shiva the destroyer – the deity mainly associated with Ayurveda is Vishnu the preserver, while some of his devotees, such as Narada can live even through destruction and creation of worlds. A following incarnation of Vishnu is said to be Kalki, the "machine man."[9])

According to the *Sushruta Samhita*, human life can be normally prolonged to 100 years. Yet, with the use of certain Rasayana remedies (such as Brahmi Rasayana and Vidanga-Kalpa), life can be prolonged to 500 or 800 years. And the use of the "Soma plant, the lord of all medicinal herbs [24 candidate plants are named], is followed by rejuvenation of the system of its user and enables him to witness ten thousand summers on earth in the full enjoyment of a new (youthful) body."

Also according to another foundational text of Ayurveda, *The Charaka Samhita* (Charaka's Compilation of Knowledge, c. 300-100 BCE), the normal human life-span is 100 years. Yet, the users of an Amalaka Rasayana could live many hundreds of years and the users of the Amalakayasa

Brahma Rasayana could reach the life-span of 1000 years. The great sages, who grasped perfectly the knowledge of Ayurveda, "attained the highest well-being and nonperishable life-span."[10]

The ancient Indian tradition abounds in medical achievements, which are perceived as positive and desirable!

In the ancient Indian epic of the *Ramayana* (often dated c. 400 BCE, and sometimes purported to relate to events occurring 4,000 and even 5000 BCE), the monkey king Hanuman uses the Sanjeevani plant (translated as "One that infuses life" and commonly identified as the lycophyte *Selaginella bryopteris*, growing at the Dunagiri (Mahodaya) mountain in the Himalayas) to revive Rama's younger brother Lakshman, severely wounded by Ravan.[11] Also according to the *Ramayana*, the mutilated nose and ears of the asura princess Surpanakha, sister of Ravan and Khara, could be restored.[12] Actual methods of skin transplantation to adhere severed earlobes and restore mutilated noses, are described in the *Sushruta Samhita*.[13] According to the epic of *Mahabharata* (commonly dated 400-500 BCE and attributed to Vyasa), the body of the Magadha king Jarasandha, could be fused from two halves and completely regenerated.[14]

Thus life-extending, rejuvenative and regenerative technologies have been vividly envisioned in Hindu tradition.

Buddhism too has a strong connection to the pursuit of longevity.

The Great Buddha who grants Longevity is Amitābha, the Buddha of Infinite Light, also known as Amitāyus, the Buddha of Infinite Life. Those who invoke him will reach longevity in this realm, and will be reborn in Amitabha's Pure Land (Sukhāvatī or Dewachen in Tibetan Buddhism) where they will enjoy virtually unlimited longevity. This pure and egalitarian land of longevity was created by Amitabha's avowed devotion and perseverance. One of the mantras in Amitabha's praise is "Om amrita teje hara hum" (Om save us in the glory of the Deathless One hum). Many Buddhist mantras for longevity are recited, dedicated to the great healers of old, so that a portal to their wisdom may be opened and, through their compassion, suffering will be abolished and health and longevity reached in this world.

Yet also, material means for rejuvenation and life extension have been developed by Buddhist physicians.[15] Of course many methods of traditional and Ayurvedic medicine currently practiced yet require thorough testing.[16]

Crucially, the vision of advanced medical technology and the idea of a significant, even radical extension of healthy life-span, in this world, are deeply entrenched in Indian cultural tradition. These positive tendencies need to be recalled and reawakened, so the vision of the golden age of extended health and longevity will be implemented in the present time using advances of modern science. The pursuit of healthy longevity is not an "all or nothing" pursuit, but any incremental improvement in this direction may be expected to be beneficial for India and its population.

The research of aging and longevity will be required to find the path toward the practical achievement of healthy longevity, and the original inspiration for this pursuit may come from Indian cultural heritage.

In summary, one can but agree with Prof. Kalluri Subba Rao's conclusion, regarding the importance of aging and longevity research for India:

"YES. India must in its own interest promote research on aging and associated diseases in a big way. There are always some discordant, perverted voices projecting the distorted Indian Wisdom. India's march towards becoming a global leader should not be allowed to be disturbed by vested and disgruntled arguments."

Several practical measures were proposed by Prof. Kalluri Subba Rao to advance the goals of healthy longevity in India. Once again, a person interested in promoting this objective in India can only agree and endeavor to support this initiative.

"Concrete steps and inputs are necessary. One such step is to establish one or more (in view of the vastness and diversity of the country) Institutes or Centers for a multidisciplinary scientific study of the phenomenon of aging and the associated diseases/problems. Such Institutes would also prepare a database for the clinical and biological profiles of the populations around particularly of the senior citizens to begin with."

One of the missions of the proposed Centers/Institutes would be to "conduct high quality research on the process of aging – at genetic, molecular, clinical, biochemical and behavioral levels" as well as study "disabilities and diseases, including neurological disorders, associated with age and more prevalent in the aged"; in addition to "psychosocial aspects of the aged with a special emphasis on the special and peculiar needs of the aged," and finally, "connectivity between the laboratory findings and the community to promote health among the aged and to make use of the healthy 'aged' to the societal needs."

Similar goals are now promoted all across the world.[17] Let us hope that with our joint efforts, healthy longevity for all will be advanced in India and everywhere.[18]

References and notes

1. Janani Sampath, "Life expectancy in India goes up by 5 years in a decade," *Times of India*, January 29, 2014, http://timesofindia.indiatimes.com/india/Life-expectancy-in-India-goes-up-by-5-years-in-a-decade/articleshow/29513964.cms;
Miriam Leis (Jisun), "India – High-Biotech, IT-Hub, DIY-Science and 8-Armed Cyborgs with a Third Eye," Institute for Ethics and Emerging Technologies (IEET), February 2, 2012, http://ieet.org/index.php/IEET/more/leis20120201;
Shreerupa Mitra-Jha, "Life expectancy in India on the rise, but quality health care services inadequate," *First Post*, May 20, 2016, http://www.firstpost.com/india/life-expectancy-in-india-on-the-rise-but-quality-health-care-services-inadequate-2790442.html.
2. International Longevity Center India, http://ilcindia.org.
3. Kites India, "The advances of Indian research in the new millennium," 2011,
http://web.archive.org/web/20141130221823/http://www.kitesindia.org/the-advances-of-indian-research-in-the-new-millennium.php.
4. Badithe T. Ashok, Rashid Ali, "Aging research in India," *Experimental Gerontology*, 38(6), 597-603, 2003, www.ncbi.nlm.nih.gov/pubmed/12814794.
5. Kalluri Subba Rao, "Should India Promote Scientific Research on Aging?" IEET, March 20, 2016 (first published in 2008), http://ieet.org/index.php/IEET/more/rao20160320.
6. *The Hymns of the Rigveda*, translated by Ralph T.H. Griffith, E.J. Lazarus and Co., Benares, 1891, Book 9, pp. 361-412, the 1896 edition is reprinted at http://www.sacred-texts.com/hin/rigveda/.
7. "Avesta: Khorda Avesta, 9. Gosh Yasht," translated by James Darmesteter, from *Sacred Books of the East*, American Edition, 1898, http://www.avesta.org/ka/yt9sbe.htm.
8. *An English translation of the Sushruta samhita, based on original Sanskrit text, Edited and published by Kaviraj Kunja Lal Bhishagratna*, Calcutta, 1907, 1911, 1916, Vol. 1, "Sutrasthanam" (Fundamental principles), Ch. 1, p. 8, Vol. 2, "Chikitsasthanam" (Therapeutics), Ch. 27, p. 518, Ch. 28, p. 525, Ch. 29, pp. 530, 536, available at http://chestofbooks.com/health/india/Sushruta-Samhita/index.html#.Uag6GNKnxvA and http://archive.org/details/englishtranslati03susr.
9. "Narada" http://en.wikipedia.org/wiki/Narada; "Kalki" http://en.wikipedia.org/wiki/Kalki.
10. *Charaka Samhita. Handbook on Ayurveda*, Gabriel Van Loon (Ed.), Durham NC, 2003, vol. 1, "Cikitsasthana" 1.1.75, p. 446, "Cikitsasthana" 1.3.3-6, p. 455, "Sutrasthana" 1.27-29, p. 107, https://ayurinfo.files.wordpress.com/2011/09/charak-samhita-handbook-vol-i-edited-by-gabriel-van-loon.pdf;

178

http://hinduonline.co/DigitalLibrary/SmallBooks/CharakaSamhitaVol2Eng.pdf;
Caraka Samhita, Text with English Translation, Complete in Four Volumes, Priyavrat V. Sharma (Editor-Translator), Chaukhambha Orientalia, Varanasi, 2014, Vol. 1, http://archive.org/details/CharakaSamhitaHindiVolume1.

11. *Ramayan of Valmiki, Translated Into English Verse by Ralph T. H. Griffith*, 1870-1874, Book 6, Canto CII "Lakshman Healed," reprinted at http://www.sacred-texts.com/hin/rama/index.htm.

12. *Ramayan of Valmiki, Translated Into English Verse by Ralph T. H. Griffith*, 1870-1874, Book 3, Cantos XVIII-XIX, reprinted at http://www.sacred-texts.com/hin/rama/index.htm. Also in Kampan's version of the Ramayana, according to Kathleen M. Erndl, "The Mutilation of Surpanakha," in Paula Richman (Ed.), *Many Rāmāyaṇas: The Diversity of a Narrative Tradition in South Asia*, University of California Press, Berkeley, 1991, p. 75, http://publishing.cdlib.org/ucpressebooks/.

13. *An English translation of the Sushruta samhita, based on original Sanskrit text, Edited and published by Kaviraj Kunja Lal Bhishagratna*, Calcutta, 1907, Vol. 1, Ch. 16, pp. 141-154.

14. *The Mahabharata, Book 2: Sabha Parva*, Kisari Mohan Ganguli, tr., 1883-1896, "Rajasuyarambha Parva," Section 17, "Jarasandhta-badha Parva," pp. 40-41, Section 24, pp. 53-54, http://www.sacred-texts.com/hin/m02/index.htm.

15. On Buddhist perspective, see for example: *Medicine Buddha. Teachings on the Medicine Buddha Sadhana and Medicine Buddha Sutra given by Ven. Thrangu Rinpoche*, http://www.dharma-haven.org/thrangu-medicine-buddha.htm. See also: Derek F. Maher, "Two Wings of a Bird: Radical Life Extension from a Buddhist Perspective," in Calvin Mercer and Derek F. Maher (Eds.), *Religion and the Implications of Radical Life Extension*, Macmillan Palgrave, New York, 2009, pp. 111-121; Luis O. Gomez, *The Land of the Bliss: The Paradise of the Buddha of Measureless Light*, Motilal Banarsidass Publishers, Delhi, 1996. On other religious perspectives of India, see: Jeffrey Lidke and Jacob W. Dirnberger, "Churning the Ocean of Milk: Imaging the Hindu Tantric Response to Radical Life Technologies," in Calvin Mercer and Derek F. Maher (Eds.), *Religion and the Implications of Radical Life Extension*, Macmillan Palgrave, New York, 2009; Sherry Fohr, "Austerity, and Time-Cycles: Jainism and Radical Life Extension," in Calvin Mercer and Derek F. Maher (Eds.), *Religion and the Implications of Radical Life Extension*, Macmillan Palgrave, New York, 2009.

16. Anand Chaudhary, Neetu Singh, Neeraj Kumar, "Pharmacovigilance: Boon for the safety and efficacy of Ayuvedic formulations," *Journal*

of Ayurveda and   *Integrative*   *Medicine*, 1(4),   251-256,   2010, https://www.ncbi.nlm.nih.gov/pmc/articles/PMC3117316/.

17. For example, see the activities and advocacy for aging and longevity research by International Society on Aging and Disease, http://isoad.org/; International Longevity Alliance, http://longevityalliance.org/; Longevity for All, http://www.longevityforall.org/; SENS Research Foundation, http://www.sens.org/ and many more.

18. Further on the history of the pursuit of healthy life extension, see: Ilia Stambler, *A History of Life-Extensionism in the Twentieth Century*, Longevity History, 2014, http://www.longevityhistory.com/.

12. Longevity in the Ancient Middle East and the Islamic Tradition

The Middle East has often been perceived as a constantly belligerent area, where human life has been held cheap, since the time of despots and tribal wars well to the present. Yet, in fact, the Middle East would be more appropriately seen as a cradle of civilization, where many ideas of human development had their roots, where many technological and scientific concepts were first formulated, and where the goals of preserving and extending human life, even ideas of radically extended longevity, have been pronounced among the earliest. Hopefully, the few examples below will help to see the Middle East not chiefly as an arena of ruthless confrontation, but as it has mostly been – a fertile ground for creativity and pursuit of life.

Thus one of the earliest known works of literature is in fact also one of the earliest representations of the pursuit of life, rejuvenation and life extension, and it stems from the Middle East. This is the Sumero-Babylonian *Epic of Gilgamesh*, a story about the hero's struggle with death. (The most complete version has been dated from circa 1300 BCE to 650 BCE, but the story possibly originated as early as about 3000 BCE.) According to the *Epic of Gilgamesh*: "There is a plant like a thorn with its root [deep down in the ocean], Like unto those of the briar (in sooth) its prickles will scratch [thee], (Yet) if thy hand reach this plant, [thou'lt surely find life (everlasting)]."[1] The plant has been sometimes likened to box-thorn and dog-rose.

There are striking parallels between the description of the immortalizing plant and the story of the extremely long-lived Utnapishtim in the *Epic of Gilgamesh*, and the biblical stories (with the composition sometimes dated c. 1300 BCE to 450 BCE) about the "tree of life," the original potential physical immortality of human beings and its loss due to ill will and negligence, as well as about the extreme and admirable longevity of antediluvian patriarchs (Genesis 2:9, 3:22-24, 5:1-32).

In the *Avesta*, the sacred text of the Iranian Zoroastrian religion (with estimated dates of origin ranging from 1200 BCE to 200 BCE), during the rule of the mythical king Jamshid (Yima), people knew no disease, aging and death.[2] The legendary "cup of Jamshid" was said to be a container for the elixir of immortality and at the same time a means for information retrieval (scrying/remote viewing). According to the Persian poet Ferdowsi (940-1020, CE), as told in the epic poem *Shah Nameh*, Jamshid became proud and his reign of prosperity and longevity was terminated by the demonic king Zahhak.[3]

Also in ancient Egypt, longevity and rejuvenation were celebrated. It may even be argued that many of the pioneering technologies of ancient Egypt, from pyramid construction to embalming and surgery, emerged in the pursuit of life preservation, balance, constancy or immortality.

In one of the earliest known Egyptian medical papyruses, "The Edwin Smith Surgical Papyrus" (commonly dated to the period of the New Kingdom of Egypt, c. 1500 BCE), there is a "Recipe for Transforming an Old Man into a Youth." The recipe involved the external use of bruised and dried hemayet-fruit (with recent identifications varying from fenugreek to almond). The remedy would not only have a cosmetic anti-aging effect – remove wrinkles, beautify the skin, remove blemishes, disfigurements, and "all signs of age" – but it would also have a true rejuvenating effect, as it would remove "all weaknesses which are in the flesh."[4]

And in yet another ancient Egyptian medical papyrus, "The Ebers Papyrus" (c. 1500-1600 BCE), there are anti-aging cosmetic remedies to prevent the graying of hair (for example by the use of honey, onion water, donkey liver and crocodile fat), and to stimulate hair growth (for example by the use of flaxseed oil, gazelle excrements and snake fat). Yet, actual treatment of aging was also mentioned: "When you examine a person," the book advised, "whose heart is weak as when old age comes upon him, you say: 'This is an accumulation of diseased juices,' the person should not arrogantly dismiss the disease or trust in weak remedies."[5]

The legendary chief minister to the Egyptian pharaoh Djoser, and the reputed builder of the first step pyramid, Imhotep (c. 2650-2600 BCE), too was said to be skilled in the art of rejuvenation. Also, according to the "Turin Papyrus" and other sources, the ruling periods of Egyptian kings in the first and second dynasty (up to c. 2500 BCE) were allegedly very long (up to 100 years) and the kings' life-spans were believed to reach into hundreds.[6] The vitality and longevity were revered.

Egypt was also apparently the birthplace of alchemy, aiming at the manipulation of matter generally, and improvement of health and longevity in particular. And alchemy's growth and maturation took place broadly in the Middle East.

The world "al-kimia" is of Arabic origin, "al" being the Arabic definite article, and the etymology of "kimia" being very uncertain, with hypotheses ranging from the Greek "Khemeioa" (appearing c. 296 CE in the decree of the Roman Emperor Diocletian banning the "old writings" of Egyptian "makers" or counterfeiters of gold and silver); "Khemia" ("the land of black earth" - the old name of Egypt); or some other Greek etymology of the Hellenic Middle East: e.g. "khymatos" (pouring/infusing in Greek) or "khymos (the Greek word for juice), etc. In either case, clearly Egypt was a hotbed of this pursuit.[7]

The term "alchemy" apparently took root in Europe only in the 12th century, and was apparently borrowed from the Middle East. The first European alchemical text was translated from Arabic, presumably by Robert of Chester in 1144 and was entitled *Liber de compositione alchimiae* (The book of alchemical composition). This was allegedly a translation from Arabic into Latin of an epistle of the Egyptian-Greek-Christian alchemist Marianos to the Arab alchemical adept, the Umayyad prince Khalid ibn Yazid (665-704 CE).[8] Also the word "elixir" comes from the Arabic "al-iksir" (dry medicinal powder), as well as many other terms currently found in modern science and born in the pursuits of Islamic alchemists, such as realgar ("raj al-har"), nushadir, alcohol ("al-kuhul") and many more.

Many Islamic alchemists spoke very explicitly about the possibility of radical life extension, which according to their views did not contain any contradiction with the Koran.

Thus one of the founding figures of alchemy is considered to be the Baghdad scholar and physician Abu Mūsā Jābir ibn Hayyān (also known as Jabir in Arabic and Geber in Latin, c. 721-815) whose theory of elements profoundly influenced both the Islamic and European (Latin-Christian) alchemy. In one of his treatises Jabir stated:[9]

"If you could take a man, dissect him in such a way as to balance his natures [qualities] and then restore him to life, he would no longer be subject to death. ... This equilibrium once obtained, they will no longer be subject to change, alteration or modification and neither they nor their children ever will perish."

Also according to the alchemist Ibn-Bishrun (c. 1000 CE), quoted by the Tunisian historian Ibn Khaldoun (1332-1406): "Man suffers from the disharmony of his component elements. If his elements were in complete harmony and thus not effected by accidents and inner contradictions, the soul would not be able to leave his body."[10]

Indeed, Islam has been sometimes presented as somehow intrinsically antagonistic to the idea of life extension. Often the story about the "70 virgins" hopefully awaiting the martyrs in Heaven (a loose paraphrase on Hadith 2687) and similar ones are regurgitated, aiming to demonstrate the alleged denigration of this worldly life in Islam.

Yet, in fact, Islamic thought has not been inherently opposed to the idea of life extension or even to radical life extension! There are strong currents favoring this pursuit.

Thus, the book *Al-Imam al-Mahdi, The Just Leader of Humanity* by Ayatollah Ibrahim Amini (b. 1925, a foremost Islamic scholar, since 1999 Vice President of the Assembly of Experts of the Leadership of the Islamic Republic of Iran), includes the chapter "The Research About Longevity." In the chapter, the necessity to pursue longevity research is largely derived from the desire to explain and emulate the remarkable longevity of Al-Mahdi – مهدي – the messianic "Last Imam" who, in the belief of the Twelver Shi'a Muslims (the largest branch of Shi'a Islam) will come to protect mankind and, together with Jesus, will bring peace and justice to the world.

According to this tradition, the Last Twelfth Imam, Muhammad al-Mahdi, was born c. 869 CE (255 AH - Anno Hegirae), and has not died but lives in "occultation." Biological science is required to explain this fact and make such great longevity a gift to humanity. As the book states:[11]

"There is no such age fixed for human life the transgression of which would be impossible. .... All the above observations in the medical and biological sciences make it possible for human beings to expect to discover the secret of longevity and overcome old age one day. Moreover, it has prompted them to continue their research until the goal is reached. There is hope that scientific research into understanding the mystery of longevity will also lead to uncovering the secret of the long life of the Qa'im [al-Mahdi] from the Family of the Prophet (peace be upon him and his progeny). Let us hope that day will come soon."

These were the words of Dr. Abu Turab Nafisi, Professor and Chair of the School of Medicine, University of Isfahan, Iran, and they were cited approvingly.

Other Islamic scholars agree. Thus according to the article "The Long Life Span of Imam Mahdi (A.S.)" at the Imam Reza website (affiliated to the Ahlul Bayt – 'People of the House' – Global Center for Information), the Islamic tradition acknowledges the possibility of extended life spans, such as those of Noah, Jesus, Khidhr ("the green one"), or Dajjal. Hence, "There is no dispute amongst theists and followers of Divine Religions about the possibility of extended longevity and that there is no limitation on the human life span."

The views of great Islamic thinkers on the subject, as quoted in the article, are unambiguous:

The Persian scientist and philosopher Khwajah Nasir al Deen Tusi (1201-1274 CE) said: 'Extended life spans have occurred for other than al-Mahdi (p.b.u.h.) and been recorded, and for this very reason it is pure ignorance to consider his longevity as improbable.'

The great Tajik-Persian physician, Avicenna (Abū Alī al-Husayn ibn Abd Allāh ibn Sīnā, c. 980-1037 CE) said: 'Consider as possible whatever you hear about the strange things until you have no reason to reject it.'

And more recently, the Azerbaijan-Iranian philosopher and theologian Allamah Tabataba'i (1904-1981 CE) stated: 'There are no intellectual reasons or rules to denote the impossibility of an extended life span; therefore, we cannot deny it.'

The article continues:[12]

"As we have seen, the Holy Qur'an, the noble traditions, intellect, and history, provide proof of the possibility and the existence of extended longevity. ...

From a biological, medical or scientific point of view, the human life span does not have a specific time frame where exceeding it would be considered impossible. No scientist up to now has stated that a specified amount of years is the maximum limit of the human life span after which death would be certain. Indeed some scientists, from the east and west, old and new, have stipulated that the human life span is not limited and in fact humans can have power over their deaths by delaying it and thus extending their life spans. This scientific hypothesis encourages scientists to research and administer tests day and night in hope of success. Through these tests they have proved that death, is similar to other illnesses because it is an effect of natural causes which, if they could be discovered and altered, death can be delayed. Just as scientists have been able to discover remedies for different illnesses through research, they can do the same for death."

Thus, clearly, extended longevity is considered as theoretically possible, ethically desirable and practically and scientifically feasible by the Islamic tradition.

However, according to Aisha Y. Musa's article "A Thousand Years, Less Fifty: Toward a Quranic View of Extreme Longevity" (2009), the idea of physical immortality, of a complete defeat of death, would be incompatible with an Islamic view. According to the author: "The Qur'an declares unambiguously that 'whenever you are death will find you,' and 'every soul will taste death.' These verses have always been understood to preclude the possibility of earthly immortality."[13] Still, according to the author, by reinterpreting certain key concepts of Islam, such as Heaven ("Jannah") and Hell ("Jahannam") understood not as physical places but as states of the soul; the concept of "the first death" understood not as a transition to unearthly paradise, but as a radical spiritual change in this world (e.g. the death of old and harmful habits); and the notion of Thereafter ("akhira") understood not as an afterlife but as a new stage of evolution – then even the idea of "practical immortality" (that is to say, not actual, but potential or biological immortality) would be acceptable by Islam.

Yet, even without such far-reaching reinterpretations, the core Islamic values clearly favor the pursuit of life extension and even radical life extension. And these values are equally shared also by representatives of other religions as well as non-religious denominations of the Middle East. Thus according to the Iranian-American philosopher, one of the chief founders of the transhumanist intellectual movement, Fereidoun M. Esfandiary (pseudonym FM-2030, 1930-2000), "More than ever therefore it is urgent to overcome death. The conquest of death is the single transcendent triumph which in one sweep will defuse all other human problems."[14]

That was an extremely optimistic forecast. The conflicts in the Middle East and in the area generally known as the "Islamic World" are real. Yet the issue of protecting and extending life needs to be raised again with great force, to overcome the destructive tendencies, to leverage the tremendous economic and human potential of the area, to work toward the practical realization of the noble intellectual tradition, to achieve healthy longevity for all.[15]

References and notes

1. *The Epic of Gilgamesh*, translated by R. Campbell Thompson, 1928, Tablet 11: The Flood, lines 268-270, "The magic gift of restored youth," reprinted at Sacred Texts, http://www.sacred-texts.com/ane/eog/index.htm.
2. "Avesta: Venidad. Fargard 2. Yima (Jamshed) and the deluge," translated by James Darmesteter, from *Sacred Books of the East*, American Edition, 1898, http://www.avesta.org/vendidad/vd2sbe.htm.
3. Ferdowsi, *The Epic of Kings*, translated by Helen Zimmern, 1883, "The Shahs of Old," http://www.sacred-texts.com/neu/shahnama.txt.
4. James Henry Breasted (Translator and Editor), *The Edwin Smith Surgical Papyrus*, The University of Chicago Press, Chicago, Illinois, 1930, XXI9-XXII10, pp. 506-507.
5. H. Joachim (Translator and Editor), *Papyrus Ebers. Das Älteste Buch Über Heilkunde* (The Ebers Papyrus, The Oldest Book on Medicine), Georg Reimer, Berlin 1890, pp. 105-107, 43-44.
6. Alan H. Gardiner, *The Royal Canon of Turin*, Oxford, 1959.
For lists of mythical longevity cases, see for example, the compilation: Craig Paardekooper, *Records of Human Longevity from Other Nations*, 2001, mentioning the Turin papyrus and other sources, http://s8int.com/phile/page44.html;
http://saturniancosmology.org/files/kings/turin5.txt.
See also the Wikipedia article "Longevity Myths" http://en.wikipedia.org/wiki/Longevity_myths.
7. Douglas Harper, *Online Etymology Dictionary*, 2012, http://www.etymonline.com/index.php?search=alchemy;

Alchemy Academy Archive, June 2006, "Diocletian's Edict against alchemy," http://www.levity.com/alchemy/a-archive_jun06.html.

8. Alchemy Academy Archive, January 2002, "Maryanus," http://www.levity.com/alchemy/a-archive_jan02.html.

9. Quoted in Gerald Joseph Gruman, *A History of Ideas about the Prolongation of Life. The Evolution of Prolongevity Hypotheses to 1800, Transactions of the American Philosophical Society*, Volume 56(9), Philadelphia, 1966, "Arabic Alchemy: The Missing Link?" p. 60.

10. Quoted in Gerald Joseph Gruman, *A History of Ideas about the Prolongation of Life. The Evolution of Prolongevity Hypotheses to 1800, Transactions of the American Philosophical Society*, Volume 56(9), Philadelphia, 1966, "Arabic Alchemy: The Missing Link?" p. 60; "Alchemy in Ibn Khaldun's Muqaddimah," edited and prepared by Prof. Hamed A. Ead, Cairo University, Giza, 1998, http://www.levity.com/alchemy/islam20.html.

11. Ayatollah Ibrahim Amini, *Al-Imam al-Mahdi, The Just Leader of Humanity*, Ch. 9 "The Research About Longevity," translated by Dr. Abdulaziz Sachedina, 1996, reprinted at "Al-Islam" – The Ahlul Bayt Digital Library Project, Spring Lake Park, MN, USA – a repository of Islamic cultural resources, https://www.al-islam.org/al-imam-al-mahdi-just-leader-humanity-ayatullah-ibrahim-amini; http://www.ibrahimamini.com/en.

12. "The Long Life Span of Imam Mahdi (A.S.)" Imam Reza, 2012, http://www.imamreza.net/eng/imamreza.php?id=7127.

13. Aisha Y. Musa, "A Thousand Years, Less Fifty: Toward a Quranic View of Extreme Longevity," in Calvin Mercer and Derek F. Maher (Eds.), *Religion and the Implications of Radical Life Extension*, Macmillan Palgrave, New York, 2009, pp. 123-131.

14. Fereidoun M. Esfandiary (FM-2030), *Up-wingers. A futurist manifesto*, Popular Library, Toronto, 1977, p. 177.

15. The text of the article "Longevity in the Ancient Middle East and the Islamic Tradition" is also available in Arabic (translated by Ahmed Adel Ibrahim, a longevity research activist from Egypt)

إطالة الحياة في التراث الإسلامي و الشرق الاوسط القديم

http://www.longevityforall.org/longevity-middle-east-arabic/

And Persian (translated by Ali Yahyaei, a longevity research activist from Iran)

تاریخچه واژه "تمدید حیات" در خاورمیانه باستان و عرف اسلامی

http://www.longevityforall.org/longevity-middle-east-persian/

The initial material for this article was presented in Ilia Stambler, *A History of Life-Extensionism in the Twentieth Century*, Longevity History, 2014, http://www.longevityhistory.com/.

See also: Ilia Stambler, "The pursuit of longevity – The bringer of peace to the Middle East," *Current Aging Science*, 6, 25-31, 2014.

13. Longevity and the Jewish Tradition

In the quite famous essay of 2001, "L'Chaim ["To Life"] and Its Limits: Why Not Immortality?" the American bioethicist Leon Kass notoriously placed a limit on the possibility and desirability of life extension, claiming that "the finitude of human life is a blessing for every human individual, whether he knows it or not." He presented such a view as truly and pristinely Jewish. Speaking in the name of true wisdom and true Judaism, he claimed that "the unlimited pursuit of longevity cannot be the counsel of wisdom, and, therefore, should not be the counsel of Jewish wisdom. L'Chaim, but with limits."[1]

Yet, I would argue that this is only one of many possible interpretations of the Jewish tradition with relation to life extension, and interpretations other than Kass's may be both better grounded in Jewish sources and more beneficial for individual and social well-being.

In fact, the pursuit of life extension, and even radical life extension, has strong roots in the Jewish religious tradition, insofar as in Judaism, human life has been an absolute and supreme value.

Thus the principle "ve-chai bahem" – וחי בהם – viz. the obligation to live by the commandments and not to die by them, is strongly emphasized (Leviticus 18:5; Talmud – Masechet (Tractate) Sanhedrin 74a; Talmud – Masechet Yoma 85b).[2]

The value of human life is illustrated by the saying that "whosoever preserves a single soul [any soul, according to most manuscript versions of the Talmud], scripture ascribes merit to him as though he had preserved a complete world" (Talmud – Masechet Sanhedrin 37a).

The obligation to preserve life ("pikuach nefesh") is so important that it overrides all other obligations and observances (such as Shabbat, Fast, etc.), in fact it overrides all commandments of the Torah. As the Talmud states, "there is nothing that can stand before the duty of saving life."[3]

The only exceptional cases, in which a person is said to be obliged to sacrifice one's life, but not transgress, are: idolatry, forbidden sexual practices, and murder. Yet, in some attenuating circumstances and according to some Rabbis, even the former two prohibitions can be excused to preserve life. In contrast, murder of innocent people (for example to use their body parts to sustain one's life) is prohibited under any circumstances, as it contradicts the very principle of the preservation of life (to be distinguished from the killing of an aggressor in self defense which is permitted).

A related principle is "ein dokhin nefesh mipney nefesh" – "do not reject a soul for another soul" (Mishnah – Ohalot 7:6). That is, one cannot curtail some person's life to preserve another person's life. It can be added that an implication of this is that one cannot reject the preservation of life for the aged in favor of the preservation of life in other diseases. All causes of death are equal, and one cannot reject one for another.[4]

In the Jewish religious rules of conduct – the Halakhah – "tumah" (the unholiness, evil or impurity) means simply "the negation of life," hence the prohibition of murder and of bloodshed, and the laws of "tumah ve'taharah" (or ritual purity).[5]

Moreover, the Talmud equates between evil, Satan and death: "Satan, the evil prompter, and the Angel of Death are all one" (Talmud - Baba Bathra 16a).

According to the Talmud, "the sins will cease" but not "the sinners."[6] That is to say, human sins need to be eliminated, but not people who commit the sins; the people need to keep on living.

All these concepts are directly supportive of life-extension, insofar as life-preservation, life-saving and life-extension are logical equivalents.

Reaching farther, super-longevity, rejuvenation, and even immortality and revival, are prominent concepts in the Jewish tradition:

Mortality, the main tragedy of the Fall, was not the original and inexorable destiny of humankind (Genesis 3:17-24).

The extreme longevity of antediluvian patriarchs is admired, ranging from 365 years for Enoch to 969 years for Methuselah (Genesis 5:1-32).

According to the Talmud, "Until Abraham there was no [signs of] old age" (Talmud – Masechet Sanhedrin 107b).

In the Torah, longevity is the main prize for observing the commandments (without a direct mentioning of an afterlife – Exodus 20:12, Leviticus 26:3, Deuteronomy 5:33).

In other books of the Tanakh (Torah, Neviim, Ketuvim – Torah, Prophets and Writings – the corpus of what has been sometimes called "The Old Testament"), the prophet Elijah attained physical immortality (the ascension in the chariot of fire – 2 Kings 2:11).

Ezekiel could revive the dead (the vision of the resurrection of dry bones – Ezekiel 37:1-14; also in the Talmud – Masechet Sanhedrin 92b). The prophecy continues: "And David, my servant, will be their prince forever" (Ezekiel 37:25).[7]

King David (conventionally dated c. 1040-970 BCE) practiced rejuvenation (by proximity to young maidens – 1 Kings 1:1-4).

"Tchiat Hametim" (resurrection in the flesh) is among the Thirteen Articles of Faith of Maimonides (1135-1204) – one of the greatest Jewish intellectual authorities, a theologian as well as a physician.[8]

Furthermore, resurrection is a subject of the daily prayer (Amida): "Blessed are you, O Eternal, Who Resurrects the Dead." And it is given the same weight in the prayer as "Blessed are you, O Eternal, Who Heals the Sick."

According to many great Rabbis, such as Rabbi Saadia Gaon (882-942), Rabbi Moshe ben Nachman/Nachmanides (1194-1270) and Rabbi Abraham Bibago (1446-1489), the resurrection is to be followed by physical immortality.[9]

These examples may appear far-reaching, mystical and mythical, yet they demonstrate that in the Jewish intellectual tradition (as in many others), the pursuit of life does not seem to have any limits.

Essentially, the preservation of life is not something just to pray for, but to work for.

There is a work by Maimonides – "The Responsum on Longevity" – which is definitive of the pro-active principle for the prolongation of life. Maimonides believed that there is no predetermined limit to human life, and therefore efforts toward the prolongation of life are justified.

In the "Responsum on Longevity," Maimonides stated directly: "For us Jews, there is no predetermined end point of life. The living being exists as long as replenishment is provided [for that amount of] its substantive moisture [i.e. bodily humors] that dissolves."

In agreement with the theoretical perception that if something can be broken, it can also be fixed, Maimonides appeared to be quite pro-active:[10]

> "It is written: 'When you build a new house, you should make a parapet for your roof so that you bring not bloodshed upon your house should any man fall therefrom" [Deut. 22:8]. This phrase proves that preparing oneself, and adopting precautionary measures – in that one is careful before undertaking dangerous enterprises – can prevent their occurrence.
> ...
> This demonstrates, however, that there is no firmly determined time for death. Moreover, the elimination of harmful things is efficacious in prolonging life, whereas the undertaking of dangerous things is the basis for shortening life."

Indeed this passage does not explicitly speak of immortality, but only implies the possibility of indefinite life extension.

Elsewhere in the Jewish oral tradition, the concept of potential physical immortality is explicit. There is even foreshadowing of regenerative biotechnology. Thus, for example, there is an extensive Jewish oral tradition about the "Etzem Luz" – עצם לוז – the bone of resurrection, the indestructible part of the human body from which the resurrection will proceed.

"Luz" (almond) is a very fraught mystical concept, denoting the source of resurrection and regeneration, as well as an endocrine gland and a sprout. Jacob used "Luz" (almond) rods for "bioengineering," to change the color of his sheep (Genesis 30:37-39). "Luz" is also the name of the blessed land of the immortals.

It may be sufficient to quote a remarkable article on "Luz" from Jewish Encyclopedia to illustrate how deeply rooted is the concept of potential immortality (and even its laboratory testing) in the Talmud and Midrash (orally transmitted legends):[11]

"LUZ - Name of a city in the land of the Hittites [a territory restricted to the hills of Canaan-Israel or broadly referring to Anatolia-Asia Minor], built by an emigrant from Beth-el, who was spared and sent abroad by the Israelitish invaders because he showed them the entrance to the city (Judges i. 26). "Luz" being the Hebrew word for an almond-tree, it has been suggested that the city derived its name from such a tree or grove of trees. Winckler compares the Arabic "laudh" ("asylum"). Robinson ("Researches," iii. 389) identifies the city either with Luwaizah, near the city of Dan, or (ib.iii. 425) with Kamid al-Lauz, north of Heshbon (now Hasbiyyah); Talmudic references seem to point to its location as somewhere near the Phenician coast (Sotah 46b; Sanh. 12a; Gen. R. lxix. 7).

Legend invested the place with miraculous qualities. "Luz, the city known for its blue dye, is the city which Sennacherib entered but could not harm; Nebuchadnezzar, but could not destroy; *the city over which the angel of death has no power; outside the walls of which the aged who are tired of life are placed, where they meet death*" (Sotah 46b); wherefore it is said of Luz, "the name thereof is unto this day" (Judges i. 26, Hebr.). It is furthermore stated that an almond-tree with a hole in it stood before the entrance to a cave that was near Luz; through that hole persons entered the cave and found the way to the city, which was altogether hidden (Gen. R.l.c.)."

Luz is also "Aramaic name for the os coccyx, the "nut" of the spinal column. *The belief was that, being indestructible, it will form the nucleus for the resurrection of the body.* The Talmud narrates that the emperor Hadrian, when told by R. Joshua that the revival of the body at the resurrection will take its start with the "almond," or the "nut," of the spinal column, *had investigations made and found that water could not soften, nor fire burn, nor the pestle and mortar crush it* (Lev. R. xviii.; Eccl. R. xii.).

The legend of the "resurrection bone," connected with Ps. xxxiv. 21 (A. V. 20: "unum ex illis [ossibus] non confringetur" - [one of those bones is unbreakable]) and identified with the cauda equina [horse tailbone] (see Eisenmenger, "Entdecktes Judenthum" [Judaism discovered], ii. 931-933), *was accepted as an axiomatic truth by the Christian and Mohammedan theologians and anatomists*, and in the Middle Ages the bone received the name "Juden Knöchlein" (Jew-bone; see Hyrtl, "Das Arabische und Hebräische in der Anatomie" [The Hebrew and Arabic elements in Anatomy] 1879, pp. 165-168; comp. p. 24). Averroes accepted the legend as true (see his "Religion und Philosophie," transl. by Müller, 1875, p. 117; see also Steinschneider, "Polemische Literatur," 1877, pp. 315, 421; idem, "Hebr. Bibl." xxi. 98; idem, "Hebr. Uebers." p. 319; Löw, "Aramäische Pflanzennamen" [Aramaic plant names] 1881, p. 320).

Possibly the legend owes its origin to the Egyptian rite of burying "the spinal column of Osiris" in the holy city of Busiris, at the close of the days of mourning for Osiris, after which his resurrection was celebrated (Brugsch, "Religion und Mythologie," 1888, pp. 618, 634). Bibliography: Jastrow, Dict.; Levy, Neuhebr. Wörterb. K." (Emphasis added)

The latter statement about potential immortality being "accepted as an axiomatic truth by the Christian and Mohammedan theologians and anatomists" is of particular interest, showing the compatibility of the religions with the concept of radical life extension.[12]

In more recent times, Jewish thinkers have expressed an agreement with life-extensionist goals and with biotechnological interventions generally.

Thus, in March 2000, the International Symposium "Extended Life – Eternal Life" took place in Philadelphia.[13] The Russian journalist Michael Ettinghoff thus summarized the symposium discussion: "Christians are against immortality. Jews are for it." The Conservative American Rabbi Neil Gilman is quoted as saying at the conference that he would be ready to break Shabbat and Yom Kippur, even if they occur on the same day, for the preservation of life.[14]

According to the Conservative American Rabbi Elliot N. Dorff, radical life extension ties with Jewish expectations of the Messianic Era. At the same time Dorff did express some concerns that radical life extension will make us "even more blind to the importance of other values, such as family, enjoying life, fixing the world, and connecting with God" and it will "likely bring a variety of yet unseen problems to thwart the arrival of the Messianic era" as it will exacerbate the "overpopulation" problem. Yet, ultimately, he asserted that imaginative thinking will "prompt us to exert yet more effort in achieving the ideal world, and may we succeed!"[15]

The Society of Jewish Science (a part of Reform Judaism), established in 1916-1921 by the American Rabbis Alfred Moses and Morris Lichtenstein, believing in the power of "affirmative" prayer for healing and longevity, exists to the present time.[16]

There has also been pronounced interest in physical immortality in the literature of Chabad (a branch of Orthodox Hasidic Judaism, deriving the name from Chochmah, Binah, Daat – Wisdom, Understanding, and Knowledge).[17]

Thus, as can be seen, the Jewish religious tradition is perfectly supportive of the pursuit of life extension, even radical life extension, perceiving it as a high manifestation of the valuation of life.[18] Let the works of the Jewish tradition inspire more people to become enthusiasts (Hasidim) of the rational and scientific pursuit of the prolongation of human life, among Jews and non-Jews alike!

References and notes

1. Leon Kass, "L'Chaim and Its Limits: Why Not Immortality?" *First Things*, 113, 17-24, May 2001, https://www.firstthings.com/article/2001/05/lchaim-and-its-limits-why-not-immortality.

2. The translation of the Talmud used here is *English Babylonian Talmud*, Rabbi Dr. J. H. Hertz, Rabbi Dr. I Epstein, et al. (Eds.), Talmudic Books, 2012, http://halakhah.com/.

3. Talmud – Masechet Yoma 82a; also Talmud – Masechet Yoma 84b-85b; Talmud – Masechet Sanhedrin 74a.

4. "Pikuach Nefesh" (Saving a life), in *Encyclopedia of Jewish Medical Ethics* (Hebrew), compiled and edited by Abraham Steinberg, The Shlezinger Institute, Jerusalem, 1996, vol. 5, pp. 390-392, 404-406.

5. "Tameh met" (unholiness of death), "Tumah" (unholiness), in *Talmudic Encyclopedia. A Digest of Halachic Literature and Jewish Law from the Tannaitic Period to the Present Time* (Hebrew), edited by Rabbi Meyer Berlin, Talmudic Encyclopedia Institute, Jerusalem, 1997, vol. 19, pp. 450-507.

6. Talmud [Gemara] – Masechet Berachoth [Tractate on Blessings], 10a.

7. The text used here is *The Bible: New International Version*, https://www.bible.com/versions.

8. Rabbi Moshe ben Maimon (the Rambam), *Perush Hamishna, Masechet Sanhedrin 10 - Maimonides' Commentary on the Mishna*, Tractate [Masechet] Sanhedrin, Chapter 10;
Rabbi Israel Meir Lau, *Judaism Halacha Lemaaseh [Practical Halakhah]. The Oral Tradition* (Hebrew), Dfus Pele, Givataim, Israel, 1988, pp. 370-371.

9. Dov Schwartz, *Messianism in Medieval Jewish Thought* (Hebrew), Bar-Ilan University Press, Ramat-Gan, Israel, 1997, pp. 36, 105, 142-143, 218-219.

10. Fred Rosner, "Moses Maimonides' Responsum on Longevity," *Geriatrics*, 23, 170-178, October 1968, reprinted in Fred Rosner, *The Medical Legacy of Moses Maimonides*, Ktav, Hoboken NJ, 1998, pp. 246-258, quotes on pp. 255, 258.

11. Kaufmann Kohler, "Luz," *Jewish Encyclopedia*, in 12 volumes, 1901-1906, online   reprint, http://www.jewishencyclopedia.com/view.jsp?artid=635&letter=L.

12. See also: Fred Rosner, *Medicine in the Bible and the Talmud*, Ktav, Hoboken NJ, 1995 (1977), particularly the articles "The Balm of Gilead" and "Therapeutic Efficacy of Chicken Soup," pp. 132-139; James Joseph Walsh, *Old-Time Makers of Medicine. The Story of The Students And Teachers of the Sciences Related to Medicine During the Middle Ages*, Fordham University Press, NY, 1911, Ch. III "Great Jewish Physicians," Ch. IV "Maimonides," pp. 61-108, http://www.gutenberg.org/files/20216/20216-h/20216-h.htm.

13. The International Symposium "Extended Life – Eternal Life," Philadelphia, March 2000, www.extended-eternallife.org.

14. *Argumeny I Fakty* (Arguments and Facts), 41/322, 2000, http://gazeta.aif.ru/online/health/322/z41_13.

15. Rabbi Elliot N. Dorff, "Becoming Yet More Like God: A Jewish Perspective on Radical Life Extension," in *Religion and the Implications of Radical Life Extension*, Edited by Calvin Mercer and Derek F. Maher, Macmillan Palgrave, New York, 2009, pp. 63-74.

16. Society of Jewish Science, http://www.appliedjudaism.org/; Rabbi Morris Lichtenstein – Founder Society of Jewish Science, http://www.irenedanon.com/Rabbi.htm.

17. See, for example: Prof. Yirmiyahu Branover, "The Immortality Enzyme," *Chabad World Magazine*, 10/22/2009, http://www.chabadworld.net/; Rabbi Nissan Dovid Dubov, *To Live And Live Again. An Overview of Techiyas Hameisim Based On The Classical Sources And On The Teachings Of Chabad Chassidism*, 1995 [5756], Ch. 10, "Life after the Resurrection," http://www.chabad.org/library/moshiach/article_cdo/aid/2312363/jewish/To-Live-and-Live-Again.htm.

18. Ilia Stambler, *A History of Life-Extensionism in the Twentieth Century*, Longevity History, 2014, http://www.longevityhistory.com/.

14. Longevity and the Christian Tradition

It has been a common conviction among atheist life-extensionists that religion generally, and particular branches of Christianity, are somehow intrinsically averse to far-reaching biomedical interventions or even to the idea of human life extension, placing a greater emphasis on faith-healing and life in the world to come. For example, Alan Harrington's *The Immortalist* (1969) exemplifies the attitude perceiving religion as inherently harmful to life extension: "Religious orthodoxy was invented to give everyone a chance to earn life everlasting. ... The false gods to whom the immortality-hunter formerly bowed will be reduced to artifacts. ... Our mission will be simply, first, to attack death and all of its natural causes, and, second, to prepare for immortality.... Death is an imposition on the human race, and no longer acceptable." In the chapter "Satan, Our Standard-Bearer," Harrington elaborated: "We created the Devil to express our most radical and dangerous intent. Through history he has been the host, the standard-bearer of man's aspiration to become immortal and divine."[1] For the atheist immortalist (or proponent of radical life extension), the unlimited prolongation of life (that is, life extension that is not constrained by any particular, arbitrary or ordained date) is logically equivalent to the pursuit of physical immortality, hence religion is inimical to both.

But is religion generally, or Christianity in particular, inherently an enemy of life prolongation? It is not! There are strong undercurrents supporting the pursuit of life extension, even of radical life extension, in religious traditions of India,[2] in Islam,[3] in Judaism.[4] There are such undercurrents in Christianity as well. They go to the very source of Christian teachings – the Gospel – which abounds with examples of healing, regeneration and resuscitation. Consider, for example, Jesus healing a paralyzed man at the pool of Bethesda (Beth-Hesda or Beth-Zatha – the house of mercy) in Jerusalem (John 5:1-15) and the healing of the blind at the pool of Siloam (Brechat Hashiloach – 'the sending pool' – in Jerusalem, receiving water from the Gihon Spring, John 9:1-12). These are among some 20 miraculous cures mentioned in the Gospels, such as the cures of leprosy, dropsy, palsy, bleeding, dumbness, possession, etc. Consider also Jesus reviving the dead: Jairus' daughter (Matthew 9:18-26, Mark 5:21-43, Luke 8:40-56), Widow's son at Nain (Luke 7:11-17) and Lazarus (John 11:1-44). What are these but expressions of the obligation to heal, resuscitate and prolong life? The obligation is made explicit in Jesus' commandment "Heal the sick, raise the dead, cleanse lepers, cast out demons. You received without paying; give without pay" (Matthew 10:8).[5] Not only diseases are to be battled, but "The last enemy to be conquered is death" (1 Corinthians 15:26). One may argue that these cures are "miraculous" and "spiritual" rather than "scientific" and "material." But the actual underlying process of healing is not detailed, only the outcomes of physical regeneration and resuscitation are posited as possible and as unequivocally desirable.

Indeed, there is a strong tradition in Christianity describing "miraculous" and "spiritual" cures, such as produced by the power of prayer and the laying on of hands: those produced by Christ, early saints (St. Paul, St. Jude, St. Cosmas and Damian, St. Anthony, St. Ambrose, St. Simon, etc. etc.), by the Church fathers, and by modern Christian devotees canonized for their "miracles."[6] Consider also the examples of alleged super-longevity of venerated Christian saints, such as Saint Servatius (Tongeren, current Belgium, 9-384 AD, 375 years), Saint Shenouda (Egypt, 348-466, 118 years), Saint Llywarch Hen (Wales, 350-500, 150 years), Saint Kevin of Glendalough (Ireland, 498-618, 120 years), Scolastica Oliveri (Bivona, Italy, 1448-1578, 130 years), Theodosius of Caucasus (a Pravoslav Saint, Stavropol, 1841-1948, 107 years) and others.[7] One may wonder whether the stories of "miraculous" and "spiritual" healing and life extension (by definition out of the realm of science and natural world order) do not undermine the scientific pursuit of healing and life prolongation, while relying on "miracles," perhaps "wishful thinking."

An answer may be manifold. First of all, regardless the method, the outcome of physical healing and life prolongation in this world, is clearly posited as desirable, giving the primary motivation even to seek the healing and life prolongation, and negating the impression that Christianity does not value "this worldly" existence. For example, one of the Church fathers, St. Augustine (354-420AD) was a strong believer in "miraculous cures." In the *City of God*, St. Augustine speaks of "miracles which were wrought that the world might believe in Christ, and which have not ceased since the world believed," providing detailed testimonial accounts of miraculous cures of blindness, fistulae, cancer, gout, etc. Yet, essentially, Saint Augustine postulates that healing and longevity, even resurrection and immortality, take place in this world of "substance," not in the world of "spirit" beyond. "In the Resurrection," he writes, "the substance of our bodies, however disintegrated, shall be entirely reunited," "the flesh shall then be spiritual, and subject to the spirit, but still flesh, not spirit." Such a body, combining the carnal and the spiritual, will be forever preserved as at 30 years of age, "the age of the fullness of Christ." The body will undergo a thorough reconstruction to attain ideal proportions, whereby "all bodily blemishes which mar human beauty in this life shall be removed in the Resurrection, the natural substance of the body remaining, but the quality and quantity of it being altered so as to produce beauty." Thus the ideal of physical body preservation is clearly articulated.[8]

Secondly, the so-called "spiritual" healing may be eventually attributed to psychosomatic effects, potentially within the realm of empirical science.

The "spiritual" influence for health and longevity has been a well established tenet in the Christian tradition. This approach goes back to *Summa Theologica* (1265-1274) by Thomas Aquinas (1225-1274) who saw the impurity of the soul as the major cause of mortality. Thomas Aquinas argued that "in the state of innocence man would have been immortal" (*Summa Theologica*, 1, Question 97, Article 1) and "Death and other bodily defects are the result of sin" (2:1, Question 85, Articles 5-6). The soul's weakness caused the Fall and brought about physical death, hence the soul's purification and strengthening can reverse the effect and bring forth immortality of the body. In such an ideal state of the soul, a level of a prophet can be achieved, allowing an insight into the spiritual world while in the physical body ("The manner in which prophetic knowledge is conveyed," 2:2, Question 173). One of Thomas Aquinas' spiritual suggestions for life extension is honoring one's parents: "Now we owe the favor of bodily life to our parents after God: wherefore he that honors his parents deserves the prolongation of his life, because he is grateful for that favor" (2:2 Question 122, Article 5).[9]

And thirdly, while positing the goals of healing and life prolongation as worthy of pursuit, the proposed methods of their achievement were far from being exclusively "spiritual," but very often quite practical, material and scientific. The history of Christianity abounds with examples of support for practical medicine generally, and for advanced medical science in particular. According to the Christian legend, the 3rd century physicians and saints, brothers Cosmas and Damian, living in Asia Minor and martyred c. 287-303 CE, were able to transplant legs. This operation was depicted in many paintings, most famously in the 15th-16th century works by Fra Angelico, Jaume Huguet, Meister des Stettener, and others. The evidential basis of this story is unclear, yet the aspiration to material medical intervention is manifest.[10] Starting from circa the 4th century AD especially (with the adoption of Christianity as the official religion of the Roman Empire), an array of hospitals and medical facilities were established by Christian devotees, both in the Byzantium (e.g. by St. Basil in Caesarea) and in the Latin West (e.g. by Saint Fabiola in Rome).[11]

In a later period, the Christian support for medicine and medical science continued. The American physician and writer James Joseph Walsh, in *Old-Time Makers of Medicine* and other works, makes a thorough case for the support of medical science by the Catholic Church and by the Papal Office during the Middle Ages, including such examples as the patronage by Abbot Desiderius (Pope Victor III, 1026-1087), the work of Pope John XXI the physician (1215-1277), the medical research of Cardinal Nicolas Cusanus (1401-1464), the studies of the Jesuit priest Athanasius Kircher (1602-1680) and great many other clerics and medical scholars.[12] Perhaps the most extreme case of 'interest in medicine' was that of Pope

Innocent VIII (1432-1492) who was said to drink the blood of boys for rejuvenation, as related by Stefano Infessura (1435-1500).[13]

Closer to our time, Pope Pius XII (Eugenio Marìa Giuseppe Giovanni Pacelli, 1876-1958), received "rejuvenative" cell therapy developed by the Swiss physician Paul Niehans (1882-1971), which in fact greatly enhanced the prestige of this kind of therapy. (Most commonly, Neihans's cell therapy involved fresh cell preparations from young sheep or sheep fetuses, though the exact kind of cells that was used in this particular case is not clear.) Pius XII was first administered cell therapy by Niehans in 1954, and since then resorted to Niehans's services on several occasions. In 1955, Pius XII made Niehans a fellow of the Pontifical Academy, in place of the late Alexander Fleming (1881-1955), the discoverer of penicillin. The Pope was also reported to try other rejuvenating therapies, such as royal jelly (or "bee's milk") and dishes from chick embryos.[14] The Pope's case demonstrates the accepting attitude for rejuvenating and life-extending means, even the most experimental ones, by the religious. Niehans himself, in his youth, went to a Protestant divinity school and received a doctorate in theology; though in his later life he was not particularly observant.

In more recent times, the encyclicals of Pope John Paul II (Karol Józef Wojtyła, 1920-2005) called to "reaffirm the culture of life." In the 1995 encyclical, *Evangelium Vitae*, John Paul II issued the dictum to use all modern biomedical means to prevent death, that "life may be always defended and promoted" (1995).[15] And his own struggle with death to the last days provides a testimony to following this principle (despite some journalistic allegations to the contrary).[16] Indeed, a study showed that religious people tend to be more likely to refuse a "do-not-resuscitate" status than non-religious.[17] The Pope Benedict XVI (Joseph Aloisius Ratzinger, b. 1927) addressed radical life extension, the possibility that "Sooner or later it should be possible to find the remedy not only for this or that illness, but for our ultimate destiny – for death itself" with unprecedented earnestness, with mixed sympathy and concern (2010).[18]

On April 28-30, 2016, the Vatican held a high level conference promoting regenerative medicine entitled: "Cellular Horizons: How Science, Technology, Information and Communication will Impact Society." It acknowledged "the paradigm shift toward regenerative medicine, with a particular focus on cellular therapies." Some of the conference's main goals were "to help identify a pathway to bring cellular cures to those in medical need throughout the world to reduce human suffering" including the effort to "catalyze the necessary funding to support the development of cell therapies that will cure and treat a broad range of debilitating diseases and medical conditions." The conference included a special panel discussion on "healthy aging" featuring leading contemporary researchers of aging and life extension, such Dr. Nir Barzilai (a researcher of genetics of longevity and the author of the TAME study – "Targeting Aging with Metformin" from the Albert Einstein College of Medicine in New York), Dr. Ronald DePinho (one of the pioneers of telomerase therapy against degenerative aging, from the University of Texas), Dr. Robert Hariri (Co-Founder and President of Human Longevity Cellular Therapeutics); and Dr. Pranela Rameshwar (Professor in the Department of Medicine, Hematology – Oncology at Rutgers, New Jersey Medical School). Thus the support for longevity research and regenerative medicine was explicitly embraced by the Vatican as a part of the Catholic Church's agenda to advance global healthcare and medical science.[19] In his address to the conference, Pope Francis (Jorge Mario Bergoglio, b. 1936) expressed his unequivocal support for this agenda, focusing on three goals: "increasing sensitivity" or "greater empathy in society," not remaining "indifferent to our neighbour's cry for help"; "research, seen in two inseparable actions: education and genuine scientific study" which "safeguards human life and the dignity of the person"; and "ensuring access to care," opposing "an economy of exclusion and inequality" that "victimizes people when the mechanism of profit prevails over the value of human life."[20] Thus, as of 2016, the Catholic Church posited some of the world's most progressive objectives for universal health care and rapid advancement of medical science.

Not only in the Catholic Church, but also in other Christian denominations, the undercurrents supportive of medical progress and life extension are strong. Thus, one of Russia's greatest life-extensionist visionaries was Nikolay Fedorovich Fedorov (1829-1903) – a Russian Pravoslav religious philosopher, the founder of "Russian Cosmism," respected and recognized as an influence by Lev Tolstoy, Fyodor Dostoevsky, Konstantin Tsiolkovsky (the visionary of space exploration), Vladimir Vernadsky (the author of the concept of the "noosphere"), Alexander Chizhevsky (a pioneer of electrophysiology), among many great Russian thinkers.[21] According to Fedorov's *Philosophy of the Common Task* (most of his works appeared posthumously in 1906 and 1913 under this title), the Christian doctrine of salvation dictated a practical program toward individual and social immortality, even resurrection of past generations, which, he believed, would be achieved by collective, scientific effort.[22] In setting these goals, Fedorov presented himself as a devoted Russian orthodox Christian, envisioning that "Pravoslav Christianity, that will sanctify this union, will become the common religion."[23] In present day Russia, Pravoslav Christianity, with its hope of universal salvation, has resurfaced as one of the ideological foundations for Russian life-extensionism, going back to Fedorov's original propositions, as for example expressed by the "Fedorov movement" mainly centered in Moscow.[24]

(Though of course, this is not the only ideology associated with life-extensionism in Russia.)

Also in contemporary US, several Christian groups have expressed strong life-extensionist sentiments. Some Christian groups have embraced the vision of emerging radical life-extending technologies with all their heart, such as the Christian Transhumanist Association.[25] The Mormon Transhumanist Association has been devoted to life extension and life enhancement, promoting "active faith in human exaltation through charitable use of science and technology."[26] There has been strong support from representatives of the Mormon community for life-extensionist endeavors, for example for Human Longevity Inc.[27] Strong activism for radical life extension has emerged from within the Unitarian Universalist Church.[28] And there has also been strong support for research of life extension from representatives of the Jehovah's Witnesses Church, for example for the Methuselah Foundation.[29] Further arguments in support of radical life extension have been produced from the reformed protestant, progressive protestant as well as catholic perspectives.[30]

Of course, these are just a few examples of Christian individual and communal support for life extension, even radical life extension. Many more such examples can be quoted. But of course, also many examples can be quoted of opposition by some Christians or Christian groups to the idea of physical immortality, or radical life extension, or to some particular forms of medical research, treatment or intervention. A thorough review of such cases would go beyond the scope of this article. The main purpose of this article is to argue that ideas of Christianity are very well compatible with the goals of progress of biomedical science and significant human life extension. Arguably other religions are compatible with these goals as well. Atheism and agnosticism are also compatible with these goals, even though one can still quote quite a few examples of atheist opposition to life extension and to "meddling" with human nature.[31] If there is a common ground that could unify the aspirations of the whole of humanity, regardless of their ideological, ethnic and religious backgrounds, it is the value of human life, and the derivative goal of human healthy life extension, for oneself, for the loved ones, eventually for all. Despite the many often conflicting undercurrents in every religious and ideological tradition, for and against this goal, hopefully those undercurrents that are supportive of this goal will take precedence in the public mind.

References and notes

1. Alan Harrington, *The Immortalist*, Celestial Arts, Millbrae, California, 1977, first published in 1969, pp. 3, 67, 92, 273.

2. Ilia Stambler, "Longevity and the Indian Tradition," Institute for Ethics and Emerging Technologies (IEET), March 16, 2016, https://ieet.org/index.php/IEET2/more/stambler20160316; first published June 13, 2013, http://indiafuturesociety.org/longevity-and-the-indian-tradition/; http://www.longevityhistory.com/articles/indian.php.

3. Ilia Stambler, "Longevity in the Ancient Middle East and the Islamic Tradition," IEET, January 13, 2015, http://ieet.org/index.php/IEET/more/stambler20150113.

4. Ilia Stambler, "Longevity and the Jewish Tradition," IEET, October 21, 2015, http://ieet.org/index.php/IEET/more/stambler20151021.

5. *The Bible. English Standard Version*, http://biblehub.com/matthew/10-8.htm.

6. "How Lourdes Cures Are Recognized as Miraculous," *ZENIT Daily Dispatch*, February 11, 2004, http://www.ewtn.com/library/MARY/ZLURDCUR.HTM; Pierre Merle, "Guérisons rationnellement inexplicables" (Rationally inexplicable cures), in *Médecine Officielle et Médecines Hérétiques* (Official Medicine and Heretical Medicines), Plon, Paris, 1945, pp. 255-291.

7. "Longevity Myths" http://en.wikipedia.org/wiki/Longevity_myths.

8. St. Augustine, *City of God*, translated by Marcus Dods, T&T Clark, Edinburgh, 1886, Book XXII, Chapters 8, 18-21, reprinted in Christian Classics Ethereal Library, http://www.ccel.org/ccel/schaff/npnf102.iv.XXII.html.

9. Thomas Aquinas, *Summa Theologica, Second and Revised Edition, Literally translated by Fathers of the English Dominican Province*, 1920, reprinted by The New Advent, http://www.newadvent.org/summa/1097.htm.

Consider, in particular, the Christian idea of the "seven deadly sins" or "capital vices" authorized by Pope Gregory I (c. 540-604) in 590, and also discussed in the *Summa Theologica* – pride, greed, lust, envy, gluttony, anger, and sloth. The avoidance of such sins corresponds to the spiritual pursuit of longevity, as the life-styles those sins produce may be life-shortening (bringing death). In contrast, following the corresponding "seven heavenly virtues" or "goods" – humility, liberality, chastity, kindness, abstinence, patience, diligence – can be life-prolonging. The vices (e.g. pride, gluttony, lust, greed) are seen by Thomas Aquinas as goods in excess (honor, appetite, sexual intercourse, riches).

("Summa Theologica: The cause of sin, in respect of one sin being the cause of another," Prima Secundae Partis, Q. 84, Article 4. "Whether the seven capital vices are suitably reckoned?" http://www.newadvent.org/summa/2084.htm#article4.)

10. Harry Hayes, *An Anthology of Plastic Surgery*, Aspen Publishers, NY, 1986, pp. 40-41.

11. Roy Porter, *The Greatest Benefit to Mankind: A Medical History of Humanity*, W.W. Norton & Company, NY, 1998, Ch. 4, "Medicine and Faith," pp. 87-88.

12. James Joseph Walsh, *Old-Time Makers of Medicine. The Story of The Students And Teachers of the Sciences Related to Medicine During the Middle Ages*, Fordham University Press, NY, 1911, https://archive.org/details/oldtimemakersme01walsgoog;

James Joseph Walsh, *The Popes and Science*, Fordham University Press, NY, 1908;

James Joseph Walsh, *Priests and Long Life*, J. F. Wagner, New York, 1927.

13. Mirko D. Grmek, *On Ageing and Old Age, Basic Problems and Historic Aspects of Gerontology and Geriatrics, Monographiae Biologicae*, 5, 2, Den Haag, 1958, pp. 45-46;

Stefano Infessura, *Diario della Città di Roma* (Diary of the City of Rome), Forzani, Roma, 1890, pp. 275-276.

14. Patrick M. McGrady, *The Youth Doctors*, Coward-McCann, NY, 1968, pp. 59-122.

15. Ioannes Paulus PP. II, *Evangelium Vitae, On the Value and Inviolability of Human Life*, March 25, 1995, http://www.vatican.va/holy_father/john_paul_ii/encyclicals/documents/hf_jp-ii_enc_25031995_evangelium-vitae_en.html.

16. Jeff Israely, "Was John Paul II euthanized?" *Time*, September 21, 2007, http://content.time.com/time/world/article/0,8599,1664189,00.html.

17. Maria A. Sullivan, Philip R. Muskin, Shara J. Feldman, Elizabeth Haase, "Effects of Religiosity on Patients' Perceptions of Do-Not-Resuscitate Status," *Psychosomatics*, 45, 119-128, April 2004.

18. *Easter Vigil, Homily of His Holiness Benedict XVI, Saint Peter's Basilica, Holy Saturday, 3 April 2010*, http://www.vatican.va/holy_father/benedict_xvi/homilies/2010/documents/hf_ben-xvi_hom_20100403_veglia-pasquale_en.html.

19. "The Vatican Hosts Third International Regenerative Medicine Conference Created by The Vatican's Pontifical Council for Culture and The Stem For Life Foundation, 3-day Event to Raise Global Awareness of the Promise of Cellular Therapies to Treat Disease and Reduce Global Suffering" http://celltherapyconference2016.com/wp-content/uploads/2016/05/5.6.15-THE-VATICAN-HOSTS-THIRD-INTERNATIONAL-REGENERATIVE-MEDICINE-CONFERENCE_new-version.pdf.

20. Pope's Address to Regenerative Medicine Conference "The globalization of indifference must be countered by the globalization of empathy," *ZENIT*, April 29, 2016, https://zenit.org/articles/popes-address-to-regenerative-medicine-conference/.

21. Nikolay Bedyaev, "Religia Voskreshenia. Philosophia Obshego Dela N. Fedorova" (The Religion of Resuscitative Resurrection. "The Philosophy of the Common Task" of N. Fedorov), *Russkaya Mysl*, 7, 1915, pp. 76-120; English translation by Fr. S. Janos, 2002, http://www.berdyaev.com/berdiaev/berd_lib/1915_186.html.

22. Fedorov N.F., *Sobranie Sochineniy v Chetyrekh Tomakh* (N.F. Fedorov. Collected works in four volumes), Progress, Moscow, 1995; Fedorov N.F., *What Was Man Created For? The Philosophy of the Common Task: Selected Works*, Koutiassov E. and Minto M. (Eds.), Lausanne, Switzerland, Honeyglen, 1990.

23. Fedorov N.F., *Sobranie Sochineniy v Chetyrekh Tomakh* (N.F. Fedorov. Collected works in four volumes), Progress, Moscow, 1995, vol. 3, "Vopros o Zaglavii" (Question of the title), p. 74.

24. Boris Georgievich Rezhabek (interview), "Nanoroboty, Nanobacterii i Bessmertie" (Nanorobots, Nanobacteria and Immortality), *Vzgliad Zdorovie* (Health View, April 19, 2010, http://health.vz.ru/columns/2010/4/19/521.html); Muzey-Biblioteka Nikolaya Fedorovicha Fedorova (N.F. Fedorov's Museum-Library, Moscow, http://www.nffedorov.ru/mbnff/index.html).

25. Micah Redding, "Why Christians Should Support Radical Life Extension," *Huffington Post*, February 09, 2016, http://www.huffingtonpost.com/micah-redding/why-christians-should-sup_1_b_9190470.html; James McLean Ledford, "Prepare for HyperEvolution with Christian Transhumanism," December 19, 2005, http://www.hyper-evolution.com/.

26. The Mormon Transhumanist Association, http://transfigurism.org/; Lincoln Cannon, "Mormons on Life Extension Therapy: Desecration or Glorification," August 15, 2013, http://lincoln.metacannon.net/2013/08/mormons-on-life-extension-therapy.html.

27. Marc Gunther, "We have this remarkable ability to create any kind of world we can imagine," *The Guardian*, October 15, 2015, https://www.theguardian.com/sustainable-business/2015/oct/15/bryan-johnson-os-fund-synthetic-genomics-matternet-vicarious.

28. Shannon Vyff, Member of Education Board, Lifeboat Foundation, http://lifeboat.com/ex/bios.shannon.vyff.

29. David Gobel, Co-Founder and CEO, Methuselah Foundation, http://diyhpl.us/~bryan/irc/extropians/www.lucifer.com/exi-lists/extropians.1Q99/1008.html; http://www.mfoundation.org/?pn=mj_about_who.

30. Nigel M. de S. Cameron, Amy Michelle DeBaets, "Be Careful What you Wish For? Radical Life Extension *coram Deo*: A Reformed Protestant Perspective," pp. 39-50; Ronald Cole-Turner, "Extreme Longevity

Research: A Progressive Protestant Perspective," pp. 51-61; Terence L. Nichols, "Radical Life Extension: Implications for Roman Catholicism," pp. 133-144 – in Calvin Mercer and Derek F. Maher (Eds.), *Religion and the Implications of Radical Life Extension*, Macmillan Palgrave, New York, 2009.

31. Ilia Stambler, *A History of Life-Extensionism in the Twentieth Century*, Longevity History, 2014, http://www.longevityhistory.com/.

15. Aristotle on Life and Long Life

The concept of life

The tremendous influence of Aristotle (384-322 BCE) on the development of western philosophy and science is undisputable. Volumes have been written on his philosophical, epistemological, esthetic, cognitive and ethical theories. Yet, in fact, Aristotle's corpus of treatises mainly concerns zoology and physiology, including: *History of Animals; Parts of Animals; Movement of Animals; Progression of Animals; Generation of Animals; On Plants; On the Soul; On Generation and Corruption; On Breath; Physiognomics;* and the various treatises of *Parva Naturalia* ("the short treatises on nature"), including *On Sense and Sensible Objects; On Memory and Recollection; On Sleep and Waking; On Dreams; On Prophecy in Sleep; On Length and Shortness of Life; On Youth and Old Age, Life and Death, and Respiration,* etc. However, it is the biological works of Aristotle that are less researched by modern scholars, and their relation to modern findings is underappreciated.[1] As the American philosopher Marjorie Grene stated, "biology, like all modern science, really is, and must be, un-Aristotelian."[2] The reason for this relative under-appreciation of Aristotle's physiology might be that Aristotle's esthetics and epistemology may have been perceived to be of a more perennial nature, relevant to the present time; whereas his physiological observations and theories came to be considered as largely erroneous and irrelevant to modern biomedical research, and therefore dismissed as undeserving of study. Thus, for example, one of the foremost British Aristotle's scholars and translators Walter Stanley Hett recurrently spoke of Aristotle's "errors" and deviations from "truth," and made an apology for him, basically saying that if Aristotle had better data he could have done better, but even as it is his theory is pretty impressive and consistent.[3] This commentary was published in 1941, and it might be interesting to trace how many physiological theories from the early 1940s are currently cited in the biomedical literature. And yet, it might be reasonable to assume that there might indeed be a succession from Aristotle to the present time, with respect to physiological research, as Aristotle's corpus was a major part of European university curricula through the Renaissance,[4] and remained on the curriculum well into our time, even though its repute and authority as a valid source of biological knowledge diminished drastically. Therefore, it might be of interest not just to study where Aristotle was "wrong," but where he might have been "right," or to put it in more correct terms: in what respects the succession of Aristotle's physiological theories can be traced through time, or where Aristotle's formidable power of common sense might coalesce with the sensibilia of later generations of researchers.

In Aristotle's physiological corpus, the main issue concerns, no more no less, the essence of life and death. In *De Anima* ("On the Soul"), an equation is made between the soul and life. In other words, when speaking of the soul, Aristotle in fact speaks of the "vital principle" or the distinct characteristics of living beings in contrast to inanimate matter.[5] Aristotle provides definitive answers to the questions 'What is life?' and 'how it can be maintained' as well as 'what constitutes death' and 'whether it can be avoided.' The most basic component of vitality (i.e. the soul) is the "nutritive soul," which is responsible for or characteristic of the organism's physical maintenance and growth, or what we may now call 'basic physiology.'[6] This faculty is common to all living beings and distinguishes them from inanimate things. Animals differ from plants by having a perceptive faculty, and man differs from animals by having an intellectual faculty, but all share this basic vital principle. While *De Anima* provides a rather brief definition of the nutritive faculty (most of the treatise deals with the perceptive and cognitive functions), *Parva Naturalia* examines in detail the physiological processes responsible for maintaining life or causing death. Despite their generality, the operation of these processes in human beings is given a predominant consideration. Within the *Parva Naturalia*, several short treatises provide a most concise, yet comprehensive account of human physiology: "On length and shortness of life," "On youth and old age, life and death, and respiration" and "On sleep." As the titles suggest, these works have a special relevance to the issue of life maintenance and life extension. In this paper, I would like to focus on a possible relation of these works to subsequent biomedical research, though other physiological treatises, such as *On the Soul* and *On the Generation of Animals* will be also considered.

Regarding the essence and the basic operative principles of life, of special interest is Aristotle's controversy with previous philosophers: Pythagoras of Samos (c. 569-475 BCE), Alcmeon of Crotona (a Pythagorean, who was active about 510-480 BCE), Anaxagoras of Clazomenae (c. 500-428 BCE), Empedocles of Acragas (c. 494-434 BCE), Democritus of Abdera (c. 460-370 BCE), Plato of Athens (427-347 BCE), and others. Aristotle's dispute with these philosophers, as presented in Aristotle's own works, is fundamental and may represent an early, perhaps even a ground-laying, instance of the age-old controversy between "mechanism" and "vitalism," the controversy that reverberated into modernity.[7] The first part of *On the Soul* summarizes previous conceptions of life and Aristotle's objections to them. According to Aristotle, most former philosophers agree in that the Soul is composed of elements (particles) that have a mechanical motion of their own, i.e. the "Soul moves itself."[8] In other words, the mutual arrangement of elements and their mechanical motion is what constitutes life. Thus, according to Aristotle,

Democritus believed that the particles composing the soul (the "smallest" "round" "fiery" elements of "the least corporeal" nature)[9] have an intrinsic motility (now we would call it a kinetic particle motion), and the unison and force of this motion is what creates life. Empedocles, on the other hand, placed a greater emphasis on the mutual arrangement, the "ratio" or "harmony" of the elements comprising a living body (or the soul).[10] According to Empedocles, Pythagoras and his "students," and other "traditional theories,"[11] the special harmonious organization (which can be expressed by numerical ratios) is what distinguishes the living matter. According to them, these ratios are controlled by forces of attraction/repulsion between the elements.[12] Empedocles called the unifying force *eros* / *philia* or "love." It is exactly the same term, in exactly the same sense, that Freud used in describing the synthesis of matter into a living being (*Beyond the Pleasure principle*, 1920).[13] Modern natural sciences (biology, chemistry and physics) usually employ the terms synthesis, anabolism and synergy (Schrödinger, *What is Life*, 1944).[14] But the meaning of these terms is similar to the ancient concept of the harmonious arrangement of elements by the natural forces of attraction and repulsion. Thus the 'pre-Aristotelian' philosophers may have laid the grounds for the 'atomistic-mechanistic' theory of life, with a special emphasis on the spatial kinetic motion and mutual arrangement of elements.

It is interesting to note that the "atomistic-mechanistic" concept of the soul may have been relevant not only to future scientific theories, but also to "near-scientific" or "meta-scientific" doctrines. Specifically, the idea that the Soul may be composed of a matter of its own, having a motion of its own, reverberated in subsequent "spiritualist" teachings, professing the separate existence and spatial migration of the soul (or "astral body"), and even in the attempts "to weigh" the soul exiting the dying body.[15]

Aristotle smashes these theories to pieces by ruthless logic. He counters the supposition of earlier philosophers that the soul must be composed of elements in order to be able to perceive the surrounding environment composed of the same elements (i.e. the soul must have a material affinity to the sensible objects). One of his counterarguments is that, from the principle of material affinity, it follows that "there will be nothing in the soul to recognize bone, for instance, or man, unless they too exist in it." "This is impossible" – Aristotle argues – "For who could seriously ask whether there is a stone or a man in the soul?"[16] In contrast, Aristotle accounts for sensation by the identity of the percipient sense and sensible object's activity, and not by the identity of their material composition: "The activity of the sensible object and of the sensation is one and the same, though their essence is not the same."[17] He also employs the principle of contradiction in order to counter the mechanistic theory. That is, according to Aristotle, a corporeal soul cannot be in a corporeal body, because then two bodies would occupy the same space.[18] More fundamentally, Aristotle undermines the mechanical composition theory of life by saying that the harmony or proportion of elements (that we may now refer to as a "pattern") cannot account for the movement or change inherent in all living beings.[19] Hence, in Aristotle's account of life, mechanics and material composition are of less importance than the functional state and activity of the living being. In other words, in Aristotle's view, life is a unity, which cannot be reduced to a combination of material components, but it is rather due to a special force of activity inherent in a living body.[20]

This definition of life is very close to the vitalist definition, to the idea of a special "life-force" or "spiritum vitae" permeating and animating all living bodies. The vitalist tradition dominated Western scholarship until late Renaissance,[21] as it was compatible with the spiritual doctrines of the Church. It might be, at least partly, because of this affinity to the prevailing vitalism that Aristotle's physiological teachings survived so long as a part of the European university curricula. It might be also this affiliation with vitalism that finally contributed to the demise of Aristotle's authority, when mechanistic and atomistic worldviews resurfaced in the works of Rene Descartes (1596-1650), Pierre Gassendi (1592-1655), Robert Boyle (1627-1692) and other "mechanists."[22]

In describing the properties of life, Aristotle uses a distinct set of terms which are in many respects synonymous. Life is associated with the soul, as the soul is the "source of movement [the generative cause], it is the end [the teleological cause], it is the essence [ontological nature] of the whole living body."[23] Life is also associated with the form (*eidos*) to distinguish it from the formless matter (*hyle*). Life is a state of actualization or activation of matter, or the transition from a state of potentiality (*dynamis*) to a state of actuality (*entelechia* or *energia*).[24] The latter two terms for the activated/animated state of matter are of special interest. The term *entelechia* later became synonymous with the notion of the "vital force" (the principal concept of vitalism),[25] whereas the term "energia" has been used to the present day to describe an activated state of matter, or the ability to perform work by a system.[26] Other key terms are the *symphyton pneuma* - σύμφυτον πνεῦμα (the connatural, innate or inherent spirit) and the symphyton thermon - σύμφυτον θερμόν (the connatural, innate or inherent heat). According to Aristotle, the "connatural heat" is a primary essential attribute of any living body, and it is the alterations of connatural heat that are responsible for all processes of life.[27]

There appears a striking similarity between Aristotle's terms of "form" (structure), "activation," "energy" and "heat," and the terms used in modern thermodynamics. A similarity can be observed between Aristotelian 'vitalism' and thermodynamics in that both emphasize the general state, faculty, property or activation degree of matter, rather than the mechanical and spatial interrelation of its components. In Aristotle's *On Youth and Old Age, Life and Death, and Respiration*, the distinction between the proto-thermodynamic and proto-mechanistic views becomes clear. In this treatise, Aristotle states that respiration is a necessary essential condition for maintaining human life and provides a qualitative explanation for this process. In doing so, Aristotle again cites previous theories. Sometimes, the insight of the preceding philosophers is uncanny. Thus Empedocles describes the respiratory system as a pneumatic device (analogous to the clepsydra, similar in operation to the modern pipette) based on pressure differences.[28] Democritus claimed that respiration is due to the relative weights and impetus of elements, describing a process very similar to what we would now term "particle convection" or "diffusion."[29] Moreover Anaxagoras and Diogenes posited that fishes breathe the air dissolved in water – again strikingly similar to modern accounts.[30] Aristotle, as usual, wrestles these theories to the ground, and shows by formidable rational arguments that 'particle convection' is impossible and that fishes couldn't possibly breathe.[31]

However, the physical insights provided by Aristotle himself are no less outstanding. Perhaps the most critical is the equation he makes between the processes of life maintenance and processes of combustion and heat equilibrium – the association that forms the basis of modern bioenergetics and the thermodynamic theory of metabolism. According to Aristotle, life can only continue for as long as the living body contains a necessary amount of "connatural heat" (now we might term it intrinsic energy), for as long as "life's fire" is maintained.[32] The amount of heat tends to dwindle either by "extinction" or "exhaustion."[33] "Extinction" occurs because of a damping, neutralizing influence of external antagonistic ("opposite") agents, or because of the wastes/residues produced during the combustion process that are antagonistic/opposite to the continuation of the burning process.[34] "Exhaustion," on the other hand, takes place because of internal processes, namely because of the depletion of the nutrients that sustain the combustion.[35] According to Aristotle, in order to conserve the vital heat and thus prolong life's existence, the living system needs "cooling" or "refrigeration," otherwise the vital heat will quickly use up all its nutrient, and the living body will "burn out" and cease living.[36] Respiration, accordingly, is a means for such a cooling in terrestrial sanguineous animals (the air is said to "cool" the vital heat), whereas in aquatic animals (such as fishes) cooling is performed by the surrounding water.[37]

It is now firmly established that "cooling" is a necessary process for the operation of any thermodynamic system or machine. The importance of "refrigeration" is shown in the formula for the thermal efficiency of a heat engine: $N=(Q1-Q2)/Q1$, where Q1 is the heat input and Q2 is the heat output.[38] This formula in fact describes the changes in the heat content and the "cooling" that take place during thermodynamic operation of either a living or inanimate system. It has also become firmly established that "combustion" is the most fundamental and essential process of metabolism. The combustion (or oxidation) of glucose has been shown to provide the energy needed to sustain life. The process is described by the equation: $C_6H_{12}O_6 + 6O_2 \rightarrow 6H_2O + 6CO_2 + E(energy)$.[39] In this process, the energy/heat is released that drives all body functions. Yet, the energy content of the carbohydrate ("the nutrient" in Aristotle's terms) is reduced by the interaction with oxygen (the electron acceptor/or oxidizing agent) supplied from the air by respiration. To describe the process in Aristotle's tropes: the "air" (oxygen) "cools" the "vital heat" inherent in the "nutrient" and aids in maintaining the "combustion" process or "life's fire." Thus, by simple observations and sheer power of imagination, namely by associating life with combustion, Aristotle may have foreshadowed the basic thermodynamic principles of biology.

Aristotle on aging and longevity

In Aristotle's works, the "proto-thermodynamic" principles are used to account for aging and dying. These principles bear a direct relation to the question of the possibility (or impossibility) of life extension, as well as practical suggestions for its achievement. The treatise *On Length and Shortness of Life* provides a most concise, yet comprehensive discussion of the physiology of aging. Aristotle carefully investigates the possible causes of longevity and mortality. He compares the life spans of various species of animals, various individuals or sexes of the same species, various life styles, and environmental conditions or animal habitats, and attempts to find a correlation between the various species, life styles or habitats and longevity. His method in doing so is not much different from that of modern comparative gerontology.[40] Specifically, he examines the size of animals, whether they are 'bloodless' or warm-blooded ('sanguineous'), whether they reside in a terrestrial or aquatic environment, warm or cold climate, whether they copulate frequently, or whether their life is leisurely or strenuous. He also points out to the difficulty in such a categorization, as exceptions can be found that may contradict the general theory.[41] Nevertheless, Aristotle does come up with a set of generalizations concerning the qualities, life style and environment that may be conducive to longevity.

According to Aristotle, terrestrial animals are generally longer lived than aquatic, sanguineous animals live longer than bloodless ones, larger animals live longer than smaller, and animals occupying warm habitats live longer than those who live in a cold climate.[42] From these observations, Aristotle proceeds to generalize about the animals' material and thermal constitution that may favor longevity. Briefly, long lived animals are said to be of a larger size, and have a greater degree of "humidity" and "warmth" in them. Short-lived species or aging animals, on the other hand, are characterized by "dryness" and "coldness."[43] Aristotle's conclusions sometimes coalesce with and sometimes contradict later findings. And yet, the fields of observation and comparative analysis outlined by Aristotle (viz. the species, life style and habitat) and the theoretical discussions of the material and thermal basis of animal longevity, have become central themes for a great deal of subsequent gerontological research.

Since Aristotle, the concept of "dryness" has undergone many contextual transformations, and yet the basic proposition that "dryness" (i.e. a deficit of fluid or rigidity) is detrimental to health and longevity, has remained scientifically valid. It has been firmly established that "dryness" in the simple sense of a fluid deficit or desiccation, is incompatible with life – water being the essential solvent necessary for most of the biochemical and bio-energetic processes occurring in the body, and for maintaining its homeostasis (in terms of osmosis and pressure maintenance, substance transport, electric potential, pH balance, etc.).[44] In line with Aristotle's suggestions, restoring the fluid content or fluid balance have become established life-saving therapies.[45] According to Aristotle, the body "humidity" must not be "easily dried up," and "viscous" or "oily" fluids are "not easily dried up."[46] By this theory he accounts for the greater longevity of plants (having more viscous/oily fluids) and the lesser longevity of aquatic animals (with less viscous body fluids). The importance of viscosity in fluid homeostasis has been later confirmed.[47] "Dryness" in a broader sense of body "rigidity" or "hardening" has proven to be an even more influential and productive concept in subsequent biomedical research. Tissue sclerosis (or tissue hardening) has become recognized as a major factor in aging and a major cause of death (especially arteriosclerosis).[48] Many other pathological processes have been associated with rigidity, such as muscle spasms due to calcium or ATP deficit, and its extreme form, the "rigor mortis" – or complete muscle rigidity upon death.[49] The increased tissue rigidity (or loss of elasticity) has become one of the most popular explanations of aging. Specifically, the cross-linking theory of aging accounts for the loss of protein elasticity by glycosylation cross-links between proteins.[50] At a more fundamental thermodynamic or information-theoretical level, rigidity may be associated with a lower entropy (or rigid order) of a subsystem or organ, and the subsystem's lower entropy can be in turn associated with pathology, as in the case of Parkinson's disease and other diseases associated with enhanced regularity.[51] Thus again, Aristotle's common sense, the fairly straightforward association between aging and "dryness," anticipated much of future research.

Aristotle's discussion of the thermal properties of life, the association of life with "fire," "warmth" or "connatural heat" proved to be even more seminal. As mentioned above, Aristotle believed that long lived animals are characterized by a greater degree of "intrinsic heat" and consequently, in order to prolong life's existence, the body "heat" must be conserved. According to Aristotle, the heat conservation can be achieved by countering the processes of "exhaustion" and "extinction" by "cooling" (so the internal "heat" will not be expended too quickly). The concept of body "connatural heat" can be recognized in the later concepts of body energy or metabolic rates. Among other current detection methods, Metabolic Rates (MR) have been measured simply by temperature changes or by the amount of heat emitted by the body.[52]

Recently, there has been a fundamental controversy on the correlation between the metabolic rates and longevity. The dominant "Rate of living" school posited that increased metabolic rates (manifested by an increased heat production) are detrimental for longevity, whereas a lower energy expenditure can extend the life span.[53] Excessive metabolic rates, contingent on excessive stimulation, were shown to be 'exhaustive,' to increase body 'wear and tear' and 'burn it out' (these are almost precisely Aristotelian terms), leading to an excess of toxic waste products (especially reactive free radicals). On the other hand, it has been suggested that life would be impossible without active exercise, and conditions characterized by slow metabolism, such as obesity and hypothyroidism, are dangerous and often fatal, and therefore increased metabolic rates favor healthy longevity.[54] Moreover, the "Uncouple to survive" school professed that higher metabolic rates (accompanied by a higher heat generation) are crucial for survival (which may explain the advantage of warm-blooded animals), and therefore the process of oxidative phosphorylation must be uncoupled (e.g. by tyrosine, or other means)[55] in order to achieve greater metabolic rates and heat production. [56] Both these options are covered by Aristotle's reasoning. Indeed, Aristotle argues, the higher degree of "connatural heat" is essential for health and longevity, because the larger amount of heat means a higher degree of life's actualization. And yet, the internal heat needs "cooling," needs "inhibition," in order to enable nutrient replenishment and heat recovery for further actualizations. In view of this, Aristotle may be considered the father of the homeostatic "balanced" approach to life extension. In particular, Aristotle's general emphasis on the need to "conserve" the "connatural heat" to achieve longevity, implied the need for moderation in life style, diet in particular – an idea with far-reaching ramifications for aging research, ranging from various attempted life-prolonging "moderate" diets to the experiments on life extension by calorie restriction[57] (literally, "heat restriction" as "Calor" is Latin for "heat").

212

Aristotle's provides extensive empirical evidence for his main theoretical claim that the degree of internal heat determines longevity. Notably, he reports that small size, cold climate, strenuous life style, and excessive copulation are all detrimental to longevity, since these conditions contribute to diminishing the internal heat by "exhaustion."[58] These phenomenological observations were based on the most extensive available research of Aristotle's time, and they have been a subject of scientific debate to the present day, in the framework of the "Rate of living" vs. "Exercise to survive" controversy.[59] Aristotle's conclusion that larger animals possess greater life spans (in order to contain a greater amount of fluid and heat) has been recently corroborated.[60] The observation that inhabitants of warmer terrains are longer-lived, might have been especially true at the time of Aristotle, as the warm Mediterranean area served as a cradle of civilization, whereas in colder climates the chances for survival were slimmer. And yet, there have been found abundant examples to the contrary. Thus, the renowned German hygienist Christoph Wilhelm Hufeland, in *Macrobiotics or the Art of Prolonging Human Life* (1796), suggested that colder climates are more favorable for health and longevity.[61] Also statistical evidence indicated that residents of the colder Scandinavian countries and certain mountainous areas (e.g. the Caucasus, the Alps, and the Himalayas) enjoy relatively good longevity.[62] Despite the continuous controversies and conflicting data, the very consideration of those factors as potential determinants of longevity is a pioneering contribution of Aristotle.

The claim that a strenuous life style or hard labor shorten the human life span, has also been actively debated. Certain studies showed that people leading a leisurely life style or people of sedentary professions live longer (possibly due to a reduced stress and lower energy expenditure).[63] On the other side, advocates of active exercise provided extensive evidence for the benefits of physical labor and exercise for life prolongation.[64] Sweeping generalizations still appear to be impossible. At the same time, the exact indications for the beneficial or adverse effects of specific rest and activity regimens for specific people or groups of people (the subject of the so-called "precision medicine") still appear to be uncertain. In any case, recognition is due to Aristotle as one of the initiators of this debate.

The debate concerning the life-prolonging effects of sexual moderation proceeded along similar lines. According to Aristotle, men who don't copulate frequently have a greater longevity (because they don't expend the vital heat and moisture inherent in the semen). Women, according to Aristotle, have a lesser degree of "vital heat" than men and therefore live less, provided men don't copulate frequently. If men do waste their semen, then women outlive the men. In the same line of argument, the sterile mules are said to live longer than their fertile sexual parents (the horse and the donkey).[65] Agreeing with Aristotle, the idea of life extension through sexual moderation (in other words, by conserving sexual energy) has been a cornerstone of medical science for centuries. For example, one of the ancient techniques of "Gerocomia" (from the Greek – "treatment of old age") was the proximity to young healthy individuals, or sexual stimulation without discharge, which was prescribed by Galen and practiced by King David (1 Kings 1:2); this method retained its popularity well into modernity.[66] In the eighteenth and nineteenth centuries, much ink was spilled on the dangers of masturbation.[67] In recent times, several studies evaluated the costs of reproduction and enhanced copulation for longevity in animals.[68] Such costs were indicated for humans as well.[69] However, in the past decades, these views have been increasingly challenged by studies professing that sexual activity is "good for health and longevity," that life span can be positively correlated to sexual activity.[70] Nonetheless, the exact thresholds, personal indications and tradeoffs for the benefits vs. drawbacks of increased or decreased sexual activity, for men vs. women, still remain undetermined.

The outcomes of Aristotle's comparison between the life spans of men and women have also remained disputable, as it has been found that women indeed generally have lower metabolic rates, but commonly live longer than men.[71] Still, there can be found numerous contrary showcases, and different population studies often arrive at different gender-longevity correlations.[72] In any case, Aristotle's bringing into consideration the relation between gender (sex) and longevity, or more precisely the consideration of the physiological differences of men and women in relation to their longevity, has become indispensable in gerontological research.

As it can be seen, despite numerous discrepancies and controversies, despite the large number of unaccounted thresholds and factors – the Aristotelian proto-thermodynamic account of aging, the ideas of "vital heat" and its "conservation" and "replenishment" haven't lost their appeal, and may be still considered as a part or origin of the ongoing physiological discourse. Sometimes Aristotle's specific deductions on the ways of "heat replenishment" may seem prophetically inspired, given the contemporary state of empirical observations. Thus, according to Aristotle, "viscous" or "oily" bodily fluids "are not easily dried up" and contribute to heat preservation.[73] It has become established much later that fat may indeed act as an insulator (and thus prevent heat dissipation), that viscous substances are less easily evaporated (due to adhesion), and that fatty substances have the highest content of energy and are used by the body as long-term nutrient reservoirs.[74]

Even more prophetic was Aristotle's idea that, during the processes of combustion in a living body, "wastes" or "residues" are produced that are antagonistic ("opposite") to the very process of combustion that generated

214

them, and thus act to "extinguish" the body's internal heat.[75] This general account closely describes the process of allosteric inhibition or negative biochemical feedback, where the products of a chemical reaction act as inhibitors to the reaction that produced them.[76] This formulation generally describes the production and accumulation of toxic metabolites in a living body. It is particularly relevant to the Free Radical theory of aging. In this theory, during the oxidation process in the mitochondria, nutrients are oxidized by oxygen (undergo combustion), with a concomitant production of reactive oxygen species. The reactive oxygen species, in turn, may damage the mitochondria and thus stall the very process of combustion that generated them, thereby contributing to cell damage, energy deficit and aging.[77]

Interesting proto-thermodynamic and proto-homeostatic insights can be found in Aristotle's treatise *On Sleep*. According to Aristotle's definition, sleep is a state of sensory deprivation and a form of "cooling" needed for the conservation and replenishment of vital heat, and therefore essential for life preservation.[78] In Aristotle's description of the mechanism of the "sleep-wakefulness" cycle, an excess of heat in the body triggers its "compression" or "condensation" into the "vital center" until the "nutrient" nourishing the combustion process is replenished, thus leading to a new heat "expansion" throughout the body.[79] In modern terms, this sequence describes a negative feedback process, relevant for both living systems and thermodynamic machines in general.[80] Modern studies of sleep and rest speak of "refractory periods," "potential recovery," "energy carriers replenishment," etc.[81] But the principle of negative biofeedback is the same, and the analogy of these processes to those described by Aristotle is apparent. The very critical role of sleep for life preservation generally, and its particular role for the amelioration of degenerative aging processes, has remained a fruitful field of study.[82]

According to Aristotle, "*symphyton pneuma*" (or innate spirit) animates the body and serves as the carrier of vital heat. Its movements and alterations in the body – such as expansion, condensation, flow, and changes in heat content – are responsible for body operations. In this regard, the "pneuma" is very similar to steam in a stem engine.[83] Presently, the transmission and transformation of vital energy and substance is discussed in terms of blood flow, diffusion, active transport, electro-mechano-chemical coupling, etc.[84] – but these modern descriptions seem to involve the same basic intuitions of energy flow and its homeostatic regulation.

According to Aristotle, the heart serves as the center and major "seat" of vital heat. Into that center the heat is condensed during sleep, and it is responsible for the expansion and distribution of heat throughout the body.[85] Indeed, also in modern views, the heart is seen as a vital organ, a motor of life, a most metabolically active center, which never ceases activity throughout life, a 'pump' supplying the "vital energy" and "vital substance" to the body. Heart's proper operation is most essential for life maintenance, and heart diseases are primary, widest-spread causes of death.[86] Aristotle did not speak of heart action in terms of "circulation," but rather in terms of "pulsation" and "palpitation."[87] However, the modern recognition of the primary function of the heart in life support, coalesced with Aristotle's assertions of the central role of the heart as the "seat of the vital principle."

In Aristotle, the heart has a supreme place in the hierarchy of animal life. It is the central locus and the highest form of life's actualization. However, according to Aristotle (*On the Length and Shortness of Life*), in other life forms, such as plants and certain insects, vitality is more uniformly distributed throughout the body and has a higher extent of potentiality. Therefore, if insects are cut to pieces, life continues in these parts for some time (not for long though, as vital organs are missing), and if plants are cut to pieces, each piece can produce a plant identical to the parent.[88] These observations may represent rudiments of another vast biological field: namely the study of regeneration, differentiation, asexual reproduction, and even genetics. The idea that certain organs reach a highest irreversible degree of actualization may correspond to the modern concept of differentiation (also a kind of ultimate and usually irreversible degree of development).[89] On the other hand, the observation of the ability of plant parts to regenerate the entire plant body (due to a greater degree of potentiality inherent in them) foreshadowed the concept of toti-potency (a key notion in modern research of vegetative reproduction and regeneration, as well as in embryological and stem cell research).[90] Moreover, Aristotle scholars noted the apparent similarity of the concept of a vital form (*eidos*) to genes: both confer structure to a living organism.[91] Indeed, concerning gene expression, Aristotle's terms are very relevant: potentiality corresponds to gene dormancy, while actuality corresponds to gene activation and expression.

This reasoning can be taken a step further. In *De Anima*, Aristotle claims that even though no body can be preserved in a constant state, it "strives" to preserve itself as something "similar" to its present state.[92] This seems to be precisely the function of genes: acting to replicate themselves and the original organism, but never able to produce a precise "replica." In *On the Length and Shortness of Life*, these observations are used to account for a generally greater longevity of plants as compared to animals (even though Aristotle recognizes a great number of exceptions from this general rule). According to Aristotle, the vital moisture in plants is not "easily dried up" (due to its greater viscosity), and plants' "vital heat" is not easily dissipated (due to a lesser nutrient expenditure).[93] Another part of the explanation is the above-mentioned uniform distribution of vital heat and a greater degree

216

of potentiality in plants that enable their constant regeneration.[94] Combining the proto-thermodynamic and proto-genetic terms, a contemporary-sounding paraphrase of Aristotle's theory can be obtained: Plants may generally have a greater longevity because their body constitution contains a sufficient amount of potential energy which is uniformly distributed and economically expended, enabling the continuous structure maintenance, self-organization and replication.

In this regard, a seeming contradiction must be noted in Aristotle's account of life and longevity. It is Aristotle's strong assertion that the soul or the vital principle is the same in every part of a living organism.[95] Yet, the amount of "vital heat" whereby the soul operates in the body or degrees of life "actualization" in various organs or faculties are not homogeneously distributed throughout the body, and in some organisms are more uniform than in others. This apparent contradiction can be reconciled using the modern gene metaphor: a complete set of genes is present in each and every somatic cell of the body, yet their expression varies in different organs and tissues. It can be also reconciled using the thermodynamic metaphor: each body has a single energy function and structural unity. However, the operators of this function and structural components may differ. Whatever the interpretation, Aristotle's reasoning about the observable properties of living beings is insightful, with both profound theoretical and practical implications.

Aristotle on the possibility of radical life extension and immortality

Among the chief practical implications of Aristotle's physiological theory is the question of the feasibility of increasing longevity and its limits. In particular, in considering animal longevity, Aristotle raises the crucial question of the possibility of a radical life extension or even immortality. This question has remained a major bone of contention in modern biomedical gerontology.[96] Even though Aristotle carefully investigates the causes of longevity and mortality, in order to select environmental and physiological factors that may increase human life span (such as gentle climate, economical heat expenditure, or diet rich in "heat and moisture") – eventually Aristotle states the impossibility of a significant, not to mention infinite, life extension. Aristotle believes that any physical entity is composed of opposite and conflicting elements. According to Aristotle, any such entity must be in a constant process of change, and therefore cannot be preserved "as is" for a long time. Thus, a living organism is fated for ultimate destruction, for it contains in itself antagonistic forces and elements that mutually annihilate each other, and thus destroy the entire body.[97] Moreover, the "vital heat" cannot be preserved indefinitely as it is continuously diminished by "extinction" and "exhaustion."

These views of the ultimate destructibility of any living body (in other words, the impossibility of its preservation beyond a predetermined limit), have continued through centuries. Among many instances, they resonated in the writings of Avicenna (who also stated an inevitable self-destruction of the body due to opposition of its components)[98] and even in recent bio-gerontological views positing an inherent genetically predetermined limit to the life span due to self-destruct programs and processes which, as believed, cannot be overcome by any means (e.g. Hayflick's school).[99] There has been a controversy among Aristotle scholars as to the exact meaning of Aristotle's term "opposite elements": some understood it in a more literary sense of opposite kinds of matter or opposite kinds of atoms (e.g. fire vs. water, or earth vs. air); others perceived it as a more general opposition of qualities, forces or states (hot vs. cold, active vs. non-active, etc).[100] In modern thermodynamics, the opposition of elements forms the basis for the concept of entropy (or degree of chaos). Systems with a low entropy (a greater degree of orderliness) are composed of elements with a distinct relation or juxtaposition to each other: the more distinct is the opposition of the elements or the less the number of their distinct states – the greater is the system's orderliness. On the other hand, when the amount of particles' states increases, or when their opposition or mutual relation becomes less distinct – such a system is more chaotic, with a higher degree of entropy.[101] According to the second law of thermodynamics, in any closed system, the entropy increases, and the system tends to reach a state of "heat equilibrium" or "heat death" where there is no distinct opposition between elements and all the elements are distributed chaotically. Thus Aristotle's 'pessimistic' precepts of the inevitable death due to heat dissipation and inevitable reduction in "opposition of elements" may have directly anticipated the thermodynamic concept of an inexorable "heat death" of any closed system.

Despite the assertion of the inevitability of death, Aristotle's views on life extension and immortality contain an element of hope. Even under the ultimate verdict of destruction, by conserving and renewing vital heat, life could be extended. Moreover, in Aristotle's vitalism, there is an indication for the possibility of immortality of the soul or of the "vital principle" which is not subject to the transformation and destruction of the physical body. Aristotle seems to present a border case (also chronologically) between Plato's idealism devaluing this-worldly existence and projecting the hope of immortality to the ideal world of forms[102] and Epicurus' 'thick' materialism resigning to the utter physical and mental annihilation upon death.[103] Aristotle's position may be termed 'thin' materialism. As it is seen in *De Anima*, most faculties of the soul are inseparable from the body, and disappear upon physical death. The "active mind," however, or the "thought that thinks itself" is given a privileged status, and is said to be

218

divine, "immortal and eternal."[104] However, the relation of the "active mind" to the rest of perceptive and intellectual faculties is obscure, and it is hard to imagine its separate existence, since its ideations are based on previous sensory experiences. The soul in Aristotle is not the ideal Platonic soul. It is associated with or operates through a kind of matter, though an infinitely thin (the "least corporeal") matter. This "least corporeal" energized matter is *symphyton pneuma* (σύμφυτον πνευμα) – the "innate spirit" – analogous to ether, the fifth element, which is not subject to a conflict of elements, and is therefore indestructible. It is the same substance the eternal Sun and higher spheres are made of (cf. Aristotle's *On the Heavens,*[105] *Physics,*[106] and *On the Soul*[107,108]). However, as in the case of the "active mind," the hardly destructible "pneuma" does not constitute the entirety of human being. Aristotle's concept of the "pneuma" is complex, with many possible interpretations.[109] In one sense, as discussed above, the pneuma serves as the carrier of "vital heat" (and is in many respects similar to steam in a steam engine). However, as previously mentioned, the heat content in the body is subject to change and exhaustion, therefore the constancy and indestructibility of the pneuma becomes questionable. Thus, Aristotle gives us a hope for immortality, but not too much hope.

Aristotle was, first and foremost, a great biologist who cherished life in all its forms. This field of Aristotle's study may have come to be underappreciated by modern scholars. Yet Aristotle's physiological corpus may not warrant oblivion. Far from being irrelevant to modern biomedical research, Aristotle's insightful and imaginative writings provide amazing anticipations of modern physiology, bioenergetics and gerontology. In the historicist school, any attempt to seek modern concepts in ancient texts is branded as "anachronism" and considered almost a mortal sin. Yet, there seems to be nothing wrong in trying to search for origins of modern concepts, or for similarity of concepts through history, in trying to understand the voices of great thinkers coming from the past, and not just disregard them as "untrue" or "anachronistic" or "contextually irrelevant." Aristotle is very inclusive. He may be considered an early anti-longevitist, stating the ultimate futility of attempts to achieve a radical life prolongation. And yet, despite the sense of doom, in many respects he is close to life-extensionism, studying causes of mortality and seeking practical ways for forestalling death. This subject matter can hardly ever become historically irrelevant.[110]

References and notes

1. Thus, for example, the 400 page long *Cambridge Companion to Aristotle* (Edited by Jonathan Barnes, Cambridge University Press, 1995), includes only about 10 pages related to Aristotle's biology.

A basic JSTOR search (https://www.jstor.org/) shows that out of tens of thousands of articles mentioning Aristotle, perhaps a few hundreds make any connection between Aristotle and physiology, still less discuss the relevance of Aristotle's theories to modern findings. No articles on the relation of Aristotle's teachings to modern bio-gerontology were to be found.

2. Marjorie Grene, "Aristotle and Modern Biology," *Journal of the History of Ideas*, 33(3), 395-424, 1972.

According to Grene, Aristotle's methodology is largely irrelevant to modern research. She perceives some continuity for Aristotle's fundamental ontological concepts of "telos," "eidos" and the "being what it is," but not for the actual physiological processes that Aristotle describes.

3. Walter Stanley Hett, "Introduction to Aristotle's On the Soul," in *Aristotle in Twenty-Three Volumes*, William Heinemann Ltd., London, 1975, Vol. VIII, p. vii.

4. Edward Grant, "Aristotelianism and the Longevity of the Medieval World View," *History of Science*, 16, 93-106, 1978.

5. Aristotle, *On the Soul* (translated with notes by Walter Stanley Hett), in *Aristotle in Twenty-Three Volumes*, William Heinemann Ltd., London, 1975 (hereafter referred to as *"On the Soul"* unless a different translation is specified), Book 2, Part 4, 415b9-12, p. 87.

6. *On the Soul*, Book 2, Part 4.

7. "Vitalism" seemed to be a very "viable" theory at the beginning of the 20th century, as can be seen from the following works:

Hans Driesch, *The History and Theory of Vitalism*, J.A.Barth, Leipzig, 1905, https://archive.org/details/cu31924003039330;

Walter T. Marvin, "Mechanism Versus Vitalism As a Philosophical Issue," *The Philosophical Review*, 27(6), 616-627, 1918;

Herbert Spencer Jennings, "Mechanism and Vitalism," The *Philosophical Review*, 27(6), 577-596, 1918.

Later, the scholarly prestige of "vitalism" appears to have been drastically decreased. However, "vitalism" continued to be referred to in the biological discourse. Of special interest is the adoption of vitalism in aging theory by the German gerontologist Max Bürger (1885-1966). See: Max Bürger, *Altern und Krankheit* (Aging and Disease), Zweite Auflage (2nd Edition), Veb Georg Thieme, Leipzig, 1954 (first published in 1947), "Das Altern im Lichte der vitalistischen Autonomielehre" (Aging in the light of the theory of vitalistic autonomy), pp. 39-41.

Aristotle's affinity with vitalism has been frequently asserted, for example in such works as:

Ernst Mayr, *The Growth of Biological Thought*, Harvard University Press, Cambridge MA, 1982, p. 52;

Richard J. Cameron, *Teleology and Contemporary Philosophy of Biology: An Account of the Nature of Life*, University of Colorado, 2000, pp. 33-40.

8. *On the Soul*, 1.2. 405b 12-31, pp. 29-30; 1.5. 409b19-410a3, p. 55.

9. *Ibid.* 1.2. 405a6-14, p. 27.

10. *Ibid.* 1.4. 407b28-32, p. 43; 408a10-28, pp. 45-46.

11. *Ibid.* 1.4. 407b28, p. 43.

12. *Ibid.* 1.4. 408a24, p. 45.

13. Sigmund Freud, *Beyond the Pleasure Principle* (Translated by James Strachey), Liveright, New York, 1976, p. 38.

14. Erwin Schrödinger, *What is Life?* Cambridge University Press, Cambridge, 1996, p. 67.

15. Len Fisher, *Weighing the soul: the evolution of scientific beliefs*, Weidenfeld & Nicolson, London, 2004.

16. *On the Soul*, 1.5. 410a7-14, p. 57.

17. *Ibid.* 3.2. 425b27-426a2, p. 147.

18. *Ibid.* 1.5. 409a32-409b4, p. 53.

19. *Ibid.* 1.4. 407b33-408a9, pp. 43-44.

20. *Ibid.* 1.5. 411b16-31, p. 65.

21. "Vitalism," Wikipedia, accessed June 2017, http://en.wikipedia.org/wiki/Vitalism;

Hans Driesch, *The History and Theory of Vitalism*, J.A.Barth, Leipzig, 1905, https://archive.org/details/cu31924003039330;

Philip G. Fothergill (Ed.), *Mechanism and Vitalism: Philosophical Aspects of Biology*, University of Notre Dame Press, Notre Dame, Indiana, 1962.

22. "Atomism," Wikipedia, accessed June 2017, http://en.wikipedia.org/wiki/Atomism#The_exile_of_atomism;

Robert Hugh Kargon, *Atomism in England from Hariot to Newton*, Clarendon Press, Oxford, 1966;

Joshua C. Gregory, *A Short History of Atomism: from Democritus to Bohr*, A. & C. Black Ltd., London, 1931.

23. Aristotle, *On the Soul* (Translated by John Alexander Smith), in *The Complete Works of Aristotle: The Revised Oxford Translation* (Edited by Jonathan Barnes), Princeton University Press, Princeton, 1984, Part 2, Ch. 4, 415b9-12, p. 661.
(Smith's translation of this passage seemed more comprehensive than that of Hett: "The soul is the cause and first principle of the living body." Except for this single instance, Hett's translation of *On the Soul* is referred to throughout this paper.)

24. Walter Stanley Hett, "Introduction to Aristotle's On the Soul," in *Aristotle in Twenty-Three Volumes*, William Heinemann Ltd., London, 1975, Vol. VIII, pp. xi-xii.

25. See notes 7, 21 and 22.

26. "Thermodynamics," in *Oxford Dictionary of Science*, Oxford University Press, 1999, pp. 784-785.

27. Aristotle, *On Youth, Old Age, Life and Death, and Respiration* (Translated by George Robert Thomson Ross), in *The Complete Works of Aristotle: The Revised Oxford Translation* (Edited by Jonathan Barnes), Princeton University Press, Princeton, 1984, Vol. 1, 14(8). 474a25-27, p. 754 (hereafter referred to as *On Youth and Old Age*).

28. *On Youth and Old Age*, 13(7). 473a28-473b8, p. 753.

29. *Ibid.* 10(4). 471b30-472a17, p. 751.

30. *Ibid.* 8(2). 470b27-471a5, p. 749-750.

31. *Ibid.* 13(7). 474a7-23, p. 754; 8(2). 471a6-19, p. 750.

32. *Ibid.* 14(8). 474a25-27, p. 754.

33. *Ibid.* 5. 469b21-470a4, p. 748.

34. *Ibid.* 5. 469b21-470a4, p. 748; 26(20). 479b19-20, p. 761.

35. *Ibid.* 5. 469b21-470a4, p. 748; 24(18). 479b1-5, p. 761.

36. *Ibid.* 5. 470a517, p. 748.

37. *Ibid.* 6. 470a20-470b5, p. 749.

38. "Carnot cycle," in *Oxford Dictionary of Science*, Oxford University Press, 1999, p. 130.

39. Max Fogiel (Ed.), *The Biology Problem Solver. A Complete Solution Guide to Any Textbook*, Research and Education Association, Piscataway, New Jersey, US, 1990 (republished in 2001), 3.35, p. 117 (hereafter referred to as "Fogiel, *The Biology Problem Solver*").

It must be noted that here the references to this rather well known and well disseminated textbook/problem solver, including about 800 topics "for undergraduate and graduate studies," relating to all areas of biology and physiology, are intended to show the relation and succession with the current commonly taught views (compared to original research that may be considered more partial and potentially controversial, which is nonetheless also quoted). References to other text books, scientific reference books and dictionaries are made with the same purpose in mind to show relevance to the contemporary common knowledge.

40. On the comparative gerontology approach, seeking the differential determinants of aging and longevity, see for example:

Steven N. Austad, Kathleen E. Fischer, "Mammalian aging, metabolism, and ecology: evidence from the bats and marsupials," *Journal of Gerontology: Biological Sciences*, 46(2), B47-53, 1991;

Steven N. Austad, "Comparative aging and life histories in mammals," *Experimental Gerontology*, 32(1-2), 23-38, 1997;

Virpi Lummaa, "Early developmental conditions and reproductive success in humans: Downstream effects of prenatal famine, birthweight, and timing of birth," *American Journal of Human Biology*, 15(3), 370-379, 2003;

S. Jay Olshansky, Toni Antonucci, Lisa Berkman, Robert H. Binstock, Axel Boersch-Supan, John T. Cacioppo, Bruce A. Carnes, Laura L. Carstensen, Linda P. Fried, Dana P. Goldman, James Jackson, Martin Kohli, John Rother, Yuhui Zheng, John Rowe, "Differences in life expectancy due to race and educational differences are widening, and many may not catch up," *Health Affairs*, 31(8), 1803-1813, 2012.

41. Aristotle, *On Length and Shortness of Life* (Translated by G.R.T. Ross), in *The Complete Works of Aristotle: The Revised Oxford Translation* (Edited by Jonathan Barnes), Princeton University Press, Princeton, 1984, Vol. 1 (hereafter referred to as *On Length and Shortness of Life*), Section 1, 464b20-465a11, p. 740.
Also available as Aristotle, *On Longevity and Shortness of Life* (Translated by G.R.T. Ross), at the Internet Classics Archive, http://classics.mit.edu/Aristotle/longev_short.html.

42. *On Length and Shortness of Life*, 4. 466a9-16, p. 742.

43. *Ibid.* 5. 466a17-31, p. 742.

44. Elie Metchnikoff, *Etudes On the Nature of Man* (in Russian), The USSR Academy of Sciences Press, Moscow, 1961 (first published in 1903), p. 193 (hereafter referred to as "Metchnikoff, *On the Nature of Man*");
Fogiel, *The Biology Problem Solver*, 1.15, p. 17;
"Water," *Oxford Dictionary of Science*, Oxford University Press, 1999, pp. 833-834.

45. Michael N. Sawka, Samuel N. Cheuvront, Robert Carter 3rd, "Human water needs," *Nutrition Reviews*, 63(6 Pt 2), S30-S39, 2005;
Michelle P.B. Guppy, Sharon M. Mickan, Chris B. Del Mar, Sarah Thorning, Alexander Rack, "Advising patients to increase fluid intake for treating acute respiratory infections," *Cochrane Database of Systematic Reviews*, 2011(2), CD004419, 2011;
Bell T.N., "Diabetes insipidus," *Critical Care Nursing Clinics of North America*, 6(4), 675-685, 1994;
Friedrich Manz, Andreas Wentz, "The importance of good hydration for the prevention of chronic diseases," *Nutrition Reviews*, 63(6 Pt 2), S2-S5, 2005.

46. *On Length and Shortness of Life*, 4. 466a17-24, p.742; 6. 467a6-9, p. 743.

47. H.T. Hammel, Whitney M. Schlegel, "Osmosis and solute-solvent drag: fluid transport and fluid exchange in animals and plants," *Cell Biochemistry and Biophysics*, 42(3), 277-345, 2005.

48. Metchnikoff, *On the Nature of Man*, p. 193;
Julie C. Wang, Martin Bennett, "Aging and Atherosclerosis: Mechanisms, Functional Consequences, and Potential Therapeutics for Cellular Senescence," *Circulation Research*, 111, 245-259, 2012.

49. Burkhard Madea, "Methods for determining time of death," *Forensic Science, Medicine, and Pathology*, 12(4), 451-485, 2016;

Fogiel, *The Biology Problem Solver*, 19.6, pp. 579-581; 14.6, pp. 424-425.

50. Johan Bjorksten, "The Crosslinkage Theory of Aging," *Journal of the American Geriatrics Society*, 16(4), 408-427, 1968;

Norman C. Avery, A.J. Bailey, "Enzymic and non-enzymic cross-linking mechanisms in relation to turnover of collagen: relevance to aging and exercise," *Scandinavian Journal of Medicine and Science in Sports*, 15(4), 231-240, 2005;

SENS Research Foundation, "A Reimagined Research Strategy for Aging. GlycoSENS: Breaking extracellular crosslinks," accessed June 2017, http://www.sens.org/research/introduction-to-sens-research/extracellular-crosslinks;

Richard D. Semba, Emily J. Nicklett, Luigi Ferrucci, "Does Accumulation of Advanced Glycation End Products Contribute to the Aging Phenotype?" *The Journal of Gerontology: Series A Biological Sciences Medical Sciences*, 65A(9), 963-975, 2010.

51. Lewis A. Lipsitz, Ary L. Goldberger, "Loss of 'complexity' and aging: potential applications of fractals and chaos theory to senescence," *Journal of the American Medical Association*, 267, 1806-1809, 1992;

Molly M. Sturman, David E. Vaillancourt, Daniel M. Corcos, "Effects of aging on the regularity of physiological tremor," *Journal of Neurophysiology*, 93(6), 3064-3074, 2005;

Olivier Toussaint, Martine Raes, José Remacle, "Aging as a multi-step process characterized by a lowering of entropy production leading the cell to a sequence of defined stages," *Mechanisms of Ageing and Development*, 61(1), 45-64, 1991.

52. John Reginald Brande Lighton, *Measuring Metabolic Rates: A Manual for Scientists*, Oxford University Press, Oxford, 2008;

Charlene Compher, David Frankenfield, Nancy Keim, Lori Roth-Yousey, Evidence Analysis Working Group, "Best practice methods to apply to measurement of resting metabolic rate in adults: a systematic review," *Journal of the American Dietetic Association*, 106(6), 881-903, 2006;

Fogiel, *The Biology Problem Solver*, 3.31, pp. 112-113; 17.4, pp. 510-511.

53. Raymond Pearl, *The Rate of Living*, University of London Press, London, 1928;

Denham Harman, "Aging: a theory based on free radical and radiation chemistry," *Journal of Gerontology*, 11, 298-300, 1956;

Rajindar S. Sohal, "Role of oxidative stress and protein oxidation in the aging process," *Free Radical Biology and Medicine*, 33(1), 37-44, 2002.

54. J. T. Nicoloff and J. Thomas Dowling, "Estimation of thyroxine distribution in man," *The Journal of Clinical Investigation*, 47(1), 26-37, 1968;

Daniel Rudman, Michael H. Kutner, C. Milford Rogers, Michael F. Lubin, G. Alexander Fleming, Raymond P. Bain, "Impaired growth hormone secretion in the adult population: relation to age and adiposity," *The Journal of Clinical Investigation,* 67(5), 1361-1369, 1981;

George A. Bray, David S. Gray, "Obesity I: Pathogenesis," *The Western Journal of Medicine,* 149(4), 429-441, 1988.

55. Fogiel, *The Biology Problem Solver,* 3.32, pp.113-114;

Antoine Stier, Pierre Bize, Damien Roussel, Quentin Schull, Sylvie Massemin, François Criscuolo, "Mitochondrial uncoupling as a regulator of life-history trajectories in birds: an experimental study in the zebra finch," *Journal of Experimental Biology,* 217, 3579-3589, 2014.

56. Martin D. Brand, "Uncoupling to survive? The role of inefficiency in ageing," *Experimental Gerontology,* 35, 811-820, 2000;

John R. Speakman, Darren A. Talbot, Colin Selman, Sam Snart, Jane S. McLaren, Paula Redman, Ela Krol, Diane M. Jackson, Maria S. Johnson, Martin D. Brand, "Uncoupled and surviving: individual mice with high metabolism have greater mitochondrial uncoupling and live longer," *Aging Cell,* 3(3), 87-95, 2004;

Giuseppina Rose, Paolina Crocco, Francesco De Rango, Alberto Montesanto, Giuseppe Passarino, "Further Support to the Uncoupling-to-Survive Theory: The Genetic Variation of Human UCP Genes Is Associated with Longevity," *PLoS One,* 6(12), e29650, 2011;

Karine Salin, Sonya K. Auer, Agata M. Rudolf, Graeme J. Anderson, Andrew G. Cairns, William Mullen, Richard C. Hartley, Colin Selman, Neil B. Metcalfe, "Individuals with higher metabolic rates have lower levels of reactive oxygen species in vivo," *Biology Letters,* 11(9), 20150538, 2015.

57. "Moderation" has been a prevalent mainstay in the history of the pursuit of life extension, throughout the world. In the words of Lao-Tse, the great teacher of Taoist immortalists (China, c. 6th century BCE), "For regulating the human in our constitution and rendering the proper service to the heavenly, there is nothing like moderation." The passage continues, "It is only by this moderation that there is effected an early return (to man's normal state). That early return is what I call the repeated accumulation of the attributes (of the Tao). With that repeated accumulation of those attributes, there comes the subjugation (of every obstacle to such return). Of this subjugation we know not what shall be the limit; and when one knows not what the limit shall be, he may be the ruler of a state." (*Lao-Tse. The Tao Teh King. The Tao and Its Characteristics,* Translated by James Legge, 1880, Section 59.1-2, reprinted in Project Gutenberg, http://www.gutenberg.org/ebooks/216.)

Also in the Western tradition, agreeing with Aristotle, moderation, particularly moderation in diet, has remained the prevailing life-extensionist consensus for centuries. (See, for example, a brief account: Steven Shapin, Christopher Martyn, "How to live forever: lessons of history," *British Medical Journal,* 321, 1580-1582, 2000.) However, it has never been agreed on what exactly a "moderate" measure is. And yet, despite the uncertainties regarding the exact "moderate" measure, the importance of moderation, of consuming less than people usually do, has been emphasized throughout by most researchers of aging, up to the modern period. The proponents of this view included, for example, the life-extensionist hygienists such as Luigi Cornaro (1467-1566, *Discorso sulla vita sobria* - Discourse on a sober life, 1566), Leonardus Lessius (1554-1623, *A Treatise of Health and Long Life - Hygiasticon*, 1613), Hufeland (*Macrobiotics*, 1796), and other authors. (See: *A Treatise of Health and Long Life, with the Sure Means of Attaining It. In 2 Books. The first By Leonard Lessius. The Second by Lewis Cornaro, Translated into English by Timothy Smith*, London, C. Hitch, 1743.)

The research on life-prolongation by calorie restriction may be one of the ramifications of this tradition. Some of the prominent studies of calorie restriction for life extension included:

C.M. McCay, W.E. Dilly, M.F. Crowell, "Growth rates of brook trout reared upon purified rations, upon skim milk diets, and upon combinations of cereal grains," *Journal of Nutrition*, 1, 233-246, 1929;

Clive McCay, "The Effect of Retarded Growth Upon the Length of Life Span and upon the Ultimate Body Size," *Journal of Nutrition*, 10, 63-79, 1935;

Richard Weindruch, Roy L. Walford, *The Retardation of Aging and Disease by Dietary Restriction*, Charles C. Thomas, Springfield, Illinois, 1988;

Luigi Fontana, Linda Partridge, Valter D. Longo, "Extending Healthy Life Span – From Yeast to Humans," *Science*, 328(5976), 321-326, 2010;

Eric Ravussin, Leanne M. Redman, James Rochon, et al., "A 2-Year Randomized Controlled Trial of Human Caloric Restriction: Feasibility and Effects on Predictors of Health Span and Longevity," *Journal of Gerontology: Medical Sciences*, 70(9), 1097-1104, 2015.

Perhaps one of the very few dissenters from this consensus for dietary moderation was the famous French lawyer, physician and gastronome Jean Anthelme Brillat-Savarin (1755-1826). In his *Physiologie du goût* (*The Physiology of Taste*, 1825), Brillat-Savarin spoke of the "Longevity of Gourmands" and claimed:

"I am happy, I cannot be more so, to inform my readers that good cheer is far from being injurious, and that all things being equal, gourmands live longer than other people. This was proved by a scientific dissertation recently read at the academy, by Doctor Villermet [the hygienist Louis René Villermé, 1782-1863]. ... Those who indulge in good cheer, are rarely, or never sick. ... as all portions of their organization are better sustained, nature has more resources, and the body incomparably resists destruction."

(Jean Anthelme Brillat-Savarin, *The Physiology of Taste; or, Transcendental Gastronomy* (Translated by Fayette Robinson), Lindsay & Blakiston, Philadelphia, 1854, pp. 194-196, first published in 1825, http://www.gutenberg.org/cache/epub/5434/pg5434.html.)

Still, even when asserting the value of moderation, it is now often emphasized that the meals need to be "nutritious" – that is, to provide all the necessary substances and sufficient energy. Yet in many cases those "necessities" are not well defined. Thus, the ambiguity exists, since Aristotle, regarding the exact measures of "heat" (energy) that is needed to be expended or "conserved" for life-prolongation.

58. *On Length and Shortness of Life*, 466b8-28, p. 743.

59. Since Aristotle's times, well until modernity, the concept of "innate heat conservation" had important implications for practical therapy. In the pre-chemotherapeutic era, many techniques employed by physicians/medicine-men for the conservation of the "vital heat" – such as drug-sedation, starving, blood-letting, freezing, purging, and even incantation – were designed to overcome stimulation and quiet the person down. This view was fundamentally opposed to the idea of exercise or internal stimulation as a means to counter the threat of destruction by the environment.

One instance of this controversy was the opposition between the views of the English physician John Brown (1810-1882), the proponent of physiological excitation or exercise, as opposed to the views of the French physician François-Joseph Broussais (1772-1838), the advocate of physiological inhibition as the path to conserving the vital energy and hence increasing longevity.

The French historian of medicine Charles Daremberg poignantly noted the old conflict between the Stimulation and Relaxation schools (1870):

"All of [John] Brown's patients were destined to become athletes. All of Broussais's were supposed to be reduced to the state of diaphanous bodies. One left Brown's care with a ruddy complexion, Broussais's as a pale and a winding sheet. For Brown stimulation was the remedy, for Broussais irritation was the ill."

(Charles Daremberg, *Histoire des sciences médicales*, 1870, quoted in Georges Canguilhem, "John Brown's system: An Example of Medical Ideology," in *Ideology and Rationality in the History of the Life Sciences*, translated from French by Arthur Goldhammer, Cambridge MA, The Massachusetts Institute of Technology Press, 1988, article note 11, p. 49.

See also: William Randall Albury, "Ideas of Life and Death," in *Companion Encyclopedia of the History of Medicine*, Edited by William F. Bynum and Roy Porter, Routledge, London and New York, 2001, pp. 253-254.)

Interestingly, both the stimulatory and inhibitory approaches agree with the vitalist conception of life and longevity. The vitalist perception of the lifespan as determined by a limited amount of "vital force" that can be "exhausted," even though ostensibly fatalistic, nonetheless offers several theoretical possibilities for life prolongation. A good explanation was provided by the German gerontologist Max Bürger in *Altern und Krankheit* (Aging and Disease) as recently as 1954, going back to Aristotle's original concept of entelechy. Basically, the vital force of entelechy could be enhanced by manipulating body structure. First of all, the life force can be conserved by diminishing activity (in line with the inhibitory approach). Yet, on the other hand, the body structure can be reduced – for example, by dissolving structure or by amputation – to "free the room" for a continued action of the "vital force." In this way, Bürger writes, "the catastrophic end can be postponed either by dissolving structure or by a forced regeneration after amputation." In this view, during a moderate exercise, some body structures become partly worn out, the life force receives a "new room" to operate and rebuilds the lost structures even stronger than before (that would agree with the stimulatory approach). And thirdly, the immaterial "vital force" could be directly affected by another "immaterial" entity – the mind (an "intellectual faculty" in Aristotle's terms).

(Max Bürger, *Altern und Krankheit* (Aging and Disease), Leipzig, 1954 (1947), "Das Altern im Lichte der vitalistischen Autonomielehre" (Aging in the light of the theory of vitalistic autonomy), pp. 39-41.)

Though Aristotle was not that explicit, he nonetheless pioneered the conceptual and terminological framework for this discussion. In practical terms, the relative merits and specific indications, thresholds and balances of stimulatory exercise vs. inhibitory conservation of life's energy for life prolongation, still appear to be unclear.

60. William A. Calder, *Size, Function, and Life History,* Harvard University Press, Cambridge MA, 1984;

Knut Schmidt-Nielsen, *Scaling: Why is Animal Size So Important?* Cambridge University Press, Cambridge UK, 1984;

João Pedro de Magalhães, "Comparative Biology of Aging," Senescence Info, 2004, http://www.senescence.info/comparative.html.

61. Christoph Wilhelm Hufeland, *Makrobiotik; oder, Die Kunst das menschliche Leben zu verlängern*, Sechste verbesserte Auflage, A.F. Macklot, Stuttgart, 1826 (Macrobiotics or the art of prolonging human life, the 6th improved edition), first published in 1796 in Jena for Gotthold Ludwig Fiedler, Academische Buchhandlung.

The book is available in several languages, including Russian: *Iskusstvo Prodlevat Chelovecheskuyu Zhizn (Macrobiotika)*, translated by P. Zablotsky, E. Pratz Typography, St. Petersburg, 1852, republished by Leila, St. Petersburg, 1996.

It is also available in English: *The Art of Prolonging Life*, Edited by Erasmus Wilson, Lindsay & Blakiston, Philadelphia, 1867 (the latter edition is used here, and is hereafter referred to as "Hufeland, *Macrobiotics*").

The influence of climate on longevity is considered in Hufeland's book, among other places, in Part 1, Ch. 6, Sections 4-5, p. 99-100.

62. Hufeland, *Macrobiotics,* Part 1, Ch. 6, Sections 4-5, pp. 99-100;

Zavadovskii A.F., Vavakin Iu.N., Korotaev M.M., "The effect of moderate altitude on the maintenance of a good health status and high physical work capacity in cosmonauts over the course of a long period of time," *Aviakosmicheskaya i Ekologicheskaya Medicina* (Aerocosmic and Ecologic Medicine), 26(4), 40-43, 1992 (in Russian);

Alexander Leaf, *Youth in Old Age*, McGraw-Hill Book Company, NY, 1975;

Dan Buettner, *The Blue Zones: Lessons for Living Longer From the People Who've Lived the Longest*, National Geographic, Washington DC, 2010;

Bloch K.F., "Why do the very aged become so old?" *Acta Biotheoretica*, 28(2), 135-144, 1979.

Just by looking at the world map of life-expectancy, it can be seen that countries with colder climates (e.g. the Scandinavian countries and Canada) are generally characterized by a greater life-expectancy than tropical ("hot and humid") countries (e.g. most of Africa and Latin America). Of course, there are also many other parameters at play.

http://www.who.int/gho/mortality_burden_disease/life_tables/situation_trends/en/;

http://gamapserver.who.int/gho/interactive_charts/mbd/life_expectancy/atlas.html;

http://www.mapsofworld.com/thematic-maps/world-life-expectancy-map.htm;

http://www.worldlifeexpectancy.com/world-life-expectancy-map.

Though exceptions from those "rules" are obvious, and arguments can be made both for the benefits of a "warm" or "cold" climate. Clearly, an enormous amount of factors are unaccounted for by the temptingly simple "climatic-geographic" theory of longevity. As Hufeland points out as well in the referenced sections, both extreme cold and heat, and the rapid oscillations of cold and heat, are detrimental for longevity. The question still remains regarding the exact definition of "warm" vs. "cold" climate, beyond common intuitive perception. Nonetheless, the assumption of the influence of climate, of the environment, on human and animal lifespan appears to be commonsensical and Aristotle's contribution to this field of study may have been groundbreaking.

63. Mary Shaw, Helena Tunstall, George Davey Smith, "Seeing social position: visualizing class in life and death," *International Journal of Epidemiology*, 32(3), 332-335, 2003;

Jong-In Kim, "Longevity and occupation," *Age and Ageing*, 31(6), 485-486, 2002.

64. On the benefits of physical exercise for healthy longevity, see for example:

James Rollin Slonaker, "The normal activity of the albino rat from birth to natural death, its rate of growth, and duration of life," *Journal of Animal Behavior*, 2, 20-42, 1912;

Alexander Vasilievich Nagorny, "K voprosu o faktorakh, obuslovlivayushikh dlitelnost zhizni" (On the question of factors determining the duration of life), in *Starost. Trudy Konferenzii po Probleme Geneza Starosti I Profilaktiki Prezhdevremennogo Starenia Organisma. Kiev 17-19 Decabria. 1938*, Izdatelstvo Akademii Nauk USSR, Kiev, 1939 (Aging. Proceedings of the Conference on the Problem of the Genesis of Aging and Prophylaxis of the Organism's Untimely Aging, Kiev, December 17-19, 1938, Publication of The Ukrainian Soviet Socialist Republic Academy of Sciences, Kiev, 1939), pp. 156-172;

Blain H., Vuillemin A., Blain A., Jeandel C., "The preventive effects of physical activity in the elderly," *Presse Médicale*, 29(22), 1240-1248, 2000;

I-Min Lee, Ralph S. Paffenbarger Jr., "Associations of light, moderate, and vigorous intensity physical activity with longevity. The Harvard Alumni Health Study," *American Journal of Epidemiology*, 151(3), 293-299, 2000;

Lee I.M., Paffenbarger R.S., Hennekens C.H., "Physical activity, physical fitness and longevity," *Aging* (Milano), 9(1-2), 2-11, 1997;

Matthew M. Robinson, Surendra Dasari, Adam R. Konopka, Matthew L. Johnson, S. Manjunatha, Raul Ruiz Esponda, Rickey E. Carter, Ian R. Lanza, K. Sreekumaran Nair, "Enhanced Protein Translation Underlies Improved Metabolic and Physical Adaptations to Different Exercise Training Modes in Young and Old Humans," *Cell Metabolism*, 25(3), 581-592, 2017.

Generally, physical exercise has been regarded as beneficial for longevity. Yet, there have been conflicting findings.

Thus, it was found that athletes live longer than normal insured men, but shorter than "physically underdeveloped" people. (Louis I. Dublin, "Longevity of college athletes," *Harper's Monthly Magazine*, 157, 229-238, 1928.)

It was also found that athletes live longer in general. (Martti J. Karvonen, "Endurance sports, longevity and health," *Annals of the New York Academy of Sciences*, 301, 653-655, 1977.)

And it was also found that athletes live shorter in general. (Peter V. Karpovich, "Longevity and athletics," *Research Quarterly*, 12, 451-455, 1941.)

And there were also found no significant differences. (Henry J. Montoye, et al., *The Longevity and Morbidity of College Athletes*, Indianapolis, 1957.)

The results also varied widely depending on the type of sports, level of athleticism, period of practice, and many other factors. (Anthony P. Polednak (Ed.), *The Longevity of Athletes*, Charles C. Thomas, Springfield IL, 1979.)

It was also shown that "blue-collar," physically active workers live shorter than sedentary "white-collar" workers. But this was explained by the assumption that the "white-collar" workers were able to exercise regularly, in a protected environment, and with sufficient rest. (Charles L. Rose and

Michel L. Cohen, "Relative importance of physical activity for longevity," *Annals of the New York Academy of Sciences*, 301, 671-702, 1977.)

(These works are reviewed in William G. Bailey, *Human Longevity from Antiquity to the Modern Lab*, Greenwood Press, Westport CN, 1987, "Athleticism and Exercise," pp. 98-104.)

Further complicating the picture, Howard Friedman and Leslie Martin's *The Longevity Project. Surprising Discoveries for Health and Long Life from the Landmark Eight-Decade Study*, Hudson Streen Press, Penguin Group, NY, March 2011, suggests that cheerful and relaxed people tended to live shorter than "prudent and persistent" individuals (p. 9) and that strenuous exercise does not necessarily lead to greater longevity (pp. 105-106).

65. *On Length and Shortness of Life*, 4. 466b8-17, p. 743.

66. There has been a vast, ancient tradition advising on sexual moderation in order to achieve life extension, from Aristotle, through Taoist physicians, to the Renaissance and early modern hygienists (Luigi Cornaro, Leonardus Lessius, Christoph Wilhelm Hufeland, and others). Some (rare) more recent examples of this attitude are Edwin Flatto's *Warning: Sex May Be Hazardous to Your Health* (1977) or David Pratt's *Sex and Sexuality* (2002). See:

Aristotle, *On Length and Shortness of Life*, Aristotle, *On Youth, Old Age, Life and Death, and Respiration*, translated by G.R.T. Ross, in *The Complete Works of Aristotle: The Revised Oxford Translation*, Princeton University Press, Princeton, 1984, Vol. 1, pp. 740-744, 745-763;

Aelius/Claudius Galenus (c. 129-217 CE), Galen, *De tuenda Sanitate. Gerontocomia (On the Preservation of Health. Gerontocomia)*, quoted in Sir John Floyer [1649-1734], *Medicina gerocomica, or, The Galenic art of preserving old men's healths*, J. Isted, London, 1725, p. 107;

Gabriele Zerbi (1445-1505), *Gerontocomia, scilicet de senium cura atque victu* ("Gerontocomia, or, care and nutrition for old age), Rome, 1489;

Hufeland, *Macrobiotics*, "Part 2 - Means which Shorten Life, Ch. 2 - Physical excess in youth," pp. 163-164; "Part 3 - Means which prolong life, Ch. 4 – Abstinence from physical love in youth, and a too early assumption of the married state," pp. 225-228;

A Treatise of Health and Long Life, with the Sure Means of Attaining It. In 2 Books. The first By Leonard Lessius. The Second by Lewis Cornaro, Translated into English by Timothy Smith, London, C. Hitch, 1743;

Gerald J. Gruman, *A History of Ideas about the Prolongation of Life. The Evolution of Prolongevity Hypotheses to 1800*, Transactions of the American Philosophical Society, Vol. 56(9), Philadelphia, 1966, in particular "Taoist prolongevitism in theory," pp. 28-37, and "Taoist prolongevitism in practice," pp. 37-49;

Edwin Flatto, *Warning: Sex May Be Hazardous to Your Health*, 2nd edition, Arco, New York, 1977;

David Pratt, *Sex and Sexuality*, 3.6. "Pleasure at a Price," New York, 2002.

67. Hufeland, *Macrobiotics*, "Part 2 - Means which Shorten Life, Ch. 2 - Physical excess in youth," pp. 163-164; "Part 3 - Means which prolong life, Ch. 4 – Abstinence from physical love in youth, and a too early assumption of the married state," pp. 225-228;

Thomas W. Laqueur, *Solitary sex: a cultural history of masturbation*, Zone Books, New York, 2003.

68. A series of studies showed the costs of reproduction for longevity in animal models, for example:

Jens Rolff, Michael T. Siva-Jothy, "Copulation corrupts immunity: a mechanism for a cost of mating in insects," *Proceedings of the National Academy of Sciences USA*, 99(15), 9916-9918, 2002;

Wayne A. Van Voorhies, "Production of sperm reduces nematode lifespan," *Nature*, 360, 456-458, 1992;

Casandra L. Rauser, Laurence D. Mueller, Michael R. Rose, "Aging, fertility, and immortality," *Experimental Gerontology*, 38(1-2), 27-33, 2003.

More generally, according to the "Disposable Soma" theory of aging, energy expenditures on reproduction come at the cost of energy expenditures on the maintenance of the body:

Tom Kirkwood, *Time of Our Lives. The Science of Human Aging*, Oxford University Press, Oxford, 1999.

And in the "Phenoptosis" or "programmed aging" theory, sex is considered as a trigger of the 'self-destruct' mechanism in animals:

Vladimir P. Skulachev, "Aging is a specific biological function rather than the result of a disorder in complex living systems: biochemical evidence in support of Weismann's hypothesis," *Biochemistry*, Moscow, 62(11), 1191-1195, 1997.

69. The indications for the potential life-prolonging effects of sexual moderation or abstinence in humans include the findings of the consistently higher longevity among monks:

Bartosz Jenner, "Changes in average life span of monks and nuns in Poland in the years 1950-2000," *Przeglad Lekarski*, 59(4-5), 225-229, 2002;

de Gouw H.W., Westendorp R.G., Kunst A.E., Mackenbach J.P., Vandenboucke J.P., "Decreased mortality among contemplative monks in The Netherlands," *American Journal of Epidemiology*, 141(8), 771-775, 1995;

Marc Luy, "Sex differences in mortality - time to take a second look," *Zeitschrift für Gerontologie und Geriatrie*, 35(5), 412-429, 2002;

Marc Luy, Katrin Gast, "Do Women Live Longer or Do Men Die Earlier? Reflections on the Causes of Sex Differences in Life Expectancy," *Gerontology*, 60, 143-153, 2014;

Marc Luy, *Klosterstudie zur Lebenserwartung von Nonnen und Mönchen* (The "Closter" study of life-expectancy in nuns and monks), http://www.klosterstudie.de/.

There have also been indications about the longer life span of eunuchs:

James B. Hamilton, Gordon E. Mestler, "Mortality and survival: comparison of eunuchs with intact men and women in a mentally retarded population," *Journal of Gerontology*, 24(4), 395-411, 1969;

John P. Phelan, Michael R. Rose, "Why dietary restriction substantially increases longevity in animal models but won't in humans," *Aging Research Reviews*, 4(3), 339-350, 2005;

Kyung-Jin Min, Cheol-Koo Lee, Han-Nam Park, "The lifespan of Korean eunuchs," *Current Biology*, 22(18), R792–R793, 2012.

70. Presently, even when discussing the "disposable soma theory," the "phenoptosis theory" or the "costs of reproduction" – sexual moderation in humans is hardly ever recommended. Instead, there is a common popular belief that "sex is good for longevity."

"Sex is good," for example, according to Dr. Mark Stibich http://longevity.about.com/od/lifelongrelationships/p/sex_longevity.htm; Dr. Michael Roizen http://www.scribd.com/doc/24835112/Longevity-Sex; Dr. Kevin Netto http://www.worldhealth.net/news/science-says-you-should-have-more-sex/; or the "sensual product designer" Anne Enke http://www.anneofcarversville.com/superyoung/sex-and-longevity-health-benefits-of-loving-sex.html; and many more such examples of the popular stance can be added.

A single most widely cited study in this approach is: George Davey Smith, Stephen Frankel, John Yarnell, "Sex and death: are they related? Findings from the Caerphilly cohort study," *British Medical Journal*, 315, 1641-1644, 1997, which correlated between high sexual activity and lower mortality in a group of aged men.

The majority of authors now heavily emphasize the possibility and desirability of sex for the aged, the benefits of sex with a constant partner, its positive role for the production of stress-reducing hormones, and for the improvement of self-image and connection. See for example:

Normal Aging: Reports from the Duke Longitudinal Study, 1955-1969, edited by Erdman Palmore, Duke University Press, Durham NC, 1970, pp. 266-303;

Nathan W. Shock, et al., *Normal Human Aging: The Baltimore Longitudinal Study of Aging*, NIH Publication, 1984, pp. 164-165;

Thomas H. Walz, Nancee S. Blum, *Sexual Health in Later Life*, Lexington Books, Lexington MA, 1987;

Modig K., Talbäck M., Torssander J., Ahlbom A., "Payback time? Influence of having children on mortality in old age," *Journal of Epidemiology & Community Health*, pii: jech-2016-207857, March 2017.

In animal models, the longevity benefits of mating were also found, for example:

Alexandra Schrempf, Jürgen Heinze, Sylvia Cremer, "Sexual cooperation: mating increases longevity in ant queens," *Current Biology*, 15, 267-270, 2005.

The terms "exhaustion" and "moderation," that had been prevalent among the earlier hygienists, are now hardly ever present, and at any rate the possibility of a "threshold" or "tradeoff" in sexual activity with reference to human longevity is hardly ever considered.

71. Jose Viña, Consuelo Borrás, Juan Gambini, Juan Sastre, Federico V. Pallardó, "Why females live longer than males? Importance of the upregulation of longevity-associated genes by oestrogenic compounds," *FEBS Letters*, 579(12), 2541-2545, 2005;

Marc Luy, Katrin Gast, "Do Women Live Longer or Do Men Die Earlier? Reflections on the Causes of Sex Differences in Life Expectancy," *Gerontology*, 60, 143-153, 2014.

72. Concerning gender-specific longevity, women might not have been always longer-lived than men. Female relative life spans were likely shorter in the past (due to higher mortality at childbirth):

Irvine Loudon, "Deaths in childbed from the eighteenth century to 1935," *Medical History*, 30(1), 1-41, 1986.

73. *On Length and Shortness of Life*, 5. 466a20-24; 466b3-8; 466b33-467a5; 6. 467a6-9, pp. 742-743.

74. "Fat," *Oxford Dictionary of Science*, Oxford University Press, 1999, p. 302; Fogiel, *The Biology Problem Solver*, 17.3, pp. 509-510; 2.31. p. 68.

75. *On Length and Shortness of Life*, 3. 465b17-21, p. 741; 5. 466b4-8, p. 743; *On Youth and Old Age*, 23, 479a14-27, pp. 760-761; 26. 479b18-18, p. 761.

76. "Allosteric Regulation," Wikipedia, accessed June 2017, https://en.wikipedia.org/wiki/Allosteric_regulation; Fogiel, *The Biology Problem Solver*, 3.19, p. 98; 3.3. p. 82; 24.26, p. 787.

77. Rajindar S. Sohal, "Role of oxidative stress and protein oxidation in the aging process," *Free Radical Biology and Medicine*, 33(1), 37-44, 2002; Rajindar S. Sohal, "Oxidative stress hypothesis of aging," *Free Radical Biology and Medicine*, 33(5), 573-574, 2002.

78. Aristotle, *On Sleep* (Translated by J.I. Beare), in *The Complete Works of Aristotle: The Revised Oxford Translation* (Edited by Jonathan Barnes), Vol. 1, Princeton University Press, Princeton, 1984, 1. 453b26-27, p. 721; 454a24-31, p. 722; 454b31-455a3, p.723; 455b20-22, p. 724; 457b1-6, pp. 726-727; 458a-26-32, p. 728 (hereafter referred to as "*On Sleep*").

79. *On Sleep*, 456b18457b2, pp. 725-726.

80. Alan H. Cromer, *Physics for the life sciences*, McGraw Hill Inc., New York, 1974, Ch. 6.5. "Feedback and Control," pp. 118-125 (hereafter referred to as "Cromer, *Physics*").

81. Vladimir M. Kovalzon, Tatyana V. Strekalova, "Delta sleep-inducing peptide (DSIP): a still unresolved riddle," *Journal of Neurochemistry*, 97(2), 303-309, 2006;

György Buzsáki, Andreas Draguhn, "Neuronal oscillations in cortical networks," *Science*, 304, 1926-1929, 2004;

Tarja Porkka-Heiskanen, Robert E. Strecker, Mahesh Thakkar, Alvhild A. Bjørkum, Robert W. Greene, Robert W. McCarley, "Adenosine: a mediator of the sleep-inducing effects of prolonged wakefulness," *Science*, 276, 1265-1268, 1997.

82. Karine Spiegel, Rachel Leproult, Eve Van Cauter, "Impact of sleep debt on metabolic and endocrine function," *The Lancet*, 354(9188), 1435-1439, 1999;

Mark R. Zielinski, Dmitry Gerashchenko, Svetlana A. Karpova, Varun Konanki, Robert W. McCarley, Fayyaz S. Sutterwala, Robert E. Strecker, Radhika Basheer, "The NLRP3 inflammasome modulates sleep and NREM sleep delta power induced by spontaneous wakefulness, sleep deprivation and lipopolysaccharide," *Brain, Behavior, and Immunity*, 62, 137-150, 2017;

Tatiana-Danai Dimitriou, Magdalini Tsolaki, "Evaluation of the efficacy of randomized controlled trials of sensory stimulation interventions for sleeping disturbances in patients with dementia: a systematic review," *Clinical Interventions in Aging*, 12, 543-548, 2017.

83. *On Sleep*, 457b27-458a9, p. 727.

84. David G. Nicholls, Stuart Ferguson, *Bioenergetics* (Fourth Edition), Academic Press, London, 2013;

Fogiel, *The Biology Problem Solver*, Sections 2.29-2.32, pp. 66-69; 15.2, pp. 458-9; 3.6. p. 84.

85. *On Sleep*, 455b34-456a23, pp. 724-25.

86. Valentín Fuster, "Applied Cardiological Research. Challenges for the New Millennium," *Revista Española de Cardiología* (English Edition), 55, 327-332, 2002;

Judith Meadows, Jacqueline Suk Danik, Michelle A. Albert, "Primary prevention of ischemic heart disease," in Elliott M. Antman (Ed.), *Cardiovascular Therapeutics: A Companion to Braunwald's Heart Disease*, Third edition, Saunders Elsevier, Philadelphia PA, 178-220, 2007;

Roger Yu, Kaveh Navab, Mohamad Navab, "Near term prospects for ameliorating cardiovascular aging," in Gregory M. Fahy, Michael D. West, L. Stephen Coles, Steven B. Harris (Eds.), *The Future of Aging: Pathways to Human Life Extension*, Springer, New York, 2010, pp. 279-306.

87. *On Youth and Old Age*, 26. 479b17-480a15, pp. 761-762.

88. *On Length and Shortness of Life*, 467a12-29, pp.743-744.

89. Oberley L.W., Oberley T.D., Buettner G.R., "Cell differentiation, aging and cancer: the possible roles of superoxide and superoxide dismutases," *Medical Hypotheses*, 6(3), 249-268, 1980.

90. Gretchen Vogel, "How does a single somatic cell become a whole plant?" *Science*, 309(5731), 86, 2005;

Gretchen Vogel, "How can a skin cell become a nerve cell?" *Science*, 309(5731), 85, 2005;

R. John Davenport, "What controls organ regeneration?" *Science*, 309(5731), 84, 2005.

91. Thomas C. Vinci, Jason Scott Robert, "Aristotle and Modern Genetics," *Journal of the History of Ideas*, 66(2), 201-221, 2005;

Ernst Mayr, *This is Biology: The Science of the Living World*, Harvard University Press, Cambridge, Massachusetts, 1997, p. 154;

Ernst Mayr, *The Growth of Biological Thought: Diversity, Evolution, and Inheritance*, Harvard University Press, Cambridge, Massachusetts, 1982, p. 89.

92. *On the Soul* (Translated by J.A. Smith), in *The Complete Works of Aristotle: The Revised Oxford Translation* (Edited by Jonathan Barnes), Princeton University Press, Princeton, 1984, Vol.1, 416b22-26, p. 663.

93. *On Length and Shortness of Life*, 6. 467a6-9, p. 743.

94. *On Length and Shortness of Life*, 467a12, p. 743.

95. *On the Soul* (translated by W.S. Hett), 1.5. 411b24-31, p. 65.

96. Metchnikoff, *On the Nature of Man*, pp. 227, 230;

On various concepts of the "limit" to the animal and human lifespan, see: Ilia Stambler, *A History of Life-Extensionism in the Twentieth Century*, Longevity History, 2014, Chapter 4, Section 10 - Rectifying "Discord" and conserving "Vital Capital," pp. 198-201, note 876 (on-line edition)/note 873 (print edition), pp. 409-410, http://www.longevityhistory.com/book/indexb.html#_edn876.

97. *On Length and Shortness of Life*, 3. 465b1-21, p. 741.

98. Avicenna, "On Causes of Health and Illness and the Inevitability of Death," in *The Canon of Medical Science, Selected Parts* (edited by U.I. Karimov, E.U. Hurshut), FAN Publisher of the Uzbekistan Academy of Sciences, Tashkent, 1994, Part 1, pp. 128-129 (in Russian, translated from Arabic by A. Rasulev, U.I. Karimov).

99. Leonard Hayflick, Paul S. Moorhead, "The serial cultivation of human diploid cell strains," *Experimental Cell Research*, 25, 585-621, 1961;

Leonard Hayflick, *How and Why we Age*, Ballantine Books, NY, 1994, "No More Aging: Blessing or Nightmare?" pp. 336-338.

100. Arthur Leslie Peck, "Introduction to Aristotle's *Generation of Animals*," in *Aristotle in Twenty-Three Volumes*, William Heinemann Ltd., London, 1975, Vol. XIII, p. L.

101. Cromer, *Physics*, "Entropy" Section 11.5, pp. 228-229.

102. Plato (427-347 BCE) – or Socrates (469 –399 BCE) in Plato's corpus – seemed to opt for the afterlife. In the "Allegory of the Cave" (*The Republic*, Book VII), Plato appeared to employ a perceptual stratagem to bring home the notion of the soul's immortality: if we believe that we can cast shadows, we can be also made to believe that the pure form, indestructible shadows can cast us, that shadows of the other realm constitute our essence.

(Plato, *The Republic*, Translated by Paul Shorey, in *The Collected Dialogues of Plato, Including the Letters* (Edited by Edith Hamilton and Huntington

Cairns), Princeton University Press, Princeton, New Jersey, 1961, Book VII. Allegory of the Cave, 7.514-7.518, pp. 747-750.)

103. In contrast to Plato's idealism, Epicurus (342-270 BCE) asserted the utter and final disintegration upon death. Epicurus' resignation to the finality of death is complete, as expressed in his *Letter to Menoeceus*. According to Epicurus, a person must live in "fullness of pleasure" banishing the fear of death: "The wise man neither seeks to escape life nor fears the cessation of life, for neither does life offend him nor does the absence of life seem to be any evil."

(Epicurus, *Letter to Menoeceus*, Translated by Cyril Bailey, in *The Stoic and Epicurean Philosophers. The Complete Extant Writings of Epicurus, Epictetus, Lucretius, Marcus Aurelius* (Edited by Whitney J. Oates), The Modern Library, New York, 1957, pp. 30-31.)

104. *On the Soul* (translated by J.A Smith), 5. 430a10-26.

105. Aristotle, *On the Heavens* (Translated by J.L. Stocks), in *The Complete Works of Aristotle: The Revised Oxford Translation* (Edited by Jonathan Barnes), Princeton University Press, Princeton, 1984, Book 1. Chapters 1, 2, Vol. 1, 184ª10-186ª3, pp. 315-317.

106. Aristotle, *Physics* (Translated by R.P. Hardie and R.K. Gaye), in *The Complete Works of Aristotle: The Revised Oxford Translation* (Edited by Jonathan Barnes), Princeton University Press, Princeton, 1984, Book 1. Ch. 3, Vol. 1, 270ᵇ1-270ᵇ25, pp. 450-451.

107. Aristotle, *On the Soul* (Translated with notes by Walter Stanley Hett), in *Aristotle in Twenty-Three Volumes*, William Heinemann Ltd., London, 1975, "Book 1. Ch. 2. Previous Theories as to the Nature of the Soul," Vol. VIII, pp. 19-31.

108. Walter Stanley Hett, "Introduction to Aristotle's *On the Soul*," in *Aristotle in Twenty-Three Volumes*, William Heinemann Ltd., London, 1975, Vol. VIII, pp. vi-vii.

109. Arthur Leslie Peck, "Appendix B to Aristotle's *Generation of Animals*," in *Aristotle in Twenty-Three Volumes*, William Heinemann Ltd., London, 1975, Vol. XIII, pp. 578-593.

110. Ilia Stambler, *A History of Life-Extensionism in the Twentieth Century*, Longevity History, 2014, http://www.longevityhistory.com/.

IV. LONGEVITY SCIENCE

16. Potential Interventions to Ameliorate Degenerative Aging

A long road ahead

The interventions into the degenerative aging process are still in their infancy.[1] A long effortful road will yet need to be traveled from basic research on cell cultures and animal models to effective, safe and widely available human therapies.[2] Many dangers to human health (such as overdose and overstimulation) and many unsubstantiated false claims yet await on this road, that need to be guarded against as much as possible.[3] Yet vast promising research is progressing, especially as regards potential pharmaceutical interventions into the aging process.[4,5] Below are some examples.

1. Targeting Aging with Metformin

On November 28, 2015, the FDA approved the testing of Metformin, a decades-old anti-diabetic (blood sugar reducing) medication (of the biguanide class), as the first drug to treat degenerative aging, rather than particular diseases or symptoms, as a way to prevent general age-associated multimorbidity (postponing the emergence of several age-related diseases and dysfunctions at once).[6,7] Though the study concept may be seminal, as of this writing in 2017, sufficient funding for this trial has been lacking.

2. Anti-aging adjuvant therapy

On November 25, 2015, the FDA approved an adjuvant therapy (the adjuvant MF59, made with squalene oil, developed by Novartis) for a flu vaccine to boost immune response in older persons. This development goes beyond "a drug against a disease" model, but seeks an appropriate regulatory framework to support the underlying health of older persons, using "adjuvant" (i.e. "supportive/additional") therapy.[8]

3. Rapamycin and rapalogs

The immunosuppressant drug Rapamycin, believed to mimic the healthspan-extending effects of calorie restriction (CR-mimetic), has been shown to produce improvements of energy metabolism, and to extend lifespan and delay aging in mice, and was also effective against particular aging-related diseases, such as Alzheimer's disease, in human studies. Further research is done on Rapamycin's analogs – the so-called "rapalogs," potentially with less side effects.[9]

4. Blood transfusion

By splicing the circulatory systems of animals (mice) together, via the process of "parabiosis," young blood was indicated to have rejuvenating effects on old tissues, including the heart, brain, and muscle tissues, with improved strength and cognitive ability. Some of the hypothetical rejuvenating factors included: Notch signaling activators, deactivation of the transforming growth factor (TGF)-β that blocks cell division, oxytocin, and Growth Differentiation Factor 11 (GDF11). In September 2014, a clinical trial by Alkahest in Menlo Park, California, became the first to start testing the benefits of young blood and young plasma in older people with Alzheimer's disease.[10] However, in a more recent evaluation, it was suggested that young blood does not contain rejuvenating substances, but rather the old blood contains pro-aging, growth-inhibiting substances (or toxic waste products) that can accelerate aging in younger animals, and these can be partly diluted or neutralized by the infusions of young blood. The search has begun for such pro-aging, growth-inhibiting substances and ways of their neutralization.[11]

5. Senescent cell elimination

A new class of drugs – the "senolytics" capable of eliminating senescent cells and the accompanying pathologies – are being developed, in Mayo Clinic, Rochester, Minnesota, and elsewhere.[12] Thus, the combinations of the "senolytic" drugs Dasatinib and Quercetin proved effective against senescent human cells and in a mouse model. Together these drugs were able to reduce senescent cell burden, extend healthspan and improve physical exercise capacity in old mice, reducing their osteoporosis and other age-related pathologies.[13] Senescent cells can also be eliminated by immunological means, such as vaccines, antibodies and killer T cells.[14]

6. Sirtuin activation and NAD replacement therapy

Resveratrol, a natural polyphenolic compound, among other sources found in red wine, has demonstrated the ability to up-regulate Sirtuin 1 (SIRT1) – an acknowledged prolongevity enzyme[15] – important for enhanced stress response, DNA stabilization, cardiovascular protection, improved cognitive function and synaptic plasticity, and suppressing inflammation.[16] SIRT1 expression is generally related to the levels of energy metabolism, as indicated by NAD/NADH levels, which have also become targets for diverse pharmaceutical interventions (NAD replacement therapy).[17] Additional forms of NAD replacement therapy (e.g. with nicotinamide riboside – NR – a form of vitamin B3, and nicotinamide mononucleotide – NMN)[18,19] and activators of other Sirtuin enzymes (such as SIRT6)[20,21] are being developed.

7. pH and Redox manipulation

Dichloroacetate and bicarbonate represent a class of compounds and therapies that may have systemic effects on tissue redox and pH state, with broad implications for the aging process[22] and derivative pathologies, such as cancer.[23]

8. Regenerative medicine – extracorporeal and intracorporeal cell and tissue growth and replacement

Generally, regenerative medicine, using stem cells of various origins to rebuild, "regenerate" or improve the function of worn out and aging organs and tissues, can be promising for combating the degenerative pathologies of aging.[24] Even entire "replacement organs and tissues" can be grown outside of the body – using such methods as growing tissues on biodegradable scaffolds, 3D tissue printing, bioreactors or self-organization — to "replace" the worn out and aging body parts.[25] Yet, recently a very promising direction in regenerative medicine has emerged – the induction of regeneration within the body by pharmacological means (e.g. using inhibitors of prostaglandin breakdown, thus promoting cell proliferation).[26]

9. Immune organ regeneration

Of special importance for regenerative medicine against aging-related degeneration is the ability to regenerate the thymus gland (that produces the immune T-cells that play the crucial role for the immune defense). This importance derives from the fact that such an ability could dramatically improve therapy not only for aging-related non-communicable chronic diseases (such as heart disease and neurodegenerative diseases that are strongly related to altered immune response), but also help combat infectious, communicable diseases (like AIDS, Herpes and Influenza) thanks to improved immunity. Such regenerative ability for the thymus was shown by genetic engineering interventions (e.g. using over-expression of the FOXO gene)[27] and even pharmaceutical treatments (e.g. using the FGF21 hormone).[28]

241

10. Telomere extension to increase cell replication

The extension of the telomere end points of the chromosomes, thus increasing the number of cell replications, by such means as genetically engineered overexpression of the telomere-repairing enzyme – telomerase, and even by some pharmacological stimulators of telomerase activity, have been associated with increased lifespan and reduced pathology in animal models.[29,30]

11. Improving mitochondrial function

There have been many methods investigated for improving mitochondrial function and cellular respiration. Thus anti-oxidant molecules attached to positively charged ions (cations) have been targeted into mitochondria to eliminate oxidative damage at its origin (the SkQ ions).[31] In another approach, chemical compounds (in particular suppressors of the IIIQsite of the respiratory chain in the mitochondria) have been identified that can block the production of certain free radicals in cells, without changing the energy metabolism of these cells.[32] A large additional array of boosters of mitochondrial activity and cellular respiration has been proposed, e.g. methylene blue, the naphthoquinone drug β-lapachone, supplementation with various components of the respiratory oxidative phoshorylation system – such as CoQ10, pyruvate, succinate, vitamins C and K, quercetin, various other anti-acidic, anti-toxic, and anti-oxidant substances.[33]

12. Immune-modulating substances

Anti-inflammatory medications have been widely tested to diminish aging-related degenerative pathologies, such as neurodegenerative pathologies, and to extend healthy lifespan in animal models.[34] But also pro-inflammatory effects have been shown to be important for tissue regeneration.[35]

13. Cross-link breakers

Diverse means are being developed to dissolve macro-molecular (cross-linked) aggregates that "clog" cell machinery. Some approaches include stimulation of cell autophagy that can help remove such aggregates (e.g. by introducing Beclin protein). Various "AGE-breakers" are being developed. These are, as a rule, small molecules capable of breaking "Advanced Glycation Endproducts (AGE)" that are chiefly responsible for the formation of macromolecular aggregates (such as glucosepane, one of the most common forms of cross-linked AGE products in collagen). Some of the therapeutic means against cross-linked aggregates include chelators (removing the metal ions that are important for the formation of the cross-links), enzymatic clearance (oxidoreductive depolymerization of the aggregates by enzymes), immunoclearance (using immune mechanisms, e.g. antibodies, to remove the aggregates), etc.[36,37] Yet, it needs to be noted that macromolecular aggregates, in certain amounts and under certain circumstances, may have a necessary function in the body too.[38] Removing too much of them and in wrong places may do more damage than good.

14. Nutrient balance

Keeping the body chemistry in balance is hoped to be achieved by supplementing deficient elements in the diet (e.g. vitamins, microelements, other essential nutrients), while eliminating excessive and therefore toxic elements (by such means as chelators, enterosorbents, dietary restriction, enhanced elimination).[39] But what is "the balance"? How much is "too much" or "too little"? The guiding rule is always: "The dose makes the poison."[1] Dietary interventions, that are being tested, include dietary restrictions of various kinds (mainly protein restriction and calorie restriction) that have been associated with extended lifespan in animal models and some health benefits in humans.[40] Also new ways are being sought to enrich the "microbiome" (intestinal bacteria populations) for healthy longevity,[41] for example using probiotic diets – the idea that goes back to the origins of scientific aging research, over a century ago.[42]

15. Epigenetic rejuvenation

Epigenetics (acquired or heritable changes in gene function without changes in DNA sequence), has been increasingly investigated and manipulated for its effects on aging and aging-related diseases, and their amelioration, at the level of the entire organism as well as particular tissues, for example, using demethylating agents, small interfering RNAs (siRNAs) and micronutrients as potential therapeutic agents.[43-45]

16. Nanomedicine

Interventions into degenerative aging are now beginning to reach the "nano" level (using molecular structures and devices up to several hundred nanometers). Some of the uses of nanomedicine against degenerative aging include nanoparticles, such as Buckminsterfullerene or "bucky-ball" C60, with assumed antiviral, antioxidant, anti-amyloid, immune-stimulating and other therapeutic activities, and some reported lifespan-extending results in mice.[46] Moreover, there even have been announced the first operating medical nanorobots, mainly intended to assist in precise drug delivery, acting as prototypes of artificial immune cells.[47] These nanodevices were mainly intended to eliminate cancer cells, but could also be used to eliminate other types of cells, e.g. senescent cells. In another area of development, oxygenated micro-particles seem to be very promising for life extension, especially in critical conditions, as oxygen deprivation is the main (or even the ultimate) cause of death.[48]

17. Physical interventions

Anti-aging and life-extending interventions do not necessarily need to be chemical and biological, but can also be physical, in particular as relates to various resuscitation technologies (hypothermia and suspended animation,[49,50] oxygenation,[51-53] electromagnetic stimulation[54-56]). Such technologies represent probably the most veritable means for life extension, demonstrably saving people from an almost certain death. But similar principles could perhaps be used for more preventive treatments and in less acute cases.

18. Biomarkers of aging

It seems to be impossible to speak of "treating" or "curing degenerative aging" without the ability to diagnose this condition and to reliably assess the effectiveness of interventions against it.[2,3,57-59] Hence a wide array of biomarkers and clinical end points are being sought to diagnose degenerative aging and aging-related ill health, and to determine correct "biological age."[60-63] Clinically applicable and scientifically grounded diagnostic criteria and definitions for aging may also have profound encouraging implications for the regulation and promotion of research, development, application and distribution of anti-aging and life-extending and healthspan-extending therapies.[64,65]

Acknowledgement

I thank Steve Hill and Kevin Perrott for their suggestions.

References and notes

1. Ilia Stambler, *A History of Life-Extensionism in the Twentieth Century*, Longevity History, 2014, http://www.longevityhistory.com/.
2. Ilia Stambler, "Human life extension: opportunities, challenges, and implications for public health policy," in Alexander Vaiserman (Ed.), *Anti-*

aging Drugs: From Basic Research to Clinical Practice, Royal Society of Chemistry, London, 2017, pp. 535-564.

3. Ilia Stambler, "Recognizing degenerative aging as a treatable medical condition: methodology and policy," *Aging and Disease*, 8(5), 2017, http://www.aginganddisease.org/EN/10.14336/AD.2017.0130.

4. Kunlin Jin, James W. Simpkins, Xunming Ji, Miriam Leis, Ilia Stambler, "The critical need to promote research of aging and aging-related diseases to improve health and longevity of the elderly population," *Aging and Disease*, 6, 1-5, 2015, http://www.aginganddisease.org/EN/10.14336/AD.2014.1210.

5. Ilia Stambler, "Stop Aging Disease! ICAD 2014," *Aging and Disease*, 6(2), 76-94, 2015, http://www.aginganddisease.org/EN/10.14336/AD.2015.0115.

6. "Dr. Nir Barzilai on the TAME Study," Healthspan Campaign, April 28, 2015, http://www.healthspancampaign.org/2015/04/28/dr-nir-barzilai-on-the-tame-study/ .

7. Stephen S. Hall, "A trial for the ages," *Science*, 349(6254), 1275-1278, 2015, http://www.sciencemag.org/news/2015/09/feature-man-who-wants-beat-back-aging;

Sarah Knapton, "World's first anti-ageing drug could see humans live to 120," *The Telegraph*, November 29, 2015, http://www.telegraph.co.uk/science/2016/03/12/worlds-first-anti-ageing-drug-could-see-humans-live-to-120/;

John C. Newman, Sofiya Milman, Shahrukh K. Hashmi, Steve N. Austad, James L. Kirkland, Jeffrey B. Halter, Nir Barzilai, "Strategies and Challenges in Clinical Trials Targeting Human Aging," *Journal of Gerontology: Biological Sciences*, 71(11), 1424-1434, 2016, https://academic.oup.com/biomedgerontology/article/71/11/1424/2577175/Strategies-and-Challenges-in-Clinical-Trials.

8. Robert Preidt, "FDA Approves Flu Shot to Boost Immune Response. Vaccine can be used in seniors, who are often hit hardest by illness," *WebMD News from HealthDay*, November 25, 2015, http://www.webmd.com/cold-and-flu/news/20151125/fda-approves-first-flu-shot-with-added-ingredient-to-boost-immune-response.

9. Arlan Richardson, Veronica Galvan, Ai-Ling Linc, Salvatore Oddo, "How longevity research can lead to therapies for Alzheimer's disease: The rapamycin story," *Experimental Gerontology*, 68, 51-58, 2015, http://www.sciencedirect.com/science/article/pii/S0531556514003490.

10. Megan Scudellari, "Ageing research: Blood to blood," *Nature*, 517(7535), January 21, 2015, http://www.nature.com/news/ageing-research-blood-to-blood-1.16762.

11. Brett Israel, "Young blood does not reverse aging in old mice, UC Berkeley study finds," *Berkeley News*, November 22, 2016,

http://news.berkeley.edu/2016/11/22/young-blood-does-not-reverse-aging-in-old-mice-uc-berkeley-study-finds/, based on Justin Rebo, Melod Mehdipour, Ranveer Gathwala, Keith Causey, Yan Liu, Michael J. Conboy, Irina M. Conboy, "A single heterochronic blood exchange reveals rapid inhibition of multiple tissues by old blood," *Nature Communications*, 7, 13363, 2016, http://www.nature.com/articles/ncomms13363.

12. Nicholas Wade, "Purging Cells in Mice Is Found to Combat Aging Ills," *The New York Times*, November 2, 2011, http://www.nytimes.com/2011/11/03/science/senescent-cells-hasten-aging-but-can-be-purged-mouse-study-suggests.html?_r=0, based on Darren J. Baker, Tobias Wijshake, Tamar Tchkonia, Nathan K. LeBrasseur, Bennett G. Childs, Bart van de Sluis, James L. Kirkland, Jan M. van Deursen, "Clearance of p16Ink4a-positive senescent cells delays ageing-associated disorders," *Nature*, 479(7372), 232-236, 2011, https://www.nature.com/nature/journal/v479/n7372/full/nature10600.html.

13. Yi Zhu, Tamara Tchkonia, Tamar Pirtskhalava, ..., James L Kirkland, "The Achilles' heel of senescent cells: from transcriptome to senolytic drugs," *Aging Cell*, 14, 644–658, 2015, https://www.ncbi.nlm.nih.gov/pmc/articles/PMC4531078/.

14. Yossi Ovadya, Valery Krizhanovsky, "Senescent cell death brings hopes to life," *Cell Cycle*, 16(1), 9-10, 2017, http://www.tandfonline.com/doi/full/10.1080/15384101.2016.1232088.

15. Carles Cantó, Johan Auwerx, "Targeting Sirtuin 1 to Improve Metabolism: All You Need Is NAD+?" *Pharmacological Reviews*, 64(1), 166-187, 2012, http://pharmrev.aspetjournals.org/content/64/1/166.

16. Maheedhar Kodali, Vipan K. Parihar, Bharathi Hattiangady, Vikas Mishra, Bing Shuai, Ashok K. Shetty, "Resveratrol Prevents Age-Related Memory and Mood Dysfunction with Increased Hippocampal Neurogenesis and Microvasculature, and Reduced Glial Activation," *Scientific Reports*, 5, 8075, 2015, http://www.nature.com/articles/srep08075.

17. Karen Weintraub, "The Anti-Aging Pill," *MIT Technology Review*, February 3, 2015, http://www.technologyreview.com/news/534636/the-anti-aging-pill/

18. Samuel A. J. Trammell, Mark S. Schmidt, Benjamin J. Weidemann, Philip Redpath, Frank Jaksch, Ryan W. Dellinger, Zhonggang Li, E. Dale Abel, Marie E. Migaud, Charles Brenner, "Nicotinamide riboside is uniquely and orally bioavailable in mice and humans," *Nature Communications*, 7, 12948, 2016, http://www.nature.com/articles/ncomms12948.

19. "A Study to Evaluate Safety and Health Benefits of Basis™ Among Elderly Subjects," 15BSHE, Sponsor: Elysium Health, at ClinicalTrials.gov,

First received: February 3, 2016, https://clinicaltrials.gov/ct2/show/NCT02678611; Kazuo Tsubota, "The first human clinical study for NMN has started in Japan," *NPJ Aging and Mechanisms of Disease*, 2, 16021, 2016, https://www.nature.com/articles/npjamd201621.

20. Heidi Ledford, "Sirtuin protein linked to longevity in mammals. Male mice overproducing the protein sirtuin 6 have an extended lifespan," *Nature News*, 22 February 2012, based on Yariv Kanfi, Shoshana Naiman, Gail Amir, Victoria Peshti, Guy Zinman, Liat Nahum, Ziv Bar-Joseph, Haim Y. Cohen, "The sirtuin SIRT6 regulates lifespan in male mice," *Nature*, 483, 218–221, 2012, http://www.nature.com/news/sirtuin-protein-linked-to-longevity-in-mammals-1.10074.

21. Weijie You, Dante Rotili, Tie-Mei Li, Christian Kambach, Marat Meleshin, Mike Schutkowski, Katrin F. Chua, Antonello Mai, Clemens Steegborn, "Structural Basis of Sirtuin 6 Activation by Synthetic Small Molecules," *Angewandte Chemie International Edition*, 56(4), 1007-1011, 2017.

22. Khachik Muradian, "'Pull and push back' concepts of longevity and life span extension," *Biogerontology*, 14(6), 687-691, 2013.

23. Ian F. Robey, Natasha K. Martin, "Bicarbonate and dichloroacetate: Evaluating pH altering therapies in a mouse model for metastatic breast cancer," *BMC Cancer*, 11, 235, 2011, http://www.ncbi.nlm.nih.gov/pmc/articles/PMC3125283/.

24. Jennifer L. Olson, Anthony Atala, James J. Yoo, "Tissue Engineering: Current Strategies and Future Directions," *Chonnam Medical Journal*, 47(1), 1-13, 2011, http://www.ncbi.nlm.nih.gov/pmc/articles/PMC3214857/.

25. Giuseppe Orlando, Shay Soker, Robert J. Stratta, Anthony Atala, "Will Regenerative Medicine Replace Transplantation?" *Cold Spring Harbor Perspectives in Medicine*, 3(8), a015693, 2013, https://www.ncbi.nlm.nih.gov/pmc/articles/PMC3721273/.

26. "New drug triggers tissue regeneration: Faster regrowth and healing of damaged tissues," *Science Daily*, June 11, 2015, http://www.sciencedaily.com/releases/2015/06/150611144438.htm, based on Yongyou Zhang, Amar Desai, Sung Yeun Yang, ..., Sanford D. Markowitz, "Inhibition of the prostaglandin-degrading enzyme 15-PGDH potentiates tissue regeneration," *Science*, 348(6240), aaa2340, 2015.

27. "Living organ regenerated for first time: Thymus rebuilt in mice," *Science Daily*, April 8, 2014, http://www.sciencedaily.com/releases/2014/04/140408115610.htm, based on Nicholas Bredenkamp, Craig S. Nowell, C. Clare Blackburn, "Regeneration of the aged thymus by a single transcription factor," *Development*, 141(8), 1627-1637, 2014.

28. "Life-extending hormone bolsters the body's immune function," *Science Daily*, January 12, 2016,

http://www.sciencedaily.com/releases/2016/01/160112093545.htm, based on Yun-Hee Youm, Tamas L. Horvath, David J. Mangelsdorf, Steven A. Kliewer, Vishwa Deep Dixit, "Prolongevity hormone FGF21 protects against immune senescence by delaying age-related thymic involution," *Proceedings of the National Academy of Sciences USA*, 113(4), 1026-1031, 2016.

29. Ian Sample, "Harvard scientists reverse the ageing process in mice – now for humans," *Guardian*, November 28, 2010, http://www.guardian.co.uk/science/2010/nov/28/scientists-reverse-ageing-mice-humans, based on Mariela Jaskelioff, Florian L. Muller, Ji-Hye Paik, ..., Ronald A. DePinho, "Telomerase reactivation reverses tissue degeneration in aged telomerase-deficient mice," *Nature*, 469, 102-106, 2011 (first published on line on November 28, 2010).

30. Christian Bär, Maria A. Blasco, "Telomeres and telomerase as therapeutic targets to prevent and treat age-related diseases," *F1000Research* 2016, 5 (F1000 Faculty Reviews), 89, doi:10.12688/f1000research.7020.1, http://f1000research.com/articles/5-89/v1.

31. Vladimir P. Skulachev, Vladimir N. Anisimov, Yuri N. Antonenko, Lora E. Bakeeva, Boris V. Chernyak, Valery P. Erichev, Oleg F. Filenko, Natalya I. Kalinina, Valery I. Kapelko, "An attempt to prevent senescence: a mitochondrial approach," *Biochimica et Biophysica Acta*, 1787(5), 437-61, 2009, http://www.sciencedirect.com/science/article/pii/S0005272808007573.

32. Eric Bender, "Stopping free radicals at their source," Novartis Institute for Biomedical Research, September 22, 2015, https://www.nibr.com/stories/discovery/stopping-free-radicals-their-source, based on Adam L. Orr, Leonardo Vargas, Carolina N. Turk, ..., Martin D. Brand, "Suppressors of superoxide production from mitochondrial complex III," *Nature Chemical Biology*, 11(11), 834-836, 2015.

33. Eric A. Schon, Salvatore DiMauro, "Medicinal and Genetic Approaches to the Treatment of Mitochondrial Disease," *Current Medicinal Chemistry*, 10, 2523-2533, 2003, http://homepages.ihug.co.nz/~Smconnell/Medicinal%20and%20Genetic%20Approaches%20to%20Mitochonrial%20Disease.pdf.

34. Buck Institute, "Could ibuprofen be an anti-aging medicine?" December 11, 2014, http://www.buckinstitute.org/buck-news/could-ibuprofen-be-an-anti-aging-medicine, based on Chong He, Scott K. Tsuchiyama, Quynh T. Nguyen, ..., Brian K. Kennedy, Michael Polymenis, "Enhanced Longevity by Ibuprofen, Conserved in Multiple Species, Occurs in Yeast through Inhibition of Tryptophan Import," *PLoS Genetics*, 10(12), e1004860, 2014.

35. Michael Karin, Hans Clevers, "Reparative inflammation takes charge of tissue regeneration," *Nature,* 529, 307-315,

2016, http://www.nature.com/nature/journal/v529/n7586/full/nature170 39.html.

36. SENS Research Foundation, "A Reimagined Research Strategy for Aging. GlycoSENS: Breaking extracellular crosslinks," accessed June 2017, http://www.sens.org/research/introduction-to-sens-research/extracellular-crosslinks.

37. Ryoji Nagai, David B. Murray, Thomas O. Metz, John W. Baynes, "Chelation: a fundamental mechanism of action of AGE inhibitors, AGE breakers, and other inhibitors of diabetes complications," *Diabetes*, 61(3), 549-559, 2012, https://www.ncbi.nlm.nih.gov/pmc/articles/PMC3282805/.

38. "In defense of pathogenic proteins," *Science Daily*, January 8, 2016, http://www.sciencedaily.com/releases/2016/01/160108083456.htm, based on Juha Saarikangas, Yves Barral, "Protein aggregates are associated with replicative aging without compromising protein quality control," *eLife*, 4:e06197, 2015, https://www.ncbi.nlm.nih.gov/pmc/articles/PMC4635334/.

39. Júlia Santos, Fernanda Leitão-Correia, Maria João Sousa, Cecília Leão, "Dietary Restriction and Nutrient Balance in Aging," *Oxidative Medicine and Cellular Longevity*, 2016:4010357, 2016, http://www.ncbi.nlm.nih.gov/pmc/articles/PMC4670908/.

40. Jim Dryden, "Drastically cutting calories lowers some risk factors for age-related diseases," *Healthchannel*, September 2, 2015, http://www.healthcanal.com/geriatrics-aging/66558-drastically-cutting-calories-lowers-some-risk-factors-for-age-related-diseases%E2%80%8B%E2%80%8B.html, based on Eric Ravussin, Leanne M. Redman, James Rochon, ..., Susan B. Roberts, CALERIE Study Group, "A 2-Year Randomized Controlled Trial of Human Caloric Restriction: Feasibility and Effects on Predictors of Health Span and Longevity," *Journal of Gerontology: Medical Sciences*, 70(9), 1097-1104, 2015, https://www.ncbi.nlm.nih.gov/pmc/articles/PMC4841173/.

41. Paul W. O'Toole, Ian B. Jeffery, "Gut microbiota and aging," *Science*, 350(6265), 1214-1215, 2015, http://science.sciencemag.org/content/350/6265/1214.

42. Ilia Stambler, "Elie Metchnikoff – the founder of longevity science and a founder of modern medicine: In honor of the 170th anniversary," *Advances in Gerontology*, 28(2), 207-217, 2015 (Russian) and 5(4), 201-208, 2015 (English), http://www.longevityforall.org/170th-anniversary-of-elie-metchnikoff-the-founder-of-gerontology-may-15-2015/.

43. Anne Brunet, Shelley L. Berger, "Epigenetics of aging and aging-related disease," *Journal of Gerontology: Biological Sciences*, 69 Suppl 1, S17-20, 2014, http://www.ncbi.nlm.nih.gov/pmc/articles/PMC4022130/.

44. Maria Manukyan, Prim B. Singh, "Epigenetic rejuvenation," *Genes to Cells*, 17(5), 337-343, 2012, https://www.ncbi.nlm.nih.gov/pmc/articles/PMC3444684/.

45. Mitch Leslie, "Researchers rejuvenate aging mice with stem cell genes," *Science*, December 15, 2016, http://www.sciencemag.org/news/2016/12/researchers-rejuvenate-aging-mice-stem-cell-genes, based on Alejandro Ocampo, Pradeep Reddy, Paloma Martinez-Redondo, ..., Juan Carlos Izpisua Belmonte, "In Vivo Amelioration of Age-Associated Hallmarks by Partial Reprogramming," *Cell*, 167(7), 1719-1733.e12, 2016, http://www.cell.com/fulltext/S0092-8674(16)31664-6.

46. Tarek Baatia, Fanchon Bourassetc, Najla Gharbid, Leila Njimb, Manef Abderrabbae, Abdelhamid Kerkenib, Henri Szwarcd, Fathi Moussa, "The prolongation of the lifespan of rats by repeated oral administration of [60] fullerene," *Biomaterials*, 33(19), 4936-4946, 2012, http://www.sciencedirect.com/science/article/pii/S0142961212003237.

47. Shawn M. Douglas, Ido Bachelet, George M. Church, "A Logic-Gated Nanorobot for Targeted Transport of Molecular Payloads," *Science*, 335(6070), 831-834, 2012, http://science.sciencemag.org/content/335/6070/831.

48. John N. Kheir, Laurie A. Scharp, Mark A. Borden, ..., Francis X. McGowan Jr., "Oxygen gas-filled microparticles provide intravenous oxygen delivery," *Science Translational Medicine*, 4(140), 140ra88, 2012, https://www.researchgate.net/publication/228089270_Oxygen_Gas-Filled_Microparticles_Provide_Intravenous_Oxygen_Delivery.

49. Ronald Bellamy, Peter Safar, Samuel Tisherman, ..., Harvey Zar, "Suspended animation for delayed resuscitation," *Critical Care Medicine*, 24(2Suppl), S24-47, 1996, http://www.ncbi.nlm.nih.gov/pubmed/8608704.

50. Peter Safar, "On the future of reanimatology," *Academic Emergency Medicine*, 7(1), 75-89, 2000, http://onlinelibrary.wiley.com/doi/10.1111/j.1553-2712.2000.tb01898.x/abstract.

51. Gennady G. Rogatsky, Avraham Mayevsky, "The life-saving effect of hyperbaric oxygenation during early-phase severe blunt chest injuries," *Undersea Hyperbaric Medicine*, 34(2), 75-81, 2007, http://archive.rubicon-foundation.org/xmlui/bitstream/handle/123456789/6468/17520858.pdf?sequence=1.

52. Gennady G. Rogatsky, Edward G. Shifrin, Avraham Mayevsky, "Optimal dosing as a necessary condition for the efficacy of hyperbaric oxygen therapy in acute ischemic stroke: a critical review," *Neurological Research*, 25(1), 95-98, 2003, https://www.researchgate.net/publication/10920324_Optimal_dosing_as_

a_necessary_condition_for_the_efficacy_of_hyperbaric_oxygen_therapy_in
_acute_ischemic_stroke_A_critical_review.

53. Gennady G. Rogatsky, Ilia Stambler, "Hyperbaric oxygenation for resuscitation and therapy of elderly patients with cerebral and cardio-respiratory dysfunction," *Frontiers In Bioscience* (Scholar Edition), 9, 230-243, 2017, http://www.bioscience.org/2017/v9s/af/484/2.htm; https://www.bioscience.org/special-issue-details?editor_id=1746.

54. "Paralyzed men move legs with new non-invasive spinal cord stimulation," NIH News Releases, July 30, 2015, https://www.nih.gov/news-events/news-releases/paralyzed-men-move-legs-new-non-invasive-spinal-cord-stimulation, based on Yury P. Gerasimenko, Daniel C. Lu, Morteza Modaber, ..., V. Reggie Edgerton, "Noninvasive Reactivation of Motor Descending Control after Paralysis," *Journal of Neurotrauma*, 32(24), 1968-1980, 2015.

55. Marcello Massimini, Fabio Ferrarelli, Steve K. Esser, Brady A. Riedner, Reto Huber, Michael Murphy, Michael J. Peterson, Giulio Tononi, "Triggering sleep slow waves by transcranial magnetic stimulation," *Proceedings of the National Academy of Sciences USA*, 104(20), 8496-8501, 2007, http://www.pnas.org/content/104/20/8496.full.

56. Max Schaldach, *Electrotherapy of the Heart: Technical Aspects in Cardiac Pacing*, Springer-Verlag, Berlin, 2012.

57. David Blokh, Ilia Stambler, "Information theoretical analysis of aging as a risk factor for heart disease," *Aging and Disease*, 6, 196-207, 2015, http://www.aginganddisease.org/EN/10.14336/AD.2014.0623.

58. David Blokh, Ilia Stambler, "The application of information theory for the research of aging and aging-related diseases," *Progress in Neurobiology*, S0301-0082(15)30059-9, 2016, doi: http://dx.doi.org/10.1016/j.pneurobio.2016.03.005.

59. Alexey Moskalev, Elizaveta Chernyagina, Vasily Tsvetkov, Alexander Fedintsev, Mikhail Shaposhnikov, Vyacheslav Krut'ko, Alex Zhavoronkov, Brian K. Kennedy, "Developing criteria for evaluation of geroprotectors as a key stage toward translation to the clinic," *Aging Cell*, 15(3), 407-415, 2016, https://www.ncbi.nlm.nih.gov/pmc/articles/PMC4854916/.

60. Georg Fuellen, Paul Schofield, Thomas Flatt, ..., Andreas Simm, "Living Long and Well: Prospects for a Personalized Approach to the Medicine of Ageing," *Gerontology*, 62(4), 409-416, 2016.

61. Robert N. Butler, Richard Sprott, Huber Warner, Jeffrey Bland, Richie Feuers, Michael Forster, Howard Fillit, S. Mitchell Harman, Michael Hewitt, Mark Hyman, Kathleen Johnson, Evan Kligman, Gerald McClearn, James Nelson, Arlan Richardson, William Sonntag, Richard Weindruch, Norman Wolf, "Biomarkers of aging: from primitive organisms to humans," *Journal of Gerontology. A. Biological Sciences Medical Sciences*, 59, B560-567, 2004.

62. Thomas Craig, Chris Smelick, Robi Tacutu, Daniel Wuttke, ..., João Pedro de Magalhães, "The Digital Ageing Atlas: integrating the diversity of age-related changes into a unified resource," *Nucleic Acids Research*, 43, D873-878, 2015, https://www.ncbi.nlm.nih.gov/pmc/articles/PMC4384002/.

63. David Blokh, Ilia Stambler, "The use of information theory for the evaluation of biomarkers of aging and physiological age," *Mechanisms of Ageing and Development*, 163, 23-29, 2017, doi: http://dx.doi.org/10.1016/j.mad.2017.01.003.

64. Alexander Zhavoronkov, Bhupinder Bhullar, "Classifying aging as a disease in the context of ICD-11," *Frontiers in Genetics*, 6, 326, http://journal.frontiersin.org/article/10.3389/fgene.2015.00326/full.

65. Ilia Stambler, "Degenerative Aging as a Medical Condition," Longevity for All, January 1, 2016, http://www.longevityforall.org/degenerative-aging-as-a-medical-condition/;

Ilia Stambler, "Recognizing degenerative aging as a treatable medical condition: methodology and policy," *Aging and Disease*, 8(5), 2017, http://www.aginganddisease.org/EN/10.14336/AD.2017.0130;

Ilia Stambler, "Human life extension: opportunities, challenges, and implications for public health policy," in Alexander Vaiserman (Ed.), *Anti-aging Drugs: From Basic Research to Clinical Practice*, Royal Society of Chemistry, London, 2017, pp. 535-564.

17. Methodological Problems of Diagnosing and Treating Degenerative Aging as a Medical Condition to Extend Healthy Lifespan

The need for an integrated approach to healthy lifespan extension

The task of extending the healthy lifespan for the population is urgent for the well-being of the society. Due to the fast population aging in the developed countries, the prevalence of chronic non-communicable diseases and disabilities – such as cancer, ischemic heart disease, stroke, type 2 diabetes, Alzheimer's disease, etc. – rises steeply.[1] Thus, while 66% of deaths in the world occur from chronic age-related diseases, in the developed countries, this proportion reaches 90%, dramatically elevating the costs of healthcare and human suffering.[2] Hence, it can be stated that the task of extending the healthy lifespan for the population is one of the most important healthcare, economic and humanitarian tasks.

In addition to the currently available lifestyle approaches (such as moderate exercise, moderate and balanced nutrition, and sufficient rest and sleep), the search for additional novel biomedical means and technologies for healthy lifespan extension is warranted. Moreover, insofar as the deteriorative aging process either precipitates or lies at the root of chronic age-related diseases, the search for novel means and technologies for healthy lifespan extension necessitates the maximal possible amelioration of the degenerative aging process. Such amelioration of the aging process should lead to better health and quality of life for the elderly.[3] The possibility of therapeutic intervention into degenerative aging and the consequent significant healthy lifespan extension has been proven on both theoretical-biological grounds and experimental grounds in a variety of animal models. In particular, the ability of cell-based regenerative medicine, gene therapy, pharmacological therapy and nanomedicine to affect basic aging processes and extend healthy lifespan in animal models has been demonstrated, and even some encouraging preliminary results have been achieved in human experiments.[4] This possibility has also been conclusively proven by the existence of a large and continuously growing long-lived population, including centenarians and super-centenarians, that exhibit not only a high longevity potential, but also a reduced rate of age-related diseases compared to the general population.[5]

Yet the pathway toward human healthy lifespan extension remains unclear and requires thorough elaboration, concerning many scientific problems that need to be clarified and technologies that need to be developed. There is a tremendous variety of studies and approaches toward healthy lifespan extension, and roadmaps indicating priority directions.[6] Perhaps the most critical drawback in this variety is the lack of integration of the different approaches. The existing approaches often present lists of potential research directions, rather than coherent and coordinated entities. Hence the integration of the various approaches, shortening the pathways between the various disciplines, could be highly valuable for the fundamental and comprehensive understanding of aging and longevity, as well as for the further translation of this knowledge to practical integrative medical applications. Several important "gaps" may yet need to be "bridged" in the current variety of approaches to healthy lifespan extension.

Longevity factors assessment and manipulation: Bridging the gap between "environmentalist" and "internalist" approaches

One of the main disparities in the current variety of approaches to healthy lifespan extension seems to be the perceived opposition between "external" or "environmental" factors for healthy lifespan extension, and "internal" or "genetically determined" factors. On the one hand, it is often assumed that environmental and lifestyle factors alone are sufficient to affect healthy lifespan, disregarding genetic composition, the inner structure and function of the body. On the other, there is a "genetic" or "biological deterministic" approach that assumes the strict genetic determination of the lifespan from birth that virtually cannot be influenced by environmental factors. There is a clear need to bridge this gap through the study of physiological, in particular metabolic, neuro-hormonal and epigenetic influences on the lifespan, which recognizes the vital regulatory role of the environment on gene expression and internal physiological function.

There are decisive practical implications of this gap, often producing conflicting therapeutic approaches, sometimes leading to struggle in terms of R&D priorities and funding. Thus, there is often a lack of connection between biotechnologies and biomedical technologies, on the one hand, and the so-called information and communication technologies (ICT) or assistive technologies for healthy aging, on the other. While biomedical approaches consider almost exclusively the "inside" of the aging organism, often disregarding the "outside" environmental influences, the ICT and other assistive geronto-technological applications often disregard the "inside" of the body. The study of physiological, in particular neuro-humoral regulation and homeostasis in response to changing environment can help build a bridge between those domains. The study of epigenetics (changes of gene function without changes in DNA sequence) can provide another link, due to the fact that the epigenetic signature of healthy functional longevity can be achieved not just by means of internal medicine, such as regenerative cell therapy and geroprotective small molecules, but in no lesser measure by changes of mental attitude, diet, exercise, the level of social involvement that can be induced not so much through biomedical therapies, as by external coaching and game-like ICT health applications, training the elderly subjects and prompting them to adopt a healthier life-style. The epigenetic mechanisms could provide the "internal/biological" basis for "external/environmental" interventions.[7]

"Multi-omics" and "frailty": bridging the gap between molecular-biological, energy-metabolic and functional-behavioral evaluation and intervention

Within the general need for integration, it may be particularly important to bring together the domains of the so-called "multi-omics analysis" and "frailty evaluation."

There has been an increasing discussion in the biotechnological and biomedical community about the need for "multi-omics" analysis.[8] This implies a combined analysis of information about the human organism, aimed to diagnose, and if possible predict its condition, and analyze, and if possible predict the efficacy of specific types of treatment. The aim is to collect the information in a systemic way from different levels of biological organization (or "omes"), including: genome – genetic information, as presented by DNA sequence; epigenome – the epigenetic markers of gene regulation (such as methylation, phosphorylation or acetylation markers); transcriptome – the collection of messenger RNA participating in the transcription of genetic information into proteins; proteome – information on the proteins present in the organism, or in specific cells or tissues; metabolome – information on products of the organism's metabolism (metabolites); physiome – information on the physiological, such as energetic or respiratory parameters of the organism, and other types of biomarkers. It is hoped that the information from the various levels ("omes") is correlated with each other and with the clinical history (anamnesis) and therapeutic regimen to provide systemic, precise, predictive, preventive, personalized and participatory diagnosis and therapy.

On the other hand, the most common concept in geriatric evaluation and therapy is old-age "frailty" – a "geriatric syndrome" used to assess the health state of the elderly, alongside age-related diseases and other geriatric "syndromes" such as delirium, incontinence and falls. In the basic sense, frailty is not an evaluation of a defined present state, but an evaluation of a risk of future adverse events. Thus, according to the classical definition, "Frail individuals are perceived to constitute those older adults at highest risk for a number of adverse health outcomes, including dependency, institutionalization, falls, injuries, acute illness, hospitalization, slow or blocked recovery from illness and mortality."[9] It is also admitted that "although a clinical 'sense' of frailty exists, there is still no explicitly agreed-

255

on, standard clinical definition of frailty or of failure to thrive that would assist identification of this high-risk subset of the population, *prior* to the onset of these adverse outcomes."[9] Hence, methods of predictive risk analysis can be most appropriate for the clinical definition and evaluation of old-age frailty.

A stronger alliance between these fields may be desirable. There may accrue a great therapeutic benefit from introducing "multi-omics" type of analysis, its systemic, predictive and personalized philosophy, for old-age frailty evaluation and treatment. And conversely, the researchers and developers of multi-omics biomarkers may need to be more strongly involved in the problems of aging, to realize the critical need to address fundamental degenerative aging processes in order to alleviate virtually all health conditions, including those they are currently working on. Such an alliance is yet a rather rare occasion.

Currently, functional-behavioral assessments dominate the evaluations of frailty.[10] For example, in the widely used "Study of Osteoporotic Fractures" (SOF) frailty index, there are 3 main diagnostic parameters: 1) *"Weight loss,"* 2) *"Inability to rise from a chair,"* and *3) "Poor energy"* as identified by an answer "yes" or "no" to the question "Do you feel full of energy?" on the Geriatric Depression Scale.[11] And in the even more widely used "Cardiovascular Health Study" (CHS) frailty index, the 5 parameters are: 1) *"Shrinking"* as shown by an unintentional weight loss, 2) *"Weakness"* as shown by a maximal grip strength, 3) *"Poor energy"* as determined by an answer to the question "Do you feel full of energy?" 4) *"Slowness"* as indicated by an average walk speed, and 5) *"Low physical activity level"* as identified by a Physical Activity Scale for the Elderly (PASE) score in the lowest quintile.[12] It may be seen that biological markers of aging are assigned little significance in such scores.

To improve the frailty evaluation, to provide a reliable science-based proxy or indication for the aging process, it appears necessary to include more parameters measuring this process at its fundamental biological level. For example, the organism's energy level can be objectively measured by such means as spirometry, oximetry, hemodynamic, electrochemical and spectroscopic energy metabolite measurements, etc., thus providing improved indication for therapy.[13] The energy metabolism measurements may supplement molecular-biological measurements that are commonly employed in the research of biomarkers of aging (e.g. age-related changes in telomere length, advanced glycation endproducts - AGE, DNA repair capacity, aging-associated gene expression and epigenetic markers, stem cell populations and others).[14] The more frequent and routine inclusion of old-age frailty evaluation into medical research and practice, and the greater addition of biological indicators to the common functional frailty assessments, in correlation with each other and reinforcing each other, may provide advanced diagnostic and therapeutic capabilities.

Selecting candidates for therapeutic interventions: Bridging the gap between longevity factor analysis and therapeutic interventions

Despite the wide variety of approaches, there can be outlined a few basic generic fields in the study of longevity. One is the study of "aging biomarkers" and "longevity factors" (both external and internal). Large databases are being developed to collect various physiological, environmental, lifestyle, genetic and other factors associated with extended healthy lifespan as opposed to debilitating aging.[14,15] On the other hand, there is the study of experimental "anti-aging" and "lifespan extension," mainly associated with cell-based regenerative medicine and pharmacological geroprotective substances, that work to experimentally restore the physiological and functional state of the aging organism.[16] Yet, there is often a deficit of interrelation between these approaches. The research of "biomarkers of aging" and "longevity factors" is often descriptive, with uncertain implications for clinical practice. The collected factors form large masses of data, yet it is often unclear how the different pieces of data are related to each other or to clinical outcomes, what factors or combinations of factors have the most weight in determining the healthy lifespan, or whether they can be therapeutically influenced either separately or in combinations to improve clinical outcomes. On the other hand, regenerative and geroprotective medicine approaches are often strongly empirical and "prescriptive," testing for a variety of potential interventions, without a former comprehensive factor analysis, with the aim to empirically establish potentially effective treatments.

Often, the longevity factor analysis and experimental life extension research proceed as if they occupy separate "neighboring domains." That is to say, a set of biomarkers and other diagnostic parameters of aging and longevity are being developed in one domain, and life-extending interventions in another. And then (in a part of the cases) an attempt is made to test the effects of the latter interventions domain on the former markers domain, rather than deriving the interventions directly from the markers. It may be possible to bridge this gap. It may be possible to conduct a thorough scan of "longevity factors" on a large population, including physiological, genetic, as well as environmental and epigenetic factors contributing to healthy lifespan. It will then be necessary to select the most informative factors contributing to healthy lifespan, for example, using advanced statistical, ontological and information-theoretical methodologies.[17] These methodologies may increase the interoperability between model systems, and allow a precise and weighted estimate of the influence of various risk factors and therapeutic interventions, and their combinations, on the healthspan and age-related disease patterns.

The aging and longevity factor analysis should then not remain in a purely descriptive, analytical phase, but should move immediately and simultaneously to clinically relevant experiments on cell, tissue and animal models. For example, the special genetic and epigenetic factors, including gene candidates and epigenetic loci found to be associated with extended healthy lifespan, can form the initial targets for testing and manipulation in experimental models. A hallmark of epigenetic regulation of gene expression is its reversibility by environmental factors. Epigenetic markers (such as methylation) have been strongly associated with the aging process, and diverse pharmacological and cell-therapeutic interventions have been indicated to affect the epigenetic status.[18] Moreover, various gene candidates have been associated with extended healthy longevity. Even though it may be practically difficult to directly modify those genes, their expression and activity can nonetheless be stimulated or mimicked via pharmacological and cell-based interventions.[19] In case no known mimetics or stimulators of longevity factors exist, those can be designed using methods of synthetic biology or nanomedicine.[20] Hence, by providing the input for therapeutic interventions from population-based aging and longevity factor analysis, it may be possible to provide a broad evidential database for further experimentation in regenerative and geroprotective medicine, as well as shorten the pathway between longevity factor analysis and experimentation. The results of experiments may in turn immediately feed back to refine data collection and analysis, accelerating the process of discovery.

Testing interventions: Bridging the gap between research models

Yet another source of discrepancy among approaches to healthy lifespan extension is the deficit of inter-operability between various models, which may include population, individual, human, animal, culture, cell or molecular models. Often, studies are conducted at different levels of organization, with a disregard of other levels. There is an apparent need for an integrative approach, spanning across the relevant scales, using a wide array of physiological, environmental, genetic and epigenetic parameters. The human being as a whole should be the focus, with a special attention given to personalized factors characteristic of individual subjects, and selecting the most informative factors. Other models and levels could be studied as supplementary. Thus, an attempt at reconstitution of beneficial human characteristics could be made, with experimental testing on the level of human and animal cells and cell cultures and animal organism models.

The latter tests could in turn help provide insights for further human studies.

Such interoperability is rare. Commonly, the data collected on humans remain as descriptive registers, with no transition to further experimentation. On the other hand, insights gathered at the level of cells, tissues and animal models remain at those levels, and their applicability for living human beings is unclear or even untenable. It is important to emphasize that the broadest possible collection of diverse biological, physiological and clinical human data, on every level of organization and on the widest possible populations, will be needed. And the human data will need to be compared and supplemented with the widest possible variety of animal data, also on all levels of organization. Such massive and diverse data could enable the creation of truly integrated, holistic models for predictive diagnostic evaluation and preventive therapeutic intervention. There may be a need to have a "common language" (e.g. non-dimensional measures) to describe the different model systems in common terms, for example using terms from information theory, such as entropy and normalized mutual information, that may be applicable for any system.[21]

Of course, it must be noted that the costs for such a comprehensive data collection and experimentation will likely be high, and funding will always be an issue. It may also be suspected that collecting and analyzing too much and too various data may become unwieldy (whatever the available computational power), and some simplification, abstraction and synthesis may be required. Yet, in any case, the more data can be available – the easier it will be to filter and simplify it. To paraphrase a proverb, 'it is easier to make a hat from the entire sheep skin than from its tail.'

Designing interventions: Bridging the gap between Science and Technology

The research of aging and lifespan and healthspan extension is not just a theoretical scientific or purely biological subject, but in many ways a technological subject, where the capabilities of biological research and manipulation are largely determined by technological capabilities. Virtually all technological fields can be ultimately enlisted for solving the problem of degenerative aging and for extending healthy lifespan. These would include such technological areas as novel measurement modalities (including comprehensive physiological vitality measurements, as well as a vast array of cell-based and molecular measurements), synthetic biology, nanotechnology and micro-fabrication, as well as advanced computational, modeling and visualization capabilities. "Technological convergence" and "cross-fertilization" may be key concepts for tackling the problem of aging.

But the solutions should not remain at the stage of fundamental research in the lab. Another key concept may be "clinical translation" understood as the process of translating fundamental scientific research to its application in clinical practice, creating and utilizing actual medical technologies. The translation process includes all the stages of research and development: from studies on cells and tissues, through animal studies and human trials, up to marketing, production and distribution. The future translation into clinical practice should always be kept in mind as a primary objective. The studies of aging are not just academically intriguing (and they are), but also have a clear purpose – to improve health for the elderly, eventually for all of us. The translation from fundamental research to clinical practice is often difficult, and not only due to scientific and technological hurdles, but often also because of societal constraints, such as lack of social interest and investment or inefficient regulation and distribution. Careful thought should always be given for the facilitation and optimization of the translation process to make aging-ameliorating, life and health-extending therapies and technologies available to all of us.

Social analysis: Bridging the gap between Science, Technology and Society

Indeed, biomedical aging amelioration and life and healthspan extension are often considered as just and only scientific or technological problems. Yet, in fact, the development, translation, application and access to treatments designed to ameliorate degenerative aging processes and extend healthy lifespan will involve a vast host of social issues and implications, including both hindering and facilitating impact factors that will require comprehensive analysis and debate.[22] Hence, it will be necessary to give due consideration to *social factors,* such as legislative, administrative, communal, economic, demographic, educational and even ethical factors that largely determine the *development* of lifespan and healthspan extension research and *translation* of this research into practice. Some of the issues include: regulatory requirements for the short and long-term testing and approval of potential geroprotective treatments; criteria for their efficacy and safety; administrative and organizational requirements needed for the active promotion of healthspan extension research and practice; incentives for the rapid development and translation of the results of this research into medical and clinical practice; provisions for the universal distribution of healthspan-extending technologies to the public, and much more. All these issues will yet need to become the subject of a broad and intense academic and public debate, including political debate.[23]

Knowledge dissemination: Bridging the gap between Research and Education

Within the general need for stronger social involvement, there is an urgent need to educate more specialists who will be able to contribute to the various areas of aging and healthspan extension research. There is an even prior need to educate the broader student body and wider public on the importance of such research to prepare the ground for further involvement. Thanks to such broad education, many more new promising studies may spring up. The increased knowledge of the field may increase the demand for therapies, which may in turn increase the offer. Even when the therapies are available, it should be the general public who should use them, hence their willingness to embark on and adhere to a preventive anti-aging and healthspan-improving regimen, their ability to intelligently choose and apply effective and safe therapy, will be vital for its successful application. Therefore comprehensive and wide-ranging "patient and consumer education," and moreover "citizen scientist" and "do-it-yourself maker" education in the field of aging and healthspan extension will be necessary. Such education is currently very limited. In practical terms, globally there are very few centers or dedicated structures to promote and coordinate knowledge exchange and dissemination on biology of aging and healthy lifespan extension. There are even few courses in this field in university curricula around the world. There is a need for more courses and training materials on the subject, in order to make the narrative on biology of aging and healthy lifespan extension an integral part of academic curriculum and public discourse.

The problem of clinical definition of degenerative aging: bridging the gaps in scientific understanding and communication

One of the major factors hindering the discussion of aging amelioration, lifespan and healthspan extension research, development and application may be the basic deficit of definitions. What is it exactly that we wish to ameliorate, and what is it exactly that we wish to extend? Such agreed definitions appear to be among the necessary conditions for the communication, dissemination and advancement of the field. But such agreed definitions are currently lacking.

Three is a growing realization that in order to combat the rising aging-related ill health and improve the healthy lifespan – the research, development and distribution of anti-aging and healthspan-improving therapies need to be accelerated.[24] It was suggested that one of the accelerating factors could be the general recognition of the degenerative aging process itself as a medical problem to be addressed.[25] It has been assumed that such a recognition may accelerate research, development and distribution in several aspects: 1) The general public would be encouraged to actively demand and intelligently apply aging-ameliorating, preventive therapies; 2) The pharmaceutical and medical technology industry would be encouraged to develop and bring effective aging-ameliorating therapies and technologies to the market; 3) Health insurance, life insurance and healthcare systems would obtain a new area for reimbursement practices, which would encourage them and their subjects to promote healthy longevity; 4) Regulators and policy makers would be encouraged to prioritize and increase investments of public funds into aging-related research and development; 5) Scientists and students would be encouraged to tackle a scientifically exciting and practically vital problem of aging. Here we would leave aside the question whether this medical condition should be called a "disease," a "syndrome," a "risk factor," an "underlying cause" or some other trope. Here "the aging process as a medical condition" just means a processes that can be materially intervened into, improved (treated) and even eliminated (cured) by medical means.

Yet, in order for degenerative aging process to be recognized as such a diagnosable and treatable medical condition and therefore an indication for research, development and treatment, a necessary condition appears to be the development of evidence-based diagnostic criteria and definitions for degenerative aging. So far, there are still no such commonly accepted or formal criteria and definitions. Yet without such scientifically grounded and clinically applicable criteria, the discussions about "ameliorating" or even "curing" degenerative aging processes, will be mere slogans. Indeed, how can we "treat" or "cure" something that we cannot even diagnose? It may even be found that such criteria are explicitly or implicitly required by several major international and national regulatory and policy frameworks, such as the International Classification of Diseases (ICD), the WHO Global Strategy and Action Plan on Ageing and Health (GSAP), the European Medicines Agency (EMA), the US Food and Drug Administration (FDA), and others.[23] Such frameworks are thirsting for evidence-based criteria for the effectiveness of interventions for "healthy aging." Nonetheless, nobody has yet done the necessary work of devising such comprehensive evidential criteria. It may seem that the problem has not been solved just for the lack of enough trying. But it must be admitted that the problem is not at all easy even to dare to take on. Many formidable methodological challenges may arise in attempting to develop commonly acceptable diagnostic definitions and criteria for degenerative aging. But try we must!

A major challenge is related even to the semantic understanding of the term "degenerative aging." The term "degenerative" may imply both the present state of degeneration and the process leading to the state of degeneration. This distinction may have major implications for intervention, respectively implying a curative approach to the already manifest state of degeneration (a late stage intervention) as opposed to a preventive approach to block a process leading to degeneration (an early stage intervention). It may be particularly helpful to explore "degenerative aging" in the latter sense, as a process leading to degeneration that can be prevented. Yet, many questions remain with such a definition. Obviously, not every time-related change leads to degeneration and disease, and some aging-related changes may be beneficial for the person (e.g. the proverbial "wisdom of age"[26]). Obviously also, many changes leading to age-related degeneration begin at conception, and may be necessary concomitants of the processes of growth and development. Then for which processes and at which stages is intervention warranted? In other words, which aging processes can be considered truly "degenerative" (leading to degeneration) that would require preventive intervention? Several sets of such candidate processes have been proposed,[6] yet there is still little empirical evidence that intervention into them will have clinical benefits. The potential interrelation and regulation of these various processes are also uncertain. In this regard, a practical worry is that under the title of "prevention" and "early intervention" – drugs and other treatments will be sold to young and relatively healthy individuals without a real need and without proven benefits in actually preventing degenerative states and/or extending healthy lifespan. A more thorough, quantitative and formal understanding of old-age degeneration (frailty) as a physiological state is required as well. Should it be measured as a lack of function and adaptation to the environment, an impairment of homeostatic or homeodynamic stability?[27] Should it be presented as an index or as physiological age?

Each of these options would raise a host of questions of its own, whose mere mentioning would go far beyond the scope of this work. To provide evidence-based answers to those questions, vast empirical and theoretical research yet appears to be needed to establish diverse age-related changes as predictors of adverse age-related outcomes (such as multi-morbidity and mortality) as well as evaluate the effects of various preventive and curative treatments on those outcomes. Based on such data, better formal, clinically applicable models and criteria of degenerative aging as a process and as a state can be developed.

It may be stated that the development of clinical definitions and criteria for degenerative aging, and the corresponding definitions and criteria for the effectiveness of anti-aging and healthspan-extending therapies would be the penultimate "gap" in the common scientific understanding of the problem that needs to be "bridged" before proceeding toward its practical solution. This would in fact mean bridging multiple "gaps" between multiple conceptions and approaches to the problem of aging amelioration and healthspan improvement, to achieve a good level of mutual understanding and agreement. With the current diversity of theories, approaches, models and prospective remedies, it may be yet a long road ahead before such a level of common understanding and agreement is reached. It may not be necessary that every researcher should accept a standard universal metrics and agree on most of the fundamental concepts and processes (as it has been accomplished in mathematics and physics), but at least some degree of commensurability for the field may be desirable. Such commensurability would not mean dictating the same approach to all, or even worse, prescribing the same measures and treatments for all, but rather providing a common language that would enrich general discourse and creativity in the field. The continuous active consultation and debate on these issues may be key to progress.

Some research areas to address in devising clinical diagnostic criteria for degenerative aging and for the effectiveness and safety of anti-aging and healthspan-improving interventions

The present work could not presume to even begin to provide any definitive answers for the above methodological problems. It does not provide any specific building blocks for the bridges between the various areas that may need to come into closer, more powerful synergistic contact. This work is only intended to attempt to emphasize some of those potential problems and stimulate their discussion (in addition to any discussions of these issues that may take place anywhere else). If it succeeds to enhance this discussion and improve this knowledge even slightly, then it has fulfilled its purpose.

As a way of a conclusion, which is not a conclusion at all, but just an attempt to raise further discussion, a few particular challenges may be listed, including some of the earlier points, problems and gaps. This list includes some of the major concerns for the development of diagnostic and treatment criteria against degenerative aging and for healthy lifespan extension. These can be tentatively classified as follows: 1) establishing definitions, 2) minimizing confounding factors, 3) improving informative value, and finally 4) improving the practical utility of the criteria. This could also be the putative priority order at which the problems can be tackled. (It must be reemphasized that these propositions are only intended to stimulate academic and public debate.)

I. Establishing definitions:

1) *Establishing basic terms and definitions.* These may include the questions above. For example, should "degenerative aging" be understood as a process or as a state? Or is "healthy aging" a helpful term for developing clinical measurements of aging, considering that most aging processes increase morbidity? Should we instead speak in terms of "healthy longevity" as opposed to "degenerative aging"?

2) *Defining clinical benefits.* Just and only biomarkers of aging may not be sufficient to provide clinically applicable diagnostic criteria for "degenerative aging" or for interventions against it. For example, as many studies of Alzheimer's disease have shown, treatments can modify

264

"biomarkers" of the disease very well (in some types of models), but do little or nothing clinically beneficial for actual human patients.[28] Hopefully, this problem can be avoided when addressing general aging as a medical condition. There is a need to precisely define measurable *clinical* end points, demonstrating evidential clinical benefits, especially for the reduction of age-related multimorbidity. The combination of structural biological and functional behavioral parameters may increase diagnostic capabilities. In practical terms, the establishment of clinical benefits would also mean more direct and fast transitions between descriptive measurements and experiments (in both directions), "bridging the gap between longevity factor analysis and therapeutic interventions."

II. Minimizing confounding factors:

1) *Focus on older persons.* The clinical benefits need to be evaluated in the primary target population – the older frail persons, rather than the younger and healthier ones who may exhibit entirely different biological responses.[29]

2) *Long term consideration.* The clinical criteria and biomarkers, as well as resources available to the organism, need to be considered *for the long term.* Thanks to long-term evaluation it may be possible to control for effects of over-stimulation, as well as rule out transient compensatory and psychosomatic effects and seeming short-term benefits that may arrive at the expense of long-term deterioration. In particular, seeming short-term "rejuvenation effects" may increase mortality and shorten the actual lifespan.[30]

III. Improving informative value:

1) *Selection.* As almost any age-related biological parameter may be considered a "biomarker of aging," there is a need to select the most predictive and economic biomarkers, for the population as well as for individuals.[31]

2) *Integration.* Criteria for degenerative aging may not be only molecular and cellular, but at every level of biological organization – from the molecular to cellular to tissues and organs, to the entire organism and to the organism's interrelation with the environment – that need to be integrated.[32] Moreover, these criteria may not necessarily be chemical and biological, but can also be physical, in particular as relates to various resuscitation technologies as applied to the elderly, such as hypothermia and suspended animation,[33] oxygenation and energy metabolism,[34] electromagnetic stimulation.[35] Social (engagement) and psychological (motivation) criteria also need to be added. Among other implications, this drive for integration would also mean "bridging the gaps" between "environmental" and "internal" evaluations and interventions, between "multi-omics" and "frailty," and between different, currently often incomparable "research models."

Individual biomarkers may not be indicative of the process or state of degeneration, and need to be considered in combinations, or ideally in a systemic balanced way – otherwise interventions on particular biomarkers and pathways may exacerbate other biomarkers and pathways, and disrupt the system as a whole. The general methodology for the evaluation of the effects of multiple integrated therapeutic agents and risk factors (including biomarkers of aging) on multiple integrated adverse effects and age-related diseases (multimorbidity) need to be improved, to allow the evaluation of non-linear, cumulative or synergistic effects.[36]

IV. Improving practical utility:

1) *Pluralism and rigor.* Particular batteries of assays and interventions are usually related (and potentially biased) to particular theories, research agendas, academic schools and commercial interests. There is an apparent need to allow pluralism of investigation, discovery and application, while maintaining standards of the scientific method. Consensus standards often emerge as a result of data-sharing,[37] which may become a practical challenge of its own.

2) *Affordability.* Costs of diagnostic biomarkers assays and therapeutic interventions may become prohibitive or even impractical for use by most people in the world. There is a need to focus on such therapies, biomarkers and functional assays that may be most cost-effective, especially those that are already routinely used in clinical practice, while still encouraging the development of more sophisticated assays and therapies, that may become more accessible in time, and specifically devising means to increase their accessibility.[38]

The issue of "affordability" actually involves most of the problems and "gaps" between "science and technology" (the problem of translating fundamental research to practical affordable therapies), between "science, technology and society" (making the therapies widely available, and not only "for the rich and powerful"), as well as between "research and education" (making the knowledge of the field more accessible and wider spread, to catalyze even more knowledge generation). The main overarching question to ask in this regard is: "How can we make the best, most effective therapies available (affordable) as fast as possible to as many as possible?" The details are to be established in a broad academic, public and political discussion.

Motivation for further discussion

All these issues must become a subject of massive and pluralistic consultation, involving scientists, policy makers and other stakeholders. Thanks to such a consultation it may be possible to develop agreeable scientific clinical criteria for degenerative aging that could improve diagnostic capabilities and allow better informed clinical decisions, as well as stimulate further research and development of effective, evidence-based anti-aging and healthspan-extending therapies, treating the underlying processes of aging-related diseases rather than their particular symptoms. In such a broad consultation, various diagnostic and therapeutic approaches to aging amelioration and healthy lifespan extension may be brought together, their relative merits and drawbacks may be compared, and points of their convergence may be clarified. Such a discussion may facilitate the creation of a comprehensive and actionable roadmap toward healthy lifespan extension. It is hoped that the present work will contribute to raising the demand to expand such discussion and research.

References and notes

1. Kunlin Jin, James W. Simpkins, Xunming Ji, Miriam Leis, Ilia Stambler, "The critical need to promote research of aging and aging-related diseases to improve health and longevity of the elderly population," *Aging and Disease*, 6, 1-5, 2015, http://www.aginganddisease.org/EN/10.14336/AD.2014.1210.
2. Rafael Lozano, Mohsen Naghavi, Kyle Foreman, Stephen Lim, Kenji Shibuya, Victor Aboyans, et al., "Global and regional mortality from 235 causes of death for 20 age groups in 1990 and 2010: a systematic analysis for the Global Burden of Disease Study 2010," *Lancet*, 380, 2095-2128, 2012.
3. Nathan Keyfitz, "Improving life expectancy: An uphill road ahead," *American Journal of Public Health*, 68, 954-956, 1978, https://www.ncbi.nlm.nih.gov/pmc/articles/PMC1654068/;
Michael J. Rae, Robert N. Butler, Judith Campisi, Aubrey D.N.J. de Grey, Caleb E. Finch, Michael Gough, George M. Martin, Jan Vijg, Kevin M. Perrott, Barbara J. Logan, "The demographic and biomedical case for late-life interventions in aging," *Science Translational Medicine*, 2, 40cm21, 2010, http://stm.sciencemag.org/content/2/40/40cm21.full.
4. Gregory M. Fahy, Michael D. West, L. Stephen Coles, Steven B. Harris, (Eds.), *The Future of Aging: Pathways to Human Life Extension*, Springer, New York, 2010;
Alexander Vaiserman (Ed.), *Anti-aging Drugs: From Basic Research to Clinical Practice*, Royal Society of Chemistry, London, 2017.
5. Swapnil N. Rajpathak, Yingheng Liu, Orit Ben-David, Saritha Reddy, Gil Atzmon, Jill Crandall, Nir Barzilai, "Lifestyle factors of people with exceptional longevity," *Journal of the American Geriatrics Society*, 59(8), 1509-1512, 2011;

Sofiya Milman, Nir Barzilai, "Dissecting the mechanisms underlying unusually successful human health span and life span," *Cold Spring Harbor Perspectives in Medicine*, 6(1), a025098, 2015;

Natalia S. Gavrilova, Leonid A. Gavrilov, "Search for mechanisms of exceptional human longevity," *Rejuvenation Research*, 13(2-3), 262-264, 2010;

Miguel A. Faria, "Longevity and compression of morbidity from a neuroscience perspective: Do we have a duty to die by a certain age?" *Surgical Neurology International*, 6, 49, 2015.

6. Ilia Stambler, *A History of Life-Extensionism in the Twentieth Century*, Longevity History, 2014, http://www.longevityhistory.com/;

Gregory M. Fahy, Michael D. West, L. Stephen Coles, Steven B. Harris, (Eds.), *The Future of Aging: Pathways to Human Life Extension*, Springer, New York, 2010;

Alexander Vaiserman (Ed.), *Anti-aging Drugs: From Basic Research to Clinical Practice*, Royal Society of Chemistry, London, 2017.

In the quite famous SENS program (Strategies for Engineering Negligible Senescence), the priority research and intervention areas include: 1) eliminating damage from cell loss and tissue atrophy by adding stem cells and tissue engineering (RepleniSENS); 2) neutralizing nuclear (epi-) mutations leading to cancer by the removal of telomere-lengthening machinery (OncoSENS); 3) backing up mutant mitochondria by allotopic expression of 13 proteins in the nucleus (MitoSENS); 4) elimination of death-resistant cells by targeted ablation (ApoptoSENS); 5) preventing tissue stiffening by substances breaking Advanced Glycation End-products – AGE-breakers (GlycoSENS) and by tissue engineering; 6) cleaning up extracellular aggregates by immunotherapeutic clearance (AmyloSENS); 7) dissolving intracellular aggregates by novel lysosomal hydrolases (LysoSENS). See:

Aubrey D.N.J. de Grey, Michael Rae, *Ending Aging. The Rejuvenation Breakthroughs That Could Reverse Human Aging in Our Lifetime*, St. Martin's Press, New York, 2007;

SENS Research Foundation, "A Reimagined Research Strategy for Aging," accessed June 2017, http://www.sens.org/research/introduction-to-sens-research/.

As another example, at the 2013 US NIH Geroscience Summit, the following priority research areas were identified: 1) adaptation to stress, 2) epigenetics, 3) inflammation, 4) macromolecular damage, 5) metabolism, 6) proteostasis, 7) stem cells/regeneration. See:

Healthspan Campaign, "NIH Geroscience Interest Group (GSIG) Releases Recommendations from the October 2013 Advances in Geroscience Summit," 2013, http://www.healthspancampaign.org/2014/02/27/nih-geroscience-interest-group-gsig-releases-recommendations-october-2013-advances-geroscience-summit/;

Brian K. Kennedy, Shelley L. Berger, Anne Brunet, Judith Campisi, Ana Maria Cuervo, Elissa S. Epel, Claudio Franceschi, Gordon J. Lithgow, Richard I. Morimoto, Jeffrey E. Pessin, Thomas A. Rando, Arlan Richardson, Eric E. Schadt, Tony Wyss-Coray, Felipe Sierra, "Geroscience: linking aging to chronic disease," *Cell*, 59(4), 709-713, 2014, http://www.cell.com/cell/fulltext/S0092-8674(14)01366-X.

In yet another popular classificatory roadmap, the "hallmarks of aging" that need to be therapeutically addressed, include: 1) genomic instability, 2) telomere attrition, 3) epigenetic alterations, 4) loss of proteostasis, 5) deregulated nutrient sensing, 6) mitochondrial dysfunction, 7) cellular senescence, 8) stem cell exhaustion, 9) altered intercellular communication. See:

Carlos López-Otín, Maria A. Blasco, Linda Partridge, Manuel Serrano, Guido Kroemer, "The hallmarks of aging," *Cell*, 153(6), 1194-1217, 2013, http://www.cell.com/cell/fulltext/S0092-8674(13)00645-4.

7. Anne Brunet, Shelley L. Berger, "Epigenetics of aging and aging-related disease," *Journal of Gerontology: Biological Sciences*, 69 Suppl 1, S17-20, 2014, http://www.ncbi.nlm.nih.gov/pmc/articles/PMC4022130/;

Maria Manukyan, Prim B. Singh, "Epigenetic rejuvenation," *Genes to Cells*, 17(5), 337-343, 2012, https://www.ncbi.nlm.nih.gov/pmc/articles/PMC3444684/;

Alejandro Ocampo, Pradeep Reddy, Paloma Martinez-Redondo, …, Juan Carlos Izpisua Belmonte, "In Vivo Amelioration of Age-Associated Hallmarks by Partial Reprogramming," *Cell*, 167(7), 1719-1733.e12, 2016, http://www.cell.com/fulltext/S0092-8674(16)31664-6.

8. Yehudit Hasin, Marcus Seldin, Aldons Lusis, "Multi-omics approaches to disease," *Genome Biology*, 18, 83, 2017, https://genomebiology.biomedcentral.com/articles/10.1186/s13059-017-1215-1.

9. Linda P. Fried, Jeremy Walston, "Frailty and failure to thrive," in William R. Hazzard, John P. Blass, Walter H. Ettinger, Jeffrey B. Halter, Joseph G. Ouslander (Eds.), *Principles of Geriatric Medicine and Gerontology*, Fourth Edition, McGraw Hill, New York, 1999, pp. 1387-1402.

10. Frailty Net, Frailty toolkit, Diagnostic tools, http://www.frailty.net/frailty-toolkit/Diagnostic-tools/.

11. Kristine E. Ensrud, Susan K. Ewing, Peggy M. Cawthon, Howard A. Fink, Brent C. Taylor, Jane A. Cauley, Thuy-Tien Dam, Lynn M. Marshall, Eric S. Orwoll, Steven R. Cummings, the Osteoporotic Fractures in Men Research Group, "A comparison of frailty indexes for the prediction of falls, disability, fractures, and mortality in older men," *Journal of the American Geriatrics Society*, 57(3), 492-498, 2009.

12. Linda P. Fried, Catherine M. Tangen, Jeremy Walston, Anne B. Newman, Calvin Hirsch, John Gottdiener, Teresa Seeman, Russell Tracy,

Willem J. Kop, Gregory Burke, Mary Ann McBurnie, Cardiovascular Health Study Collaborative Research Group, "Frailty in older adults: evidence for a phenotype," *Journal of Gerontology: Medical Sciences*, 56(3), M146–M156, 2001.

13. Johannes H.G.M. van Beek, Thomas B.L. Kirkwood, James B. Bassingthwaighte, "Understanding the physiology of the ageing individual: computational modelling of changes in metabolism and endurance," *Interface Focus*, 6(2), 20150079, 2016, http://rsfs.royalsocietypublishing.org/content/6/2/20150079.

Gennady G. Rogatsky, Edward G. Shifrin, Avraham Mayevsky, "Physiologic and biochemical monitoring during hyperbaric oxygenation," *Undersea and Hyperbaric Medicine*, 26(2), 111-122, 1999;

Nili Zarchin, Sigal Meilin, Joseph Rifkind, Avraham Mayevsky, "Effect of aging on brain energy-metabolism," *Comparative Biochemistry and Physiology Part A: Molecular & Integrative Physiology*, 132(1), 117-120, 2002.

14. Thomas Craig, Chris Smelick, Robi Tacutu, Daniel Wuttke, Shona H. Wood, Henry Stanley, Georges Janssens, Ekaterina Savitskaya, Alexey Moskalev, Robert Arking, João Pedro de Magalhães, "The Digital Ageing Atlas: integrating the diversity of age-related changes into a unified resource," *Nucleic Acids Research*, 43, D873-878, 2015, https://www.ncbi.nlm.nih.gov/pmc/articles/PMC4384002/;

Georg Fuellen, Paul Schofield, Thomas Flatt, Ralf-Joachim Schulz, Fritz Boege, Karin Kraft, Gerald Rimbach, Saleh Ibrahim, Alexander Tietz, Christian Schmidt, Rüdiger Köhling, Andreas Simm, "Living Long and Well: Prospects for a Personalized Approach to the Medicine of Ageing," *Gerontology*, 62(4), 409-416, 2016.

15. Marian Beekman, Hélène Blanché, Markus Perola, Anti Hervonen, Vladyslav Bezrukov, Ewa Sikora, ..., Claudio Franceschi, the GEHA consortium, "Genome-wide linkage analysis for human longevity: Genetics of Healthy Aging Study," *Aging Cell*, 12(2),184-193, 2013;

Alexander Bürkle, María Moreno-Villanueva, Jürgen Bernhard, María Blasco, Gerben Zondag, Jan H.J. Hoeijmakers, Olivier Toussaint, Beatrix Grubeck-Loebenstein, Eugenio Mocchegiani, Sebastiano Collino, Efstathios S. Gonos, Ewa Sikora, ..., Richard Aspinall, "MARK-AGE biomarkers of ageing," *Mechanisms of Ageing and Development*, 151, 2-12, 2015;

Gregory K. Farber, "Can data repositories help find effective treatments for complex diseases?" *Progress in Neurobiology*, 152, 200-212, 2017.

16. John C. Newman, Sofiya Milman, Shahrukh K. Hashmi, Steve N. Austad, James L. Kirkland, Jeffrey B. Halter, Nir Barzilai, "Strategies and Challenges in Clinical Trials Targeting Human Aging," *Journal of Gerontology: Biological Sciences*, 71(11), 1424-1434, https://academic.oup.com/biomedgerontology/article/71/11/1424/2577175/Strategies-and-Challenges-in-Clinical-Trials;

Anthony Atala, "Extending life using tissue and organ replacement," *Current Aging Science*, 1(2), 73-83, 2008.

17. David Blokh, Ilia Stambler, "The application of information theory for the research of aging and aging-related diseases," *Progress in Neurobiology*, S0301-0082(15)30059-9, 2016, doi: http://dx.doi.org/10.1016/j.pneurobio.2016.03.005;

David Blokh, Ilia Stambler, "The use of information theory for the evaluation of biomarkers of aging and physiological age," *Mechanisms of Ageing and Development*, 163, 23-29, 2017, doi: http://dx.doi.org/10.1016/j.mad.2017.01.003;

Keren Yizhak, Orshay Gabay, Haim Cohen, Eytan Ruppin, "Model-based identification of drug targets that revert disrupted metabolism and its application to ageing," *Nature Communications*, 4, 2632, 2013, https://www.nature.com/articles/ncomms3632.

Georg Fuellen, Melanie Boerries, Hauke Busch, Aubrey de Grey, Udo Hahn, Thomas Hiller, ..., Daniel Wuttke, "In Silico Approaches and the Role of Ontologies in Aging Research," *Rejuvenation Research*, 16(6), 540-546, 2013, http://online.liebertpub.com/doi/abs/10.1089/rej.2013.1517.

18. Anne Brunet, Shelley L. Berger, "Epigenetics of aging and aging-related disease," *Journal of Gerontology: Biological Sciences*, 69 Suppl 1, S17-20, 2014;

Maria Manukyan, Prim B. Singh, "Epigenetic rejuvenation," *Genes to Cells*, 17(5), 337-343, 2012;

Alejandro Ocampo, Pradeep Reddy, Paloma Martinez-Redondo, ..., Juan Carlos Izpisua Belmonte, "In Vivo Amelioration of Age-Associated Hallmarks by Partial Reprogramming," *Cell*, 167 (7), 1719-1733.e12, 2016;

Shuji Kishi, Peter E. Bayliss, Jun-ichi Hanai, "A prospective epigenetic paradigm between cellular senescence and epithelial-mesenchymal transition in organismal development and aging," *Translational Research*, 165(1), 241-249, 2014;

Steve Horvath, "DNA methylation age of human tissues and cell types," *Genome Biology*, 14, R115, 2013, https://www.ncbi.nlm.nih.gov/pmc/articles/PMC4015143/;

Danny Ben-Avraham, Radhika H. Muzumdar, Gil Atzmon, "Epigenetic genome-wide association methylation in aging and longevity," *Epigenomics*, 4(5), 503-509, 2012.

19. Konrad T. Howitz, Kevin J. Bitterman, Haim Y. Cohen, Dudley W. Lamming, Siva Lavu, Jason G. Wood, Robert E. Zipkin, Phuong Chung, Anne Kisielewski, Li-Li Zhang, Brandy Scherer, David A. Sinclair, "Small molecule activators of sirtuins extend Saccharomyces cerevisiae lifespan," *Nature*, 425(6954), 191-196, 2003;

Yariv Kanfi, Shoshana Naiman, Gail Amir, Victoria Peshti, Guy Zinman, Liat Nahum, Ziv Bar-Joseph, Haim Y. Cohen, "The sirtuin SIRT6 regulates lifespan in male mice," *Nature*, 483(7388), 218-221, February 22, 2012;

271

Yan Sun, Jia Li, Na Xiao, Meng Wang, Junping Kou, Lianwen Qi, Fang Huang, Baolin Liu, Kang Liu, "Pharmacological activation of AMPK ameliorates perivascular adipose/endothelial dysfunction in a manner interdependent on AMPK and SIRT1," *Pharmacological Research*, 89, 19-28, 2014;

Laurent Mouchiroud, Laurent Molin, Nicolas Dallière, Florence Solari, "Life span extension by resveratrol, rapamycin, and metformin: The promise of dietary restriction mimetics for an healthy aging," *Biofactors*, 36(5), 377-382, 2010.

20. Weijie You, Dante Rotili, Tie-Mei Li, Christian Kambach, Marat Meleshin, Mike Schutkowski, Katrin F. Chua, Antonello Mai, Clemens Steegborn, "Structural Basis of Sirtuin 6 Activation by Synthetic Small Molecules," *Angewandte Chemie International Edition*, 56(4), 1007-1011, 2017;

Sriram Kosuri, George M. Church, "Large-scale de novo DNA synthesis: technologies and applications," *Nature Methods*, 11(5), 499-507, 2014;

Shawn M. Douglas, Ido Bachelet, George M. Church, "A Logic-Gated Nanorobot for Targeted Transport of Molecular Payloads," *Science*, 335(6070), 831-834, February 17, 2012.

21. David Blokh, Ilia Stambler, "The application of information theory for the research of aging and aging-related diseases," *Progress in Neurobiology*, S0301-0082(15)30059-9, 2016, doi: http://dx.doi.org/10.1016/j.pneurobio.2016.03.005.

22. Ilia Stambler, "The pursuit of longevity – The bringer of peace to the Middle East," *Current Aging Science*, 6, 25-31, 2014.

23. Ilia Stambler, "Recognizing degenerative aging as a treatable medical condition: methodology and policy," *Aging and Disease*, 8(5), 2017, http://www.aginganddisease.org/EN/10.14336/AD.2017.0130;

Ilia Stambler, "Human life extension: opportunities, challenges, and implications for public health policy," in Alexander Vaiserman (Ed.), *Anti-aging Drugs: From Basic Research to Clinical Practice*, Royal Society of Chemistry, London, 2017, pp. 535-564.

24. Michael J. Rae, Robert N. Butler, Judith Campisi, Aubrey D.N.J. de Grey, Caleb E. Finch, Michael Gough, George M. Martin, Jan Vijg, Kevin M. Perrott, Barbara J. Logan, "The demographic and biomedical case for late-life interventions in aging," *Science Translational Medicine*, 2, 40cm21, 2010, http://stm.sciencemag.org/content/2/40/40cm21.full;

Luigi Fontana, Brian K. Kennedy, Valter D. Longo, Douglas Seals, Simon Melov, "Medical research: treat ageing," *Nature*, 511(7510), 405-407, 2014, http://www.nature.com/news/medical-research-treat-ageing-1.15585;

Kunlin Jin, James W. Simpkins, Xunming Ji, Miriam Leis, Ilia Stambler, "The critical need to promote research of aging and aging-related diseases to improve health and longevity of the elderly population," *Aging and*

Disease, 6, 1-5, 2015, http://www.aginganddisease.org/EN/10.14336/AD.2014.1210;

Dana P. Goldman, David M. Cutler, John W. Rowe, Pierre-Carl Michaud, Jeffrey Sullivan, Jay S. Olshansky, Desi Peneva, "Substantial health and economic returns from delayed aging may warrant a new focus for medical research," *Health Affairs*, 32(10), 1698-1705, 2013, https://www.ncbi.nlm.nih.gov/pmc/articles/PMC3938188/.

25. Alex Zhavoronkov, Bhupinder Bhullar, "Classifying aging as a disease in the context of ICD-11," *Frontiers in Genetics*, 6, 326, 2015, http://journal.frontiersin.org/article/10.3389/fgene.2015.00326/full;

Sven Bulterijs, Raphaella S. Hull, Victor C.E. Björk, Avi G. Roy, "It is time to classify biological aging as a disease," *Frontiers in Genetics*, 6, 205, 2015, http://journal.frontiersin.org/article/10.3389/fgene.2015.00205/full;

Ilia Stambler, "Has aging ever been considered healthy?" *Frontiers in Genetics*, 6, 202, 2015, http://journal.frontiersin.org/article/10.3389/fgene.2015.00202/full.

26. Joshua K. Hartshorne, Laura T. Germine, "When does cognitive functioning peak? The asynchronous rise and fall of different cognitive abilities across the life span," *Psychological Science*, 26(4), 433-443, 2015.

27. Alan A. Cohen, "Complex systems dynamics in aging: new evidence, continuing questions," *Biogerontology*, 17(1), 205-220, 2016, https://www.ncbi.nlm.nih.gov/pmc/articles/PMC4723638/;

David Blokh, Ilia Stambler, "The application of information theory for the research of aging and aging-related diseases," *Progress in Neurobiology*, S0301-0082(15)30059-9, 2016, doi: http://dx.doi.org/10.1016/j.pneurobio.2016.03.005;

Alexey Moskalev, Elizaveta Chernyagina, Vasily Tsvetkov, Alexander Fedintsev, Mikhail Shaposhnikov, Vyacheslav Krut'ko, Alex Zhavoronkov, Brian K. Kennedy, "Developing criteria for evaluation of geroprotectors as a key stage toward translation to the clinic," *Aging Cell*, 15(3), 407-415, 2016, http://onlinelibrary.wiley.com/wol1/doi/10.1111/acel.12463/full;

Alexey Moskalev, Elizaveta Chernyagina, Anna Kudryavtseva, Mikhail Shaposhnikov, "Geroprotectors: a unified concept and screening approaches," *Aging and Disease*, 8(3), 354-363, 2017, http://www.aginganddisease.org/EN/10.14336/AD.2016.1022.

28. Eric M. Reiman, Jessica B.S. Langbaum, Adam S. Fleisher, Richard J. Caselli, Kewei Chen, Napatkamon Ayutyanont, Yakeel T. Quiroz, Kenneth S. Kosik, Francisco Lopera, Pierre N. Tariot, "Alzheimer's Prevention Initiative: A plan to accelerate the evaluation of presymptomatic treatments," *Journal of Alzheimer's Disease*, 26(Suppl 3), 321-329, 2011;

Jeremy Toyn, "What lessons can be learned from failed Alzheimer's disease trials?" *Expert Review of Clinical Pharmacology*, 8(3), 267-269, 2015.

29. Morrison D.H., Rahardja D., King E., Peng Y., Sarode V.R., "Tumour biomarker expression relative to age and molecular subtypes of invasive breast cancer," *British Journal of Cancer*, 107, 382-387, 2012.

30. David G. Le Couteur, Stephen J. Simpson, "Adaptive senectitude: the prolongevity effects of aging," *Journal of Gerontology: Biological Sciences*, 66, 179-182, 2011, https://academic.oup.com/biomedgerontology/article/66A/2/179/594634/Adaptive-Senectitude-The-Prolongevity-Effects-of.

31. David Blokh, Ilia Stambler, "Applying information theory analysis for the solution of biomedical data processing problems," *American Journal of Bioinformatics*, 3(1), 17-29, 2015, http://thescipub.com/abstract/10.3844/ajbsp.2014.17.29.

32. Alexander N. Khokhlov, "From Carrel to Hayflick and back or what we got from the 100 years of cytogerontological studies," *Biophysics*, 55(5), 859-864, 2010.

33. Ronald Bellamy, Peter Safar, Samuel Tisherman, ..., Harvey Zar, "Suspended animation for delayed resuscitation," *Critical Care Medicine*, 24(2Suppl), S24-47, 1996;
Peter Safar, "On the future of reanimatology," *Academic Emergency Medicine*, 7(1), 75-89, 2000.

34. Gennady G. Rogatsky, Ilia Stambler, "Hyperbaric oxygenation for resuscitation and therapy of elderly patients with cerebral and cardio-respiratory dysfunction," *Frontiers In Bioscience* (Scholar Edition), 9, 230-243, 2017, http://www.bioscience.org/2017/v9s/af/484/2.htm;
Gennady G. Rogatsky, Avraham Mayevsky, "The life-saving effect of hyperbaric oxygenation during early-phase severe blunt chest injuries," *Undersea Hyperbaric Medicine*, 34(2), 75-81, 2007;
John N. Kheir, Laurie A. Scharp, Mark A. Borden, ..., Francis X. McGowan Jr., "Oxygen gas-filled microparticles provide intravenous oxygen delivery," *Science Translational Medicine*, 4(140), 140ra88, 2012.

35. Yury P. Gerasimenko, Daniel C. Lu, Morteza Modaber, ..., V. Reggie Edgerton, "Noninvasive Reactivation of Motor Descending Control after Paralysis," *Journal of Neurotrauma*, 32(24), 1968-1980, 2015;
Max Schaldach, *Electrotherapy of the Heart: Technical Aspects in Cardiac Pacing*, Springer-Verlag, Berlin, 2012.

36. David Blokh, Ilia Stambler, "Estimation of heterogeneity in diagnostic parameters of age-related diseases," *Aging and Disease*, 5, 218-225, 2014, http://www.aginganddisease.org/EN/10.14336/AD.2014.0500218;
David Blokh, Ilia Stambler, "Information theoretical analysis of aging as a risk factor for heart disease," *Aging and Disease*, 6, 196-207, 2015, http://www.aginganddisease.org/EN/10.14336/AD.2014.0623;
David Blokh, Ilia Stambler, "The use of information theory for the evaluation of biomarkers of aging and physiological age," *Mechanisms of*

Ageing and Development, 163, 23-29, 2017, doi: http://dx.doi.org/10.1016/j.mad.2017.01.003.

37. Gregory K. Farber, "Can data repositories help find effective treatments for complex diseases?" *Progress in Neurobiology*, 152, 200-212, 2017, http://dx.doi.org/10.1016/j.pneurobio.2016.03.008.

38. Ilia Stambler, "Human life extension: opportunities, challenges, and implications for public health policy," in Alexander Vaiserman (Ed.), *Anti-aging Drugs: From Basic Research to Clinical Practice*, Royal Society of Chemistry, London, 2017, pp. 535-564.

18. The Use of Information Theory for the Evaluation of Biomarkers of Aging and Physiological Age to Predict Aging-related Diseases and Frailty

Ilia Stambler and David Blokh

Summary

This article argues for the expanded application of information-theoretical measures, such as entropy and normalized mutual information, for research of biomarkers of aging and physiological age as an early predictive measure of age-related multimorbidity and frailty. The use of information theory enables unique methodological advantages for the study of aging processes, as it allows the researchers to evaluate non-linear relations between biological parameters, showing the precise quantitative strength of those relations, both for individual and multiple parameters, demonstrating cumulative or holistic (synergistic) effects. The diagnostic models can be built based on diagnostic parameters routinely available to physicians (frailty indexes, laboratory analysis, physical evaluations) as well as more advanced biomarkers (e.g. genetic and epigenetic analysis) – in relation with age and age-related diseases and frailty. The diagnostic systems that are built in this way can be open and can include any number of additional parameters correlated with age and age-related diseases.

The use of information-theoretical methods, utilizing normalized mutual information, can reveal the exact amount of information that various diagnostic parameters or their combinations contain about the persons' physiological (or biological) age. Based on those exact diagnostic values for physiological age determination, it is possible to construct a diagnostic decision rule to evaluate a person's physiological age, as compared to chronological age. The working hypothesis is that people characterized by higher physiological age will have increased risk of age-related frailty and diseases (e.g. heart disease, cancer, type 2 diabetes, neurodegenerative diseases, fractures, falls, mental and functional decline, etc.). Utilizing information-theoretical measures, with additional data, it may be possible to create comprehensive clinically applicable information-theory-based panels of markers and models for the evaluation of physiological age, its relation to age-related diseases and its potential modifications by therapeutic interventions, such as medications and behavioral interventions.[1]

Introduction: The increasing need for anti-aging intervention and longevity medicine

With the rapidly growing aging population, and the corresponding rise in the incidence of aging-related diseases (such as heart disease, cancer, type 2 diabetes, neurodegenerative disease, chronic obstructive pulmonary diseases, etc), there emerges a special need to estimate health conditions and effectiveness of treatments for a variety of aging-related diseases, based on the evaluation of the aging processes underlying those diseases. Such evaluation is also needed to assess the effectiveness of potential anti-aging interventions and interventions against aging-related diseases. Even more importantly, it is needed for an early preventive intervention in these diseases, based on the calculated physiological age. The importance of quantifying the effects of "normal" aging as compared to "abnormal," "pathological," "accelerated" or "premature" aging cannot be overestimated. It is critically important to be able to diagnose "early aging," that is, to identify subjects in whom "biological" or "physiological age" markedly exceeds the "chronological age." Thanks to such "early diagnosis" of aging, as a pre-clinical or concomitant condition for a variety of aging-related diseases, it may be possible to solve the problems of early diagnosis of those aging-derived diseases. In other words, it may be stated that pre-clinical diagnosis of aging-related diseases (such as Alzheimer's disease, type 2 diabetes, cancer and heart disease) naturally belongs in the field of aging research, as aging can be seen as a pre-symptomatic, pre-clinical root determinant of a variety of aging-related diseases.[2]

Cancer

Of special importance, early evaluation of physiological age may facilitate the early diagnosis of cancer with a prolonged preclinical period. This may considerably improve the efficacy of treatment for oncological diseases. There have been debates regarding the usefulness or lack thereof of mammography for subjects aged 40-49, that is regarding the possibility of preclinical diagnosis.[3] It may be difficult to solve this problem in the framework of pure oncology, disregarding the factors of age or aging, but only in the framework of aging research, for which information-theoretical analysis can be meaningfully applied.

Heart disease

The same may be said for cardiovascular diseases, the main age-related cause of death in the world, including deaths due to ischemic heart disease and ischemic and hemorrhagic stroke.[4] Yet, it is also known that

277

cardiovascular diseases, and ischemic heart disease in particular, can be highly susceptible to therapeutic and lifestyle interventions, capable of dramatically extending the health and longevity of the subjects.[5] Hence it is of primary importance to be able to early assess the entire array of risk factors, as well as the effects of therapeutic interventions on the risk factors, either individually or in combinations, including both biological and chronological age.[6]

Neurodegenerative diseases

Also for neurodegenerative diseases, such as Alzheimer's disease, the vast plasticity of the brain of the aged and the feasibility of positive therapeutic interventions, or even cures, have been recognized. Yet, it has also been recognized that, in order to accomplish such interventions, the earliest possible detection and the consideration of polygenic etiologies will be necessary.[7] Here too information-theoretical statistics, capable of utilizing time series methods for prediction from an earlier, preclinical age, and employing mutual information measures to establish non-linear diagnostic correlations of multiple disease determinants, including age, can be indispensable.

Diabetes – Metabolic syndrome

Also, for type 2 diabetes, "diagnosis of aging" can be very helpful for early diagnosis of diabetes, as the diagnostic parameters relevant to diabetes, as well as the underlying biological mechanisms have a great similarity with "normal" aging.[8]

Frailty

Generally, the ability to reliably quantitatively diagnose "delayed aging" or "healthy aging" may pinpoint powerful factors facilitating healthy and productive longevity. Here "healthy aging" (or "healthy longevity") may be understood as the absence of age-related frailty, as commonly defined in geriatric medicine, that is, an active and functional state of older adults characterized by a decreased risk for future poor clinical outcomes, diminished development of disability, dementia, falls, hospitalization, institutionalization or decreased mortality.[9] The ability to provide early quantitative evaluation of frailty risks is also of great medical and economic significance.

Prospective economic benefits from the early detection of aging-related diseases thanks to improved diagnosis of aging itself

278

The humanitarian and economic importance of early detection of aging-related diseases is obvious. Early detection makes it possible to apply preventive medical interventions when the disease is in a more manageable and even curable state, ideally even before any clinical manifestations, thus significantly postponing the time it may take for the disease to progress to a severe, debilitating and more costly state. This postponement of morbidity is also the reason for the vast economic benefits of early detection, necessary for the early preventive intervention. As shown for the US, patients with chronic age-related diseases expend in their last year of life about one third of the total Medicare expenditures (~$15,000 per person).[10] Any postponement of this high morbidity period thanks to early detection and preventive interventions can produce massive net health and economic benefits.

Some of the economic benefits of early detection derive from the improvement of individual health, averting direct medical costs and entitlement payments, reducing lost productivity, disability, and employee turnover.[11] As of 2004, it was estimated that "75 percent of the $1.9 trillion spent on health care in the United States stem from preventable chronic health conditions ... but only 1 percent is allocated to protecting health and preventing illness."[12]

Specifically, regarding particular aging related diseases, such as Alzheimer's disease and Cancer, the savings from early detection per patient are commonly estimated at several thousand dollars for the developed countries: $1,000-10,000+ for Alzheimer's disease,[13] $1,000-10,000+ for various forms of cancer.[11] Comparable savings can be expected from the early detection of heart disease[14] and diabetes.[15]

The numbers of patients suffering from these conditions globally are estimated at tens of millions, and are expected to strongly increase worldwide due to the rapid population aging.[16] Thus, 36 million people worldwide are living with dementia, including ~10M in Europe and ~5M in the US, with their numbers expected to double every 20 years, reaching 66 million by 2030, and 115 million by 2050.[13] Out of the total of 56 million deaths that occurred worldwide in 2012, about 38 million were due to non-communicable (NCD) aging-related diseases, in particular: cardiovascular diseases (17.5 million deaths, or 46.2% of NCD deaths), cancers (8.2 million, or 21.7% of NCD deaths), respiratory diseases, including asthma and chronic obstructive pulmonary disease (4.0 million, or 10.7% of NCD deaths) and diabetes (1.5 million, or 4% of NCD deaths).[17]

The costs of aging-related diseases worldwide are correspondingly vast, amounting to hundreds of billions and trillions of dollars: ~US$600 billion in 2010 only for dementia worldwide,[13] approximately US$800 billion for heart disease; US$850 billion for type 2 diabetes; US$900 billion for cancer; US$300 billion for Chronic Obstructive Pulmonary Disease – COPD.[18]

Thus the healthcare benefits of even minor improvement in the ability of early diagnosis, necessary for early preventive treatments of aging-related diseases, could be immense. The economic benefits from the preventive approach, intervening in the aging processes underlying the non-communicable diseases before they take clinical forms, would be immense as well (hundreds of billions of dollars savings in health expenditures in the course of several decades just in the US, according to some models[19]). Yet, to accomplish this, improved diagnostic capabilities are needed for the aging process itself, capable to reliably estimate the person's physiological and biological age and the effects of interventions on that age.

New methodologies are needed to provide early diagnosis of aging-related ill health

In view of the pressing global social need, new methodologies are required to enable early detection of aging-related ill health. We argue that information-theory-based approaches, utilizing such measures as entropy and mutual information, may provide powerful methodological tools for the solution of these problems. First of all, information theory may allow a more reliable estimation of biological and physiological correlates (biomarkers) of aging, due to its ability to estimate non-linear correlations between parameters, utilizing mutual information measures. The *a priori* reliance on linear statistical correlations when trying to determine such biomarkers has been failing to produce practically applicable results.[20,21] Information-theoretical measures may provide new means to intensify and facilitate this search. Moreover, the preclinical diagnosis requires the simultaneous analysis of a large number of parameters of various kinds, including continuous parameters, with both Gaussian and non-Gaussian distribution, as well as discrete and ranked parameters. Presently, the only theoretically grounded method for the simultaneous analysis of multiple parameters of different kinds is information theory.[22]

Advantages of the information-theoretical methodology

Arguably, it is methodologically problematic to use the current approaches in biomarkers research and quantified health for practical assessments of physiological age and potential aging-ameliorating and healthspan-extending interventions. The methodological difficulties may derive from two major current shortcomings. Firstly, the current approaches, both in quantified health and biomarkers research, are mainly based on static or short term, average or median population values to define the norm. This makes personalization of clinical evaluations and treatments difficult. Secondly and crucially, the existing approaches commonly assume normal (Gaussian) distribution and linear relations of parameters. Hence, they mainly employ linear statistical measures of correlation, such as the correlation coefficient or linear regression. However, such measures do not correspond to physiological realities, where the relations between parameters are non-linear, including the non-linear alterations with age. Hence the currently used methods are ill suited to evaluate physiological age and aging-ameliorating and healthspan-extending interventions. The main advantage of the information-theoretical methodology is that it provides an integrated approach that can take into consideration the non-linear interrelation of a multitude of parameters – biomarkers and intervention factors, using information-theoretical measures, rather than linear statistical measures.[1]

Information theory can serve as a universal methodology to assess health and disease status, in relation to age, unifying a variety of model systems, focusing on age-related changes as the root cause of a variety of chronic age-related diseases and health impairments. Information theory may provide the following specific methodological capabilities, currently not available in any other system:

1st)   The current health metrics mainly employ statistical measures. Yet, statistical measures are often inadequate, insofar as in biological systems, the relations between parameters are often non-linear. In contrast, information-theoretical methods allow for the estimation (measurement) of complex non-linear relations between parameters, hence they allow for the inclusion of a wider range of data for making health decisions.

2nd)   Currently, the results from different study models are described in incompatible terms, that do not permit an easy mutual inference. In contrast, the common terms and measures of information theory, such as entropy and mutual information, can serve as a universal language to describe, in a unified way, any number of diverse models and results.

3rd)   Currently, the degree of mutual applicability between animal model systems and humans, as well as between diverse human samples, is uncertain. In contrast, the evaluation of mutual information between different model systems, can be used as a standardized and convenient estimate of their mutual applicability.

4th)   Currently, the effects of various treatments on human health are often examined in a disconnected manner, without knowing the precise interactions of various treatments. The information-theoretical measures of correlation (such as normalized mutual information) can be employed to test the effects of single or combinations of various treatment factors (such as drugs, genes and lifestyle factors) on the health span and the disease status. By the precise quantitative evaluation of the influence of such factors on the health span and disease status, both synergistic positive and antagonistic adverse effects of treatment interactions can be determined.

5th)   The current systems lack the formal ability to select the most informative (and hence clinically useful) parameters. Using information-theoretical methods, the most informative single parameters or groups of parameters with the highest influence on the health span and disease status can be selected. The selection of the most informative parameters, such as those that contain information about other selected parameters, will allow for a more economic, convenient and efficient diagnostic system. This can save time and expenditures on unnecessary testing, by eliminating the less informative parameters from the outset.

6th)   The current statistical systems are largely heuristic. In contrast, in the information-theoretical diagnostic systems, mutual information is able to provide the exact estimate of similarity between various model systems. Therefore it may be possible to predict the efficacy of a yet untested drug or treatment using the estimates of its similarity (mutual information) with other tested drugs and treatments along with the similarity of model systems to which they are applied. Such an approach may save on unnecessary animal and human testing and facilitate the development of new drugs and treatments.

7th)   The current health assessment systems lack a unified standard or frame of reference. The information-theory-based combined metrics for measuring health status may be based on the convenient and standardized evaluation of system stability, using information-theoretical measures, such as entropy and mutual information. The current systems are mainly based on static, average or median population values. The proposed information-theoretical measures of system stability, assessing dynamic changes in a particular system, can be self-referential, and hence truly personalized.

8th)   The current systems do not permit formal assessment of system stability due to treatments. In contrast, information theory may permit to estimate the effects of particular drugs and treatments, or their combinations, on the stability of a particular system for the short and/or long term, by calculating the system alterations at the input and output caused by the particular treatments. This may provide a common measure of health status and effects of interventions, for the short and long term.

These capabilities are based on the known abilities of information theory, such as 1) to estimate non-linear relations; 2) to describe diverse systems in common terms of entropy change; 3) to estimate the degree of similarity or difference between various systems; 4) to examine combined effects of different parameters on a parameter of choice; 5) to select the most informative parameters; 6) to predict outcomes, as was shown by the wide use of information theory in diagnosis, especially of age related diseases,[1] including cancer;[23] 7) to estimate the general system stability;[22] 8) to estimate changes in system stability, heterogeneity, regulation and information loss in response to external stimuli.

Sample selection

A critical requirement for building an information-theoretical diagnostic model of physiological age and aging-related diseases is the availability of a large range of clinical and biological data on a large population sample. The data can be as diverse as possible, any data may be of interest. The more data are available and the more diverse they are, the more interesting correlations may be discovered and the better may be the diagnostic power. The data may include biomarkers of aging and the types of data that are commonly used in quantified health applications. For example, cellular, molecular and biochemical markers for biological age may include: age-related changes in telomere length (telomere measurement), advanced glycation endproducts (AGE), 8-hydroxyguanine in DNA and amino acids with oxidized side chains as biomarkers of oxidative stress, levels of proteins that are essential for critical functions, DNA repair capacity, decrease in one or more stem cell populations, T-lymphocyte subsets, gene expression micro-array analysis (e.g. for such genes as Sirtuins, Foxo, Clotho, etc.), epigenetic markers (e.g. methylation), measures of oxidative-reductive and acid-base balance, and more. Furthermore, functional markers for aging may include: muscle strength (manual muscle-testing; dynamometer: hand-grip strength), vascular rarefaction and dysfunction (capillaroscopy; forearm blood flow techniques), gait speed, step-to-step variability, balance, functional mobility (timed-up-and-go), endurance capacity (VO2 max), cardio-respiratory indicators (PaO2; PaO2/FiO2), EEG/ECG/EMG, nutritional state/intake, cognition (tests), psychological type profiling (tests), social participation, socio-economic status (income, employment).

Diverse therapeutic influences may be factored into the model in order to evaluate the efficacy of potential aging and lifespan improving interventions and their effects on the biological, physiological and functional age.[24] Those interventions may include: pharmacological treatments (specific drugs, such as rapamycin, metformin, statins, aspirin, etc.), regenerative cell therapies, specific biomedical interventions (operations, physiotherapeutic techniques), reduction of risk factors (smoking, alcohol consumption), dietary factors (e.g. supplements, nutrients, functional foods), physical activity, exercise, rest and sleep, education.

Thus, thanks to the diversity of modeled parameters, various factors affecting aging – biological, environmental and social – can be inter-related and integrated. Of course, the costs of particular markers is an important consideration, hence it may become preferable, at least for practical applications, to use such parameters that would be routinely and inexpensively available to practicing physicians. Notably, however, the number of parameters and the amounts of data, collected, analyzed and made available to physicians and researchers, are constantly and rapidly increasing.

Another issue in selecting data to construct a diagnostic model for physiological age and aging-related ill health is the fact that there is currently no clear, formal and universally accepted clinical definition of aging that can serve as the basis for diagnosis and therapy, which can formally and reliably distinguish between "pathological/accelerated aging" as opposed to "healthy aging." Not surprisingly, the World Health Organization's "Global Strategy and Action Plan on Ageing and Health" (2015) includes "Strategic objective 5" – "Improving measurement, monitoring and research on Healthy Ageing" with such priority tasks as "Develop norms, metrics and new analytical approaches to describe and monitor Healthy Ageing" and "Develop resources, including standardized survey modules, data and biomarker collection instruments and analysis programs."[25] Such a formal understanding and measurement of healthy aging can be aided thanks to the use of standard information-theoretical measures.

An additional important issue for the diagnostic model construction may be the choice of subjects and samples. Arguably, it is preferable to rely on the long-term (longitudinal), rather than short-term (immediate benefit) analysis. Thus, for example, it may be desirable to consider a large number of medical histories of people who were, say, 65-70 a couple of decades back (say in 1990 for illustration) and who were at that time considered "clinically" healthy. From this set, we can form two subsets:

1. The set of medical histories of people who died in 1990-1995, at the age of 65-75 years, from various aging-related diseases, such as type 2 diabetes, cancer, heart disease and Alzheimer's disease.

2. The set of medical histories of people, with a comparable birth time, who are alive presently (in 2017). These persons are at the time approximately 90-100 years old. We assume that the second subset is characterized by greater resilience or delayed aging as compared to the first set. Despite the potential issues with incomplete data and changing measurement techniques, the use of such a sample selection may allow the investigators to solve the following problems:

1. To quantitatively determine the risk factors, related to the emergence and course (severity) of the aging-related diseases: diabetes, cancer, heart disease and Alzheimer's disease.

2. To quantitatively determine the influence of those factors on the emergence and course of the diseases.

3. To quantitatively estimate the combined influence of groups of factors on the diseases and reveal the factors producing cumulative effects.

4. To construct algorithms of pre-clinical diagnosis of the aging-related diseases, such as diabetes, cancer, heart disease and Alzheimer's disease.

For the solution of each of these problems, out of the two subsets, it may be possible to select further subdivisions corresponding to the particular diagnostic tasks at hand. Such a two-fold sample set may also allow the researchers to quantitatively and formally investigate the process of aging, as an underlying and common factor of these diseases, by utilizing a multi-factorial model which corresponds to the understanding of aging as a complex process depending on multiple factors of different etiology. In other words, rather than attempting to infer from the poorly defined concept of biological aging toward its derivative conditions (diseases), it may be possible to formally define pathological or early aging from these diagnosable conditions, seeking common age-related denominators between them.

It should be noted that information-theoretical models of physiological age and aging-related ill health do not need to restrict themselves from the outset to any particular kinds of parameter data or hypothesis. The information-theoretical approach may allow the researchers to utilize any kind of data, at any level, into a single diagnostic model. Thus it can, for example, combine diverse biochemical, molecular-biological, cellular, tissue, physiological, functional and other parameters related to aging. Thus the more parameters of different kinds the researchers may be able to obtain, and the larger the investigated sample they will be able to obtain – the stronger and more informative the model will be. Yet, for practical concerns, and at the initial stages, it may be preferable to strive to first utilize the parameters commonly used in the clinic, such as blood work (biochemistry and cytology). It should also be noted that the choice of the 2 subsets, as indicated above, is not restrictive either. The two subsets allow the convenient primary distinction between subjects presumably characterized by different levels of resilience in aging. Yet, with the addition of more age cohorts, including the young (e.g. across several decades of life) – the diagnostic capabilities may be improved, depending on the availability of data.

Even though the information-theoretical approach can incorporate any number of subjects into the model, improving its diagnostic capabilities, at the initial stage it may be desirable to analyze data from at least 2000 subjects, say 1000 from each subset, as this number of subjects is a putative desirable requirement to establish combined diagnostic indicators from 3 or 4 different parameters. The following rule of thumb can be applied for the selection of the sample size: In the analysis of tables of conjunction, we assume that for almost all the cells, the expected number of elements should be no less than 5 in each cell.[26] We consider discrete parameters that can assume 3 values (i.e. below, equal or above some normative of delimiting value). The rule of thumb, to fulfill the sufficiency criteria for the estimation of the sample size, is: the number of cells in the conjunction matrix (say 9 for 2 parameters - 3x3) x 5 (5 elements in each cell) x 5 (to increase the probability that there will be 5 elements in each cell, though this latter number can be more). Thus for a correlation between 2 single parameters, it is 9x5x5=225 (~200-250), for a correlation of 2 parameters with a third one: 27x5x5=675 (~500-700), for a correlation of 3 combined parameters with a fourth one: 81x5x5=2025 (~2000), etc. 2000 subjects is also the typical number involved in FDA phase 3 clinical trials.[27] However, with further increasing the sample size, the diagnostic value will be further increased. The sample sizes will also depend on the nature of the relations examined. For example, when the parameters are strongly mechanistically related, the sample size could be less. And once again, costs of analysis need to be considered, obviously increasing with a greater sample size.

Evaluation of age-related multimorbidity

Using information-theoretical methodology, it may be possible to establish diagnostic decision rules not just for individual diseases,[22] or for physiological age,[28] but also for combined age-related diseases (age-related multimorbidity). Out of several individual disease variables, a single "multimorbidity" variable can be established composed of several diseases (e.g. diabetes and heart disease and dementia, etc.). And this new composite variable can be correlated to individual or combined risk factors by normalized mutual information. Based on the values of normalized mutual information (strength of correlations), the decision rule could be constructed for the entire multimorbidity variable, or for different types of multimorbidities.

The added value and even necessity of estimating physiological age and age-related multimorbidity, in addition to diagnosing individual diseases, is due to the following reasons:

1) Knowing chronological and physiological age is necessary for diagnosis. It is necessary to accomplish early diagnosis also for individual diseases. The degenerative aging process is the main contributor to age-related diseases. Hence, not being able to evaluate it, discards one of the

main, most informative diagnostic parameters. Moreover, the corresponding inability to intervene into degenerative aging, discards one of the most promising therapeutic targets.

2) There is a need for an integrative, time-related approach. Evaluation of only single diagnostic parameters and risk factors, or only single diseases, without their connection to each other and to the patients' age, without considering their dynamic changes in time, their long-term and synergistic effects, can produce misleading results in diagnosis, and ineffective and even unsafe therapy. The various diagnostic parameters, including age and period, should be evaluated together and intervened together.

3) Evidence-based criteria for physiological age and multimorbidity are needed to develop new therapies and interventions. Furthermore, establishing quantitative and holistic criteria for healthy aging/longevity can help validate the new treatments. The currently existing therapies and interventions are not always effective. There is a critical need to advance novel biomedical research of aging and aging-related diseases, to develop and test new treatments, to improve the healthspan of the elderly. The development of diagnostic criteria for healthy longevity (healthspan), like physiological age or multimorbidity, can help gauge the effects of new treatments and interventions.

It is hoped that information-theoretical methodology will contribute to the advancement of these tasks.

References and notes

1. David Blokh, Ilia Stambler, "Estimation of heterogeneity in diagnostic parameters of age-related diseases," *Aging and Disease*, 5, 218-225, 2014, http://www.aginganddisease.org/EN/10.14336/AD.2014.0500218; David Blokh, Ilia Stambler, "Information theoretical analysis of aging as a risk factor for heart disease," *Aging and Disease*, 6, 196-207, 2015, http://www.aginganddisease.org/EN/10.14336/AD.2014.0623; David Blokh, Ilia Stambler, "Applying information theory analysis for the solution of biomedical data processing problems," *American Journal of Bioinformatics*, 3(1), 17-29, 2015, http://thescipub.com/abstract/10.3844/ajbsp.2014.17.29; David Blokh, Ilia Stambler, "The application of information theory for the research of aging and aging-related diseases," *Progress in Neurobiology*, S0301-0082(15)30059-9, 2016, doi: http://dx.doi.org/10.1016/j.pneurobio.2016.03.005; David Blokh, Ilia Stambler, "The use of information theory for the evaluation of biomarkers of aging and physiological age," *Mechanisms of*

Ageing and Development, 163, 23-29, 2017, doi: http://dx.doi.org/10.1016/j.mad.2017.01.003;

David Blokh, Ilia Stambler, "Quantified Longevity Guide (QLG)," Comorbidity Detection Technologies, 2017, https://ec.europa.eu/eip/ageing/commitments-tracker/a3/quantified-longevity-guide-qlg_en, http://www.longevityisrael.org/comorbidity-detection.html, http://www.qlongevityguide.com/.

2. Michael J. Rae, Robert N. Butler, Judith Campisi, Aubrey DNJ de Grey, Caleb E. Finch, Michael Gough, George M. Martin, Jan Vijg, Kevin M. Perrott, Barbara J. Logan, "The demographic and biomedical case for late-life interventions in aging," *Science Translational Medicine*, 2, 40cm21, 2010, http://stm.sciencemag.org/content/2/40/40cm21.full;

Luigi Fontana, Brian K. Kennedy, Valter D. Longo, Douglas Seals, Simon Melov, "Medical research: treat ageing," *Nature*, 511(7510), 405-407, 2014, http://www.nature.com/news/medical-research-treat-ageing-1.15585;

Kunlin Jin, James W. Simpkins, Xunming Ji, Miriam Leis, Ilia Stambler, "The critical need to promote research of aging and aging-related diseases to improve health and longevity of the elderly population," *Aging and Disease*, 6, 1-5, 2015, http://www.aginganddisease.org/EN/10.14336/AD.2014.1210;

Ilia Stambler, "Recognizing degenerative aging as a treatable medical condition: methodology and policy," *Aging and Disease*, 8(5), 2017, http://www.aginganddisease.org/EN/10.14336/AD.2017.0130;

Ilia Stambler, "Human life extension: opportunities, challenges, and implications for public health policy," in Alexander Vaiserman (Ed.), *Anti-aging Drugs: From Basic Research to Clinical Practice*, Royal Society of Chemistry, London, 2017, pp. 535-564, http://pubs.rsc.org/en/content/ebook/978-1-78262-435-6#!divbookcontent.

3. Bonnie N. Joe, "Risk-based screening misses breast cancers in women in their forties," Radiological Society of North America, 2014, http://www.rsna.org/;

Hakan Jonsson, Lars-Gunnar Larsson, Per Lenner, "Detection of breast cancer with mammography in the first screening round in relation to expected incidence in different age groups," *Acta Oncologica*, 42, 22-29, 2003.

4. Rafael Lozano, et al. (189 authors), "Global and regional mortality from 235 causes of death for 20 age groups in 1990 and 2010: a systematic analysis for the Global Burden of Disease Study 2010," *Lancet*, 380, 2095-2128, 2012.

5. Judith Meadows, Jacqueline Suk Danik, Michelle A. Albert, "Primary prevention of ischemic heart disease," in Elliott M. Antman (Ed.), *Cardiovascular Therapeutics: A Companion to Braunwald's Heart Disease*, Third edition, Saunders Elsevier, Philadelphia PA, 2007, pp. 178-220.

6. David Blokh, Ilia Stambler, "Information theoretical analysis of aging as a risk factor for heart disease," *Aging and Disease*, 6, 196-207, 2015, http://www.aginganddisease.org/EN/10.14336/AD.2014.0623.

7. Zaven S. Khachaturian, "Perspectives on Alzheimer's disease: past, present and future," *Advances in Biological Psychiatry*, 28, 179-188, 2012.

8. David Blokh, Ilia Stambler, "Estimation of heterogeneity in diagnostic parameters of age-related diseases," *Aging and Disease*, 5, 218-225, 2014, http://www.aginganddisease.org/EN/10.14336/AD.2014.0500218; Diane Chau, Steven V. Edelman, "Clinical management of diabetes in the elderly," *Clinical Diabetes*, 19, 172-175, 2001.

9. Linda P. Fried, Jeremy Walston, "Frailty and failure to thrive," in William R. Hazzard, John P. Blass, Walter H. Ettinger, Jeffrey B. Halter, Joseph G. Ouslander (Eds.), *Principles of Geriatric Medicine and Gerontology*, 4th Ed., McGraw Hill, New York, 1999, pp. 1387-1402.

10. Amber E. Barnato, Mark B. Mcclellan, Christopher R. Kagay, Alan M. Garber, "Trends in inpatient treatment intensity among medicare beneficiaries at the end of life," *Health Services Research*, 39(2), 363-376, 2004.

11. C-Change: Collaborating to Conquer Cancer, *Making the Business Case: How Engaging Employees in Preventive Care Can Reduce Healthcare Costs*, 2008, http://c-changetogether.org/Websites/cchange/images/Risk_Reduction/C-Change_Business_Case_White_Paper_(1).pdf.

12. National Committee for Quality Assurance, *Executive Summary. The State of Health Care Quality 2004*, National Committee for Quality, Washington DC, 2005, quoted in C-Change: Collaborating to Conquer Cancer, *Making the Business Case: How Engaging Employees in Preventive Care Can Reduce Healthcare Costs*, 2008, http://c-changetogether.org/Websites/cchange/images/Risk_Reduction/C-Change_Business_Case_White_Paper_(1).pdf.

13. Alzheimer's Disease International, *World Alzheimer Report 2011. The benefits of early diagnosis and intervention*, Martin Prince, Renata Bryce, Cleusa Ferri (Eds.), Institute of Psychiatry, King's College, London, 2011, https://www.alz.co.uk/research/world-report-2011.

14. National Association of Chronic Disease Directors, "Why we need public health to improve healthcare," 2015, http://www.chronicdisease.org/?page=WhyWeNeedPH2impHC.

15. WHO Media Center, "Diabetes: the cost of diabetes," Fact sheet N°236, 2015, http://www.who.int/mediacentre/factsheets/fs236/en/.

16. Stephen S. Lim, et al., "A comparative risk assessment of burden of disease and injury attributable to 67 risk factors and risk factor clusters in 21 regions, 1990–2010: a systematic analysis for the Global Burden of Disease Study 2010," *Lancet*, 380, 2224-2260, 2012;

Rafael Lozano, et al., "Global and regional mortality from 235 causes of death for 20 age groups in 1990 and 2010: a systematic analysis for the Global Burden of Disease Study 2010," *Lancet*, 380, 2095-2128, 2012.

17. World Health Organization, *Global Status Report on Noncommunicable diseases 2014*, http://www.who.int/nmh/publications/ncd-status-report-2014/en/.

18. David E. Bloom, et al., *The Global Economic Burden of Non-Communicable Diseases: A report by the World Economic Forum and the Harvard School of Public Health*, World Economic Forum, Geneva, 2011, http://www3.weforum.org/docs/WEF_Harvard_HE_GlobalEconomicBurdenNonCommunicableDiseases_2011.pdf.

19. Dana P. Goldman, David M. Cutler, John W. Rowe, Pierre-Carl Michaud, Jeffrey Sullivan, Jay S. Olshansky, Desi Peneva, "Substantial health and economic returns from delayed aging may warrant a new focus for medical research," *Health Affairs*, 32(10), 1698-1705, 2013, https://www.ncbi.nlm.nih.gov/pmc/articles/PMC3938188/;
Dana P. Goldman, "The economic promise of delayed aging," in Stuart Jay Olshansky, George M. Martin, James L. Kirkland (Eds.), *Aging: The Longevity Dividend*, Cold Spring Harbor Laboratory Press, 2016.

20. Robert N. Butler, Richard Sprott, Huber Warner, Jeffrey Bland, Richie Feuers, Michael Forster, Howard Fillit, S. Mitchell Harman, Michael Hewitt, Mark Hyman, Kathleen Johnson, Evan Kligman, Gerald McClearn, James Nelson, Arlan Richardson, William Sonntag, Richard Weindruch, Norman Wolf, "Biomarkers of aging: from primitive organisms to humans," *Journal of Gerontology. A. Biological Sciences Medical Sciences*, 59, B560-567, 2004.

21. Arthur K. Balin (Ed.), *Practical Handbook of Human Biologic Age Determination*, CRC Press, Boca Raton FL, 1994.

22. David Blokh, Ilia Stambler, "The application of information theory for the research of aging and aging-related diseases," *Progress in Neurobiology*, S0301-0082(15)30059-9, 2016, doi: http://dx.doi.org/10.1016/j.pneurobio.2016.03.005; http://www.sciencedirect.com/science/article/pii/S0301008215300599.

23. David Blokh, Elena Afrimzon, Ilia Stambler, Eden Korech, Yana Shafran, Naomi Zurgil, Mordechai Deutsch, "Breast cancer detection by Michaelis-Menten constants via linear programming," *Computer Methods and Programs in Biomedicine*, 85, 210-213, 2006;
David Blokh, Ilia Stambler, Elena Afrimzon, Yana Shafran, Eden Korech, Judith Sandbank, Ruben Orda, Naomi Zurgil, Mordechai Deutsch, "The information-theory analysis of Michaelis–Menten constants for detection of breast cancer," *Cancer Detection and Prevention*, 31, 489-498, 2007;
David Blokh, Naomi Zurgil, Ilia Stambler, Elena Afrimzon, Yana Shafran, Eden Korech, Judith Sandbank, Mordechai Deutsch, "An information-

theoretical model for breast cancer detection," *Methods of Information in Medicine*, 47, 322-327, 2008;

David Blokh, Ilia Stambler, Elena Afrimzon, Max Platkov, Yana Shafran, Eden Korech, Judith Sandbank, Naomi Zurgil, Mordechai Deutsch, "Comparative analysis of cell parameter groups for breast cancer detection," *Computer Methods and Programs in Biomedicine*, 94, 239-249, 2009.

David Blokh, "Information-theory analysis of cell characteristics in breast cancer patients," *International Journal on Bioinformatics & Biosciences (IJBB)*, 3(1), 2013.

24. Imre Zs.-Nagy, Denham Harman, Kenichi Kitani (Eds.), *Pharmacology of Aging Processes: Methods of Assessment and Potential Interventions*, Annals of the New York Academy of Sciences, Volume 717, 1994;

Alexander Vaiserman (Ed.), *Anti-aging Drugs: From Basic Research to Clinical Practice*, Royal Society of Chemistry, London, 2017.

25. World Health Organization, *Global Strategy and Action Plan on Ageing and Health*, World Health Organization, Geneva, November 2015, http://who.int/ageing/global-strategy/en/.

26. Solomon Kullback, *Information Theory and Statistics*, John Wiley & Sons, New York, 1958;

John H. Pollard, *A Handbook of Numerical and Statistical Techniques. With Examples Mainly From The Life Sciences*, Cambridge University Press, Cambridge, 1977.

27. US Food and Drug Administration, "The Drug Development Process. Step 3: Clinical Research," accessed June 2017, http://www.fda.gov/ForPatients/Approvals/Drugs/ucm405622.htm.

28. David Blokh, Ilia Stambler, "The use of information theory for the evaluation of biomarkers of aging and physiological age," *Mechanisms of Ageing and Development*, 163, 23-29, 2017, doi: http://dx.doi.org/10.1016/j.mad.2017.01.003.

19. Physical Means for Healthy Life Extension

Introduction

Various means of therapeutic intervention into degenerative aging processes are now gaining increasing interest. The interest is largely due to the mounting challenges of the rapidly aging world population and the correspondingly strengthening desire to seek solutions.[1] Yet, when searching for means to intervene into degenerative aging processes, the emphasis is often placed either on traditional means of life-style improvement (rest, exercise, moderate and balanced nutrition) or various pharmacological means (the so-called geroprotective or anti-aging drugs)[2] or gene-therapeutic or cell-therapeutic means (the so-called regenerative medicine).[3] Yet, additional classes of potential interventions may be possible. Anti-aging and life-extending interventions do not necessarily need to be behavioral, biochemical or biological, but can also be physical, in particular as relates to various resuscitation technologies for the elderly, for example hypothermia and suspended animation,[4] electromagnetic stimulation,[5] or oxygenation (also in a sense a "biochemical" intervention, but with a stronger emphasis on physical energy metabolism and physical properties, such as gas pressure). Such technologies represent some of the most veritable means for life extension, demonstrably saving people from an almost certain death in severe acute conditions. But similar principles could perhaps be used for more preventive treatments and in less acute cases.

This work will focus on means of oxygenation, in particular hyperbaric (high pressure) oxygenation. It may be stated that 100% cases of death, including aging-related deaths, ultimately are caused by a lack of oxygen supply. Hence, various means of oxygenation may be considered as anti-aging means. On the other hand, oxidative damage has been long associated with the aging process.[6] From early times, human life has been likened to a burning candle: too much and too fast burning (oxygenation) could lead to an early death.[7] Hence efficient oxygen supply management may be essential for maintaining healthy longevity. This article draws attention to the issue of oxygenation, in particular the use of hyperbaric oxygen therapy. It is not intended as a clinical guideline, but as a reflection on a potentially important issue and an invitation for further consideration of physical, energy-modulating means for anti-aging and life extension, in particular oxygen management by such means as hyperbaric oxygenation therapy.[8] Some other physical means, such as temperature manipulation and electromagnetic stimulation, are also briefly considered with the same purpose to stimulate further interest.

Insofar as many (perhaps ultimately all) of the cases of death are ultimately due to various forms of oxygen deficit, a powerful means of life extension may be by improving oxygen supply. One way of oxygen supply can be in the form of Hyperbaric Oxygenation (using Oxygen Pressure Chamber or Barochamber). Such therapy was indicated as beneficial against a variety of life-threatening acute conditions, such as traumas and injuries, including severe brain and chest injuries, and could also improve a variety of degenerative and aging-related conditions, from neurological impairments, such as cerebral palsy and strokes, to diabetes.[9]

However, in high concentrations, oxygen can be cytotoxic. On the positive side, oxygen toxicity against bacteria may partly explain beneficial effects of hyperbaric oxygenation for treating acute infections, as well as wound, burn and fracture healing, where infections can be a major obstacle to effective healing.[10] The cytotoxic effects may be also involved in anti-cancer treatment, to destroy cancer cells by high oxygen concentrations.[11] Yet, the oxygen cytotoxic effect can be problematic, when either the oxygen dose or the time of exposure to oxygen exceed a desirable physiological threshold.[12] Oxygen can lead to excessive cell and tissue stimulation, exhausting cell replicative potential, increasing the amount of reactive oxygen species and hastening the transition to apoptotic cell death via mitochondria activation.[13] The thresholds of oxygen toxicity have been uncertain even regarding single time applications of hyperbaric oxygenation.[14] And long-term effects of hyperbaric oxygenation on human life span apparently have not been studied.

Mechanisms of action of hyperbaric oxygenation against aging-related conditions

The mechanisms of potential general protective and/or anti-aging (geroprotective) effects of hyperbaric oxygenation, if such are indeed present, are yet to be elucidated. The question of dosages may be also critical for determining the mechanisms of such anti-aging effects. High dosages of hyperbaric oxygen should intuitively induce oxidative stress, with high reactive oxygen species (ROS) production, which has been long seen as one of the major sources of molecular damage in aging.[6] Indeed, oxidative damage has been observed under hyperbaric oxygen treatment, among other effects potentially contributing to cataract development.[15] Yet, it is also appreciated that, at certain levels, ROS may stimulate tissue regeneration.[16] And yet at certain dosages, hyperbaric oxygen may produce stimulatory "hormetic" effects (i.e. stimulation by a low dose, as opposed to inhibition by a high dose of the same factor), which may in fact increase anti-oxidant protection, via stimulation of anti-oxidant defense systems.[17] In other words, under a certain non-dangerous threshold, ROS generated due to hyperbaric oxygenation may stimulate the body's anti-ROS defense.

The protective effects of hyperbaric oxygen by stimulating heat shock protein expression[18] and stem cell mobilization[19] have also been suggested. In a related way, chronic systemic inflammation has been long implicated as a major source of aging-related damage.[20] Furthermore, excessive neuro-inflammation has been a sustained therapeutic target.[21] Hyperbaric oxygenation has been commonly reported to produce an anti-inflammatory effect, which has been suggested as one of its major therapeutic mechanisms, for both age-related chronic and acute conditions (like acute ischemic stroke).[22] Yet, there is also a growing realization that pro-inflammatory effects may be essential for tissue regeneration, including neuro-regeneration.[23]

Closely related to the phenomenon of hormesis (low dose stimulation), hyperbaric oxygenation may exert protective anti-ischemic effects through ischemic preconditioning, that is applying a certain sub-threshold dosage of hyperbaric oxygen that would induce a transient, mild ischemia that would create tolerance to subsequent, more severe ischemia.[24] This mechanism opens the possibility for using hyperbaric oxygenation as a preventive therapy for the elderly. Some of the mechanisms of preconditioning were associated with enhanced expression of protective enzymes, such as Sirtuins,[25] enhanced mitogen-activated protein kinases (MAPKs) and autophagy,[26] and inhibiting the mechanistic target of rapamycin (mTOR) enzyme pathway.[27] Thus, the mechanisms of preconditioning by hyperbaric oxygenation may be similar with the application of other geroprotective medicines (e.g. Sirtuin-stimulating or mTOR-inhibiting drugs),[28] producing a general improvement of energy metabolism, yet potentially with fewer pharmacogenic side effects. However, this possibility will yet require extensive investigation, necessitating a very careful consideration of the dosages. The short vs. long term effects should be considered when studying the mechanisms of action of hyperbaric oxygenation.[29] Indeed, there may be a need for a systemic, long-term evaluation of oxygen therapy effects, as a part of a whole-organism whole-life-course model of energy resources expenditures. Such models are currently only emerging,[30] and are in great need of elaboration, both experimental and theoretical.

Supplementing Hyperbaric Oxygenation with additional treatment modalities

Hyperbaric Oxygenation can be seen as a potentially effective therapeutic or stimulating means, but it is unclear to which extent it can serve as a lifespan-extending means. Hence, the therapeutic modality of Hyperbaric Oxygenation may be supplemented or followed by additional modalities particularly designed to serve life-prolonging, rejuvenative and reparative functions. Pressure chamber could in principle provide a convenient environment to implement such modalities, insofar as it provides a protected, isolated and enclosed space unit, which can be easily manipulated and monitored for a variety of purposes. Some of the potential reparative applications can be as follows.

O_2/CO_2 Balance

For the life-span and health-span extension, rather than applying hyperbaric oxygenation, actually reducing oxygen partial pressure may be beneficial. Thus people living at high altitudes (with reduced oxygen pressure) are noted for high longevity, presumably due to either reduced metabolic rate or long-term adaptations to improve oxygen supply. Some of the potential beneficial adaptations may include increased production of red blood cells, formation of new capillaries and increase in respiratory enzymes, and other mechanisms.[31]

Also, increased CO_2 can be beneficial, insofar as persistent hypercapnia (enhanced CO_2 level) has been associated with an increased life-span in animal models. This may presumably be due to increasing blood alkalinity (through liberating bicarbonate reserves) which may in turn positively affect proteins' isoelectric stability.[32]

Interestingly and seemingly paradoxically, both hyperbaric oxygenation therapy and its apparent opposite – therapeutic hypoxia or hypoxic training (for example intermittent hypoxia) have been suggested to produce positive preconditioning effects against ischemic aging-related conditions, such as heart disease and neurodegenerative diseases.[33] The apparent paradox may be once again explained by the phenomenon of "hormesis" – namely the activation of anti-hypoxic/anti-ischemic protective mechanisms by certain extents of both deficit and excess of oxygen (in the latter case possibly increasing reactive oxygen species levels to induce a protective counter-effect), as well as possibly by other mild stressors (chemical, mechanical or electrical). The precise dosages and thresholds of such similar protective effects by seemingly diverse means, as well as their potential common central neuro-humoral regulatory mechanisms, yet require elucidation.

Besides hyperbaric oxygen therapy, normobaric (normal pressure) oxygen therapy, or just oxygen therapy generally (increasing oxygen supply) has been a widely practiced means of therapy and resuscitation.[34] While hyperbaric oxygenation (using a pressure chamber) may be more effective to achieve rapid oxygen delivery to deep vital tissues, normobaric oxygenation (e.g. using an oxygen mask) may be more conveniently applicable and less expensive. Yet for normobaric oxygenation too, the appropriate balance of O_2/CO_2 levels may be critical. The pressure chamber may provide an ideal environment to control both O_2 and CO_2 levels and pressures, for acute therapeutic or prolonged restorative regimens. Still, with regard to CO_2 manipulation, its exact therapeutic dosages, long-term effects, as well as its effects on immediate daily performance, will yet need to be established.

The issue of optimal thresholds or O_2/CO_2 balance will be vital, insofar as excessive O_2 application may lead to a "burnout," while excessive CO_2 application may lead to a "death zone." Both acidosis and alkalosis may be produced by O_2/CO_2 imbalance. Perhaps the most beneficial therapeutic regimen may be maintaining and/or rapidly restoring the physiological O_2/CO_2 balance. The normal (balanced) concentration of alveolar CO_2 is sometimes assumed to be about 6.5%, yet may vary according to particular metabolic requirements of every individual.[35]

Monitoring

In order to personalize the therapy, and to ensure its safety and efficacy, the treatment modalities should be related with a thorough array of monitoring and evaluation modalities, in particular for the evaluation of the organism's energy metabolism, before, during and after the treatment. In performing oxygen therapy (in particular hyperbaric oxygenation), reference needs to be made for Oxygen and CO_2 balance (supply vs. demand), as well as for the supply and demand of macroergic (energy-rich) substances, in the entire organism and particular organs.[36] Measurement modalities may include oxygen measurement by mitochondrial cytochrome a,a3 reflectance spectrophotometry, mitochondrial NADH redox state by NADH fluorometry, tissue blood flow by Laser Doppler Flowmetry, hemoglobin oxygen saturation by reflectometry, Direct Current potential and various ionic levels by micro-electrodes, gas partial pressure (O_2, CO_2, NO, etc.) and pH levels by micro-electrodes and optodes, up to more advanced methods such as functional magnetic resonance imaging (fMRI) or using sequential single photon emission computerized tomography (SPECT) scans, etc.[37]

The monitoring of the gas composition (PaO_2 and $PaCO_2$) of the arterial blood may be seen as a necessary condition to perform effective hyperbaric oxygen therapy against life-threatening situations in patients with deteriorating cardio-respiratory functions, especially for the elderly patients.[8] This is necessary in order to control and maintain adequate levels of lung gas exchange, with regulated parameters of oxygen supply and controlled oxygen concentration. The speed of the blood flow and blood pressure in vital organs are also among the critical vital signs that need to be known. The basic parameters of cardio-respiratory function need to be monitored, such as: PaO_2 mmHg – arterial partial pressure of oxygen; $PaCO_2$ – arterial partial pressure of CO_2; PaO_2/FiO_2 – the ratio of the partial pressure of oxygen to the fraction of inspired oxygen; SVI ml/m^2 – stroke volume index; CI L/min/m^2 – cardiac index; pH – blood acidity level. Such measures of cardio-respiratory function can help reference the normal balanced O_2/CO_2 levels in the blood and favorable blood electric charge and hemodynamic conditions.

The anatomical and physiological effects of aging on the heart and lungs are also vitally important parameters, including such indicators as the rise of arterial pressure and resistance with aging due to the increasing arterial stiffness, reduced contractility and relaxation of the heart, a reduction of lung vital capacity, impairment of gas mixture in the lungs, and other harmful anatomical and physiological effects of aging. All the deteriorative changes in the cardio-respiratory system generally show in the reduction of maximal oxygen uptake (VO$_2$max) which has been considered one of the most informative parameters for biological age evaluation.[38]

The above parameters of cardio-respiratory function are practically indispensable in emergency and intensive care medicine, when treating acute and often life-threatening conditions. Yet, arguably, the cardio-respiratory parameters routinely employed in emergency and intensive care medicine may be good candidates for biomarkers of aging as they have proved their utility as real-time indicators of the organism's vitality and energy. Often, in general frailty assessments, energy levels in the elderly are evaluated simply by asking the question "Do you feel full of energy?"[39] Yet, there may be more objective measures of the aging organism's energy level, by such means as spirometry, oximetry, hemodynamic, electrochemical and spectroscopic energy metabolite measurements, as well as other structural and functional parameters of the cardio-respiratory system, that can provide improved indication for therapy.[40] Arguably, such cardio-respiratory "physiomic" parameters or markers of aging may be clinically valuable and conveniently interpretable for a practicing physician, alongside the many "biomarkers of aging" based on predominantly molecular-biological, e.g. genetic, epigenetic and other "omic" age-related alterations that are currently investigated.[41]

The main clinical utility of biomarkers or diagnostic parameters of aging is that their changes can help evaluate the effectiveness of particular therapeutic regimens, especially the effectiveness of particular therapeutic dosages. Yet curiously, in hyperbaric oxygen therapy, the concept of dosage is only rudimentary and there is no commonly agreed way to define the dosage. Moreover, there is no agreed way to evaluate the effects of this kind of therapy, and correspondingly no agreed way to correlate between the dose and the effect. The same may be said regarding other potential "energy-modulating" interventions into aging, whose definition is yet very nebulous.

In certain studies, it was suggested to define the dose of hyperbaric oxygen therapy as the product of intra-barochamber pO_2 (ATA), the duration of a single hyperbaric oxygenation exposure (hours), and the number of hyperbaric oxygenation treatments, yielding the dose unit: (ATA*h*N).[8,12] In those studies, the efficacy of hyperbaric oxygenation therapy was evaluated according to the number of patients who showed a significant clinical improvement in their neurological state in the course of the treatment (the percent of the total number of patients). The level of the therapy efficacy was compared with a corresponding value of the dose. For the treatment of acute ischemic stroke, a higher efficacy was indicated with increasing the average total hyperbaric oxygenation dose, reaching the maximum efficacy with the average doses of no less than 30 units (ATA*h*N).[12]

However, such a definition of the dosages has not become consensus, and the definitions of the therapy effects and of the dose-effect relations are rather vague and yet require a thorough elaboration and clarification. Hopefully, thanks to refinement of the definitions and massive additional data collection on dose-effect relations, including the evaluation of long-term effects and differential personalized effects in different patient groups (e.g. the elderly vs. the young) – oxygen therapy, hyperbaric oxygen therapy particularly, or "energy-modulating therapy" more generally, can become efficient means to alleviate aging-related conditions and increase healthy and productive life.

It is also necessary to note that the obtained datasets of biomarkers, diagnostic parameters, and dose-effect relations, will be not only necessary for monitoring and personalizing treatment regimens, but will also be able to provide invaluable information for many yet unforeseen "quantified health" and "quantified longevity" applications – collecting a vast amount of health data on aging-related changes and their possible improvements, to enable planning better informed therapeutic and life-style regimens and strategies to achieve healthy longevity.[42]

Comprehensive physiological manipulation unit

Enhancing blood supply: The main purpose of oxygenation therapy (in particular hyperbaric oxygen therapy) is to directly enhance the supply of potentially deficient oxygen to the tissues that need it (while necessarily watching out against "burning out" and "oxygen toxicity"). However, oxygen supply can be improved by more indirect means, such as improving

298

blood supply to the tissues. Historically, improved blood supply to the tissues (also for the purposes of rejuvenation) has been persistently sought. For example, the whole-body increase of the blood flow (hyperemia) has been achieved by various means ranging from hormone replacement therapy (by supplements, tissue transplants, and even operations on the endocrine organs) through diathermy (tissue heating), massage, exercise and baths.[1] The problems of oxygen delivery to the vital tissues have been also tackled with additional approaches, such as oxygenated micro-particles and "artificial blood,"[43] various forms of heart-lung machines, artificial hearts and other assisted circulation devices,[44] or pharmacological means to improve energy metabolism.[28] The blood flow can be also stimulated by electromagnetic devices.

As briefly mentioned above, recording electrodes and magnetic resonance devices may be employed for monitoring (for example during the course of oxygen therapy). Yet, in addition, stimulation electrodes may be also used for physiological manipulation purposes, in particular to stimulate nervous activity and blood flow, even to stimulate tissue regeneration, in particular blood vessels growth (angiogenesis – another potential means to improve tissue blood supply and oxygenation, but also requiring caution to avoid uncontrolled growth).[45] Such electromagnetic therapeutic devices have been sometimes termed "electroceuticals."[46] They can be incorporated into the therapeutic regimens, either within the pressure chamber or as a part of accompanying regimens.

The incorporation or fitting of the additional therapeutic modalities within the pressure chamber can provide cumulative benefits. The ability allowed by the pressure chamber to control and manipulate pressure, gas concentrations and temperature, can produce a convenient environment for physiological manipulation. Furthermore, with the addition of an infusion apparatus for delivering medications, including various regenerative and anti-aging medications (depending on the costs involved), this can become a multifunctional treatment unit. Some of its functions can be as follows.

"Resting state" induction: One possibility may be inducing a restorative "resting state" through a variety of environmental means (pressure, temperature, oxygen and carbon dioxide concentration) as well as by electromagnetic and pharmacological means. Thus both reversible hypothermic and pharmacological resting states (reversible coma) are already becoming widely used clinical methods for recuperation and resuscitation, and can be incorporated into the chamber.[47] Just by using such physical manipulation means that are available in the pressure chamber – such as pressure, temperature, O_2 and CO_2 concentrations – a resting state can be induced, insofar as rest and sleep are characterized by particular breathing and temperature patterns.[48] Temperature control can be another powerful means of physical manipulation. Thus, lower core body

temperature has been correlated with longer lifespans.[49] In particular, lowering the body temperature (hypothermia) during hyperbaric oxygenation treatment could reduce energy (oxygen) demand by the organism and thus potentially lower oxygen toxicity. On the other hand, increased blood flow through heating may be used for therapeutic stimulation purposes. Within the chamber, temperature can be manipulated in both directions. The electric charge of the breathing mixture (e.g. negative ionization) can be also significant for recuperation vs. stimulation.[50]

Sleep enhancement: Sleep enhancement can be yet another promising restorative modality (in fact a form of "resting state"). In particular, slow-wave or deep sleep (Stage 3, with synchronized EEG activity, showing slow "delta" waves with a frequency of less than 1 Hz) has been known to be vital for recuperation, presumably due to enhanced growth hormone production[51] or synchronization of physiological functions.[52] The restorative effects of sleep generally, and deep sleep in particular, may be also possibly due to activation of the immune response during sleep, or elimination of toxins, or other mechanisms.[53] This stage can be induced by a variety of methods, including: transcranial direct current stimulation (tDCS) and transcranial magnetic stimulation (TMS),[54] other forms of sensory sleep stimulation[55] and a variety of slow-wave sleep enhancing drugs.[56] Sleeping in a hyperbaric chamber has already been practiced, and this combination of therapeutic modalities can be further explored and expanded, if proven safe and effective.

All such technologies are yet extremely experimental, dose responses have not been thoroughly studied, hence side effects may be unpredictable. Both their short and long-term effects are largely unknown, and the introduction of such additional technologies may become prohibitively expensive and unwieldy. They are mentioned here only as possibilities that can be further investigated and prospectively included within a potential "comprehensive restorative chamber" or "survival chamber."

References and notes

1. Ilia Stambler, *A History of Life-Extensionism in the Twentieth Century*, Longevity History, 2014, http://www.longevityhistory.com/.
2. Ilia Stambler, "Human life extension: opportunities, challenges, and implications for public health policy," in Alexander Vaiserman (Ed.), *Anti-aging Drugs: From Basic Research to Clinical Practice*, Royal Society of Chemistry, London, 2017, pp. 535-564, http://pubs.rsc.org/en/content/ebook/978-1-78262-435-6#!divbookcontent;
Alexander Vaiserman, Oleh Lushchak, "Anti-aging drugs: where are we and where are we going?" in Alexander Vaiserman (Ed.), *Anti-aging Drugs: From*

Basic Research to Clinical Practice, Royal Society of Chemistry, London, 2017, pp. 3-10, http://pubs.rsc.org/en/content/ebook/978-1-78262-435-6#!divbookcontent.

3. Anthony Atala, "Extending life using tissue and organ replacement," *Current Aging Science*, 1(2), 73-83, 2008, http://www.eurekaselect.com/95101/article;

Giuseppe Orlando, Shay Soker, Robert J. Stratta, Anthony Atala, "Will Regenerative Medicine Replace Transplantation?" *Cold Spring Harbor Perspectives in Medicine*, 3(8), a015693, 2013, https://www.ncbi.nlm.nih.gov/pmc/articles/PMC3721273/.

4. Ronald Bellamy, Peter Safar, Samuel Tisherman, ..., Harvey Zar, "Suspended animation for delayed resuscitation," *Critical Care Medicine*, 24(2Suppl), S24-47, 1996, http://www.ncbi.nlm.nih.gov/pubmed/8608704.

5. Yury P. Gerasimenko, Daniel C. Lu, Morteza Modaber, ..., V. Reggie Edgerton, "Noninvasive Reactivation of Motor Descending Control after Paralysis," *Journal of Neurotrauma*, 32(24), 1968-1980, 2015, http://online.liebertpub.com/doi/abs/10.1089/neu.2015.4008;

Max Schaldach, *Electrotherapy of the Heart: Technical Aspects in Cardiac Pacing*, Springer-Verlag, Berlin, 2012.

6. Denham Harman, "Aging: a theory based on free radical and radiation chemistry," *Journal of Gerontology*, 11, 298-300, 1956, http://www.uccs.edu/Documents/rmelamed/harman_1956_13332224.pdf ;

Rajindar S. Sohal, "Role of oxidative stress and protein oxidation in the aging process," *Free Radical Biology and Medicine*, 33(1), 37-44, 2002, http://www.sciencedirect.com/science/article/pii/S0891584902008560;

Rajindar S. Sohal, "Oxidative stress hypothesis of aging," *Free Radical Biology and Medicine*, 33(5), 573-574, 2002, http://www.sciencedirect.com/science/article/pii/S0891584902008857;

Toren Finkel, Nikki J. Holbrook, "Oxidants, oxidative stress and the biology of ageing," *Nature*, 408(6809), 239-247, 2000, https://www.nature.com/nature/journal/v408/n6809/full/408239a0.html.

7. Gerald J. Gruman, *A History of Ideas about the Prolongation of Life. The Evolution of Prolongevity Hypotheses to 1800*, Transactions of the American Philosophical Society, Vol. 56(9), Philadelphia, 1966.

8. Gennady G. Rogatsky, Ilia Stambler, "Hyperbaric oxygenation for resuscitation and therapy of elderly patients with cerebral and cardio-respiratory dysfunction," *Frontiers In Bioscience* (Scholar Edition), 9, 230-243, June 1, 2017, http://www.bioscience.org/2017/v9s/af/484/2.htm, https://www.bioscience.org/special-issue-details?editor_id=1746, https://www.ncbi.nlm.nih.gov/pubmed/28410116.

9. The standard indications for the use of hyperbaric oxygenation, as established by the US-incorporated Undersea and Hyperbaric Medicine

Society (UHMS), include: 1. Air or Gas Embolism, 2. Carbon Monoxide Poisoning, 3. Clostridial Myositis and Myonecrosis (Gas Gangrene), 4. Crush Injury, Compartment Syndrome and Other Acute Traumatic Ischemias, 5. Decompression Sickness, 6. Arterial Insufficiencies, 7. Severe Anemia, 8. Intracranial Abscess, 9. Necrotizing Soft Tissue Infections, 10. Osteomyelitis (Refractory), 11. Delayed Radiation Injury (Soft Tissue and Bony Necrosis), 12. Compromised Grafts and Flaps, 13. Acute Thermal Burn Injury; 14. Idiopathic Sudden Sensorineural Hearing Loss.

(Undersea and Hyperbaric Medicine Society (UHMS), "Indications for Hyperbaric Oxygen Therapy," https://www.uhms.org/resources/hbo-indications.html.)

Yet, there is good evidence for the possible use of this treatment against other severe and chronic conditions. See for example:

Gennady G. Rogatsky, Avraham Mayevsky, "The life-saving effect of hyperbaric oxygenation during early-phase severe blunt chest injuries," *Undersea and Hyperbaric Medicine*, 34(2), 75-81, 2007, http://archive.rubicon-foundation.org/xmlui/bitstream/handle/123456789/6468/17520858.pdf?sequence=1;

Ning Gu, Fumiko Nagatomo, Hidemi Fujino, Isao Takeda, Kinsuke Tsuda, Akihiko Ishihara, "Hyperbaric oxygen exposure improves blood glucose level and muscle oxidative capacity in rats with type 2 diabetes," *Diabetes Technology & Therapeutics*, 12(2), 125-133, 2010, http://online.liebertpub.com/doi/abs/10.1089/dia.2009.0104;

Majid Kalani, Gun Jörneskog, Nazanin Naderi, Folke Lind, Kerstin Brismar, "Hyperbaric oxygen (HBO) therapy in treatment of diabetic foot ulcers: Long-term follow-up," *Journal of Diabetes and its Complications*, 16(2), 153-158, 2002, http://www.jdcjournal.com/article/S1056-8727(01)00182-9/fulltext;

Michael H. Bennett, Jan P. Lehm, Nigel Jepson, "Hyperbaric oxygen therapy for acute coronary syndrome," *Cochrane Database of Systematic Reviews*, 2015(7), CD004818, 2015, http://onlinelibrary.wiley.com/doi/10.1002/14651858.CD004818.pub4/full;

Peter Kranke, Michael H. Bennett, Marrissa Martyn-St James, Alexander Schnabel, Sebastian E. Debus, "Hyperbaric oxygen therapy for chronic wounds," *Cochrane Database of Systematic Reviews*, 2015(6), CD004123, 2015, http://onlinelibrary.wiley.com/doi/10.1002/14651858.CD004123.pub3/abstract;

Michael H Bennett, Barbara Trytko, Benjamin Jonker, "Hyperbaric oxygen therapy for the adjunctive treatment of traumatic brain injury," *Cochrane Database of Systematic Reviews*, 2012(12), CD004609, 2012, http://onlinelibrary.wiley.com/doi/10.1002/14651858.CD004609.pub2/abstract;

Richard A. Neubauer Research Institute, "Resources," www.ranri.org/resources.html.

10. Escobar S.J., Slade J.B., Hunt T.K., Cianci P., "Adjuvant hyperbaric oxygen therapy (HBO2) for treatment of necrotizing fasciitis reduces mortality and amputation rate," *Undersea and Hyperbaric Medicine*, 32(6), 437–43, 2005, http://dspace.rubicon-foundation.org/xmlui/bitstream/handle/123456789/4061/16509286.pdf?sequence=1.

11. Ingrid Moen, Linda E. B. Stuhr, "Hyperbaric oxygen therapy and cancer – a review," *Targeted Oncology*, 7, 233–242, 2012, https://www.ncbi.nlm.nih.gov/pmc/articles/PMC3510426/.

12. Gennady G. Rogatsky, Edward G. Shifrin, Avraham Mayevsky, "Optimal dosing as a necessary condition for the efficacy of hyperbaric oxygen therapy in acute ischemic stroke: a critical review," *Neurological Research*, 25(1), 95-98, 2003, http://www.tandfonline.com/doi/abs/10.1179/016164103101201003; https://www.researchgate.net/publication/10920324_Optimal_dosing_as_a_necessary_condition_for_the_efficacy_of_hyperbaric_oxygen_therapy_in_acute_ischemic_stroke_A_critical_review.

13. Elena Afrimzon, Naomi Zurgil, Yana Shafran, Pnina Leibovich, Maria Sobolev, Larissa Guejes, Mordechai Deutsch, "The use of sequential staining for detection of heterogeneous intracellular response of individual Jurkat cells to lysophosphatidylcholine," *Journal of Immunological Methods*, 387(1-2), 96-106, 2013, http://www.sciencedirect.com/science/article/pii/S0022175912002992.

14. Serguei N. Efouni, et al., "Hyperoxia. Patofiziologicheskie aspekty lechebnogo i toxicheskogo vozdeystvia hyperbaricheskogo kisloroda (Hyperoxia. Pathophysiological aspects of therapeutic and toxic effects of hyperbaric oxygenation), in Serguei N. Efouni (Ed.), *Rukovodstvo po Hyperbaricheskoy Oxygenazii. Teoria I Praktika Klinicheskogo Primenenia* (Hyperbaric Oxygenation: a manual. The theory and practice of clinical application), Akademia Medizinskikh Nauk SSSR (Academy of Medical Sciences of the USSR), Medizina, Moscow, 1986, pp. 29-56;
Richard D. Vann, *Oxygen Toxicity Risk Assessment*, Office of Naval Research, Arlington VA, 1988, https://www.researchgate.net/publication/235051634_Oxygen_Toxicity_Risk_Assessment;
Noemi Bitterman, "CNS oxygen toxicity," *Undersea and Hyperbaric Medicine*, 31(1), 63-72, 2004, http://dspace.rubicon-foundation.org/xmlui/bitstream/handle/123456789/3991/15233161.pdf?sequence=1.

15. Yi Zhang, Shan OuYang, Lan Zhang, XianLing Tang, Zhen Song, Ping Liu, "Oxygen-induced changes in mitochondrial DNA and DNA repair

enzymes in aging rat lens," *Mechanisms of Ageing and Development*, 131(11-12), 666-673, 2010, http://www.sciencedirect.com/science/article/pii/S0047637410001740.

16. Carole Gauron, Christine Rampon, Mohamed Bouzaffour, Eliane Ipendey, Jérémie Teillon, Michel Volovitch, Sophie Vriz, "Sustained production of ROS triggers compensatory proliferation and is required for regeneration to proceed," *Scientific Reports*, 3, 2084, 2013, https://www.nature.com/articles/srep02084.

17. Cassandra A. Godman, Rashmi Joshi, Charles Giardina, George Perdrizet, Lawrence E. Hightower, "Hyperbaric oxygen treatment induces antioxidant gene expression," *Annals of the New York Academy of Sciences*, 1197, 178-183, 2010, http://onlinelibrary.wiley.com/doi/10.1111/j.1749-6632.2009.05393.x/abstract.

18. Jeysen Zivan Yogaratnam, Gerard Laden, Levant Guvendik, Mike Cowen, Alex Cale, Steve Griffin, "Can hyperbaric oxygen be used as adjunctive heart failure therapy through the induction of endogenous heat shock proteins?" *Advances in Therapy*, 24(1), 106-118, 2007, https://oxfordrecoverycenter.com/wp-content/uploads/2017/02/Can-Hyperbaric-Oxygen-Be-Used-as-Adjunctive-Heart-Failure-Therapy-Through-the-Induction-of-Endogenous-Heat-Shock-Proteins.pdf.

19. Stephen R. Thom, Veena M. Bhopale, Omaida C. Velazquez, Lee J. Goldstein, Lynne H. Thom, Donald G. Buerk, "Stem cell mobilization by hyperbaric oxygen," *American Journal of Physiology - Heart and Circulatory Physiology*, 290(4), H1378-1386, 2006, http://ajpheart.physiology.org/content/290/4/H1378.long.

20. Claudio Franceschi, Judith Campisi, "Chronic inflammation (inflammaging) and its potential contribution to age-associated diseases," *The Journals of Gerontology Series A, Biological Sciences and Medical Sciences*, 69 (Supplement 1), S4-9, 2014, https://academic.oup.com/biomedgerontology/article-lookup/doi/10.1093/gerona/glu057.

21. Joaquin Jordan, Tomas Segura, David Brea, Maria F. Galindo, Jose Castillo, "Inflammation as therapeutic objective in stroke," *Current Pharmaceutical Design*, 14, 3549-3564, 2008, http://www.eurekaselect.com/68189/article.

22. Zheng Ding, Wesley C. Tong, Xiao-Xin Lu, Hui-Ping Peng, "Hyperbaric oxygen therapy in acute ischemic stroke: a review," *Interventional Neurology*, 2(4), 201-211, 2014, https://www.ncbi.nlm.nih.gov/pmc/articles/PMC4188156/.

23. Michael Karin, Hans Clevers, "Reparative inflammation takes charge of tissue regeneration," *Nature*, 529(7586), 307-315, 2016, http://www.nature.com/nature/journal/v529/n7586/full/nature17039.html;

Kuti Baruch, Aleksandra Deczkowska, Neta Rosenzweig, Afroditi Tsitsou-Kampeli, Alaa Mohammad Sharif, Orit Matcovitch-Natan, Alexander Kertser, Eyal David, Ido Amit, Michal Schwartz, "PD-1 immune checkpoint blockade reduces pathology and improves memory in mouse models of Alzheimer's disease," *Nature Medicine*, 22, 135-137, 2016, http://www.weizmann.ac.il/neurobiology/labs/schwartz/sites/weizmann.ac.il.neurobiology.labs.schwartz/files/2016_natmed.pdf.

24. Qin Hu, Anatol Manaenko, Nathanael Matei, Zhenni Guo, Ting Xu, Jiping Tang, John H. Zhang, "Hyperbaric oxygen preconditioning: a reliable option for neuroprotection," *Medical Gas Research*, 6(1), 20-32, 2016, https://www.ncbi.nlm.nih.gov/pmc/articles/PMC5075679/;

Zheng Ding, Wesley C. Tong, Xiao-Xin Lu, Hui-Ping Peng, "Hyperbaric oxygen therapy in acute ischemic stroke: a review," *Interventional Neurology*, 2(4), 201-211, 2014, https://www.ncbi.nlm.nih.gov/pmc/articles/PMC4188156/;

Gerd Heusch, Hans Erik Bøtker, Karin Przyklenk, Andrew Redington, Derek Yellon, "Remote Ischemic Conditioning," *Journal of the American College of Cardiology*, 65(2), 177-195, 2015, https://www.ncbi.nlm.nih.gov/pmc/articles/PMC4297315/.

25. Wenjun Yan, Zongping Fang, Qianzi Yang, Hailong Dong, Yan Lu, Chong Lei, Lize Xiong, "SirT1 mediates hyperbaric oxygen preconditioning-induced ischemic tolerance in rat brain," *The Journal of Cerebral Blood Flow & Metabolism*, 33(3), 396-406, 2013, https://www.ncbi.nlm.nih.gov/pmc/articles/PMC3587810/.

26. Xiao-qian Liu, Rui Sheng, Zheng-hong Qin, "The neuroprotective mechanism of brain ischemic preconditioning," *Acta Pharmacologica Sinica*, 30(8), 1071-1080, 2009, https://www.ncbi.nlm.nih.gov/pmc/articles/PMC4006675/.

27. Mikhail V. Blagosklonny, "Hormesis does not make sense except in the light of TOR-driven aging," *Aging (Albany NY)*, 3(11), 1051-1062, 2011, http://www.aging-us.com/article/100411/text.

28. Valter D. Longo, Adam Antebi, Andrzej Bartke, Nir Barzilai, Holly M. Brown-Borg, Calogero Caruso, Tyler J. Curiel, Rafael de Cabo, Claudio Franceschi, David Gems, Donald K. Ingram, Thomas E. Johnson, Brian K. Kennedy, Cynthia Kenyon, Samuel Klein, John J. Kopchick, Guenter Lepperdinger, Frank Madeo, Mario G. Mirisola, James R. Mitchell, Giuseppe Passarino, Karl L. Rudolph, John M. Sedivy, Gerald S. Shadel, David A. Sinclair, Stephen R. Spindler, Yousin Suh, Jan Vijg, Manlio Vinciguerra, Luigi Fontana, "Interventions to slow aging in humans: Are we ready?" *Aging Cell*, 14(4), 497-510, 2015, http://www.ucl.ac.uk/~ucbtdag/Longo_2015.pdf;

Ilia Stambler, "Stop Aging Disease! ICAD 2014," *Aging and Disease*, 6(2), 76-94, 2015, http://www.aginganddisease.org/EN/10.14336/AD.2015.0115;

Ilia Stambler, "Human life extension: opportunities, challenges, and implications for public health policy," in Alexander Vaiserman (Ed.), *Anti-aging Drugs: From Basic Research to Clinical Practice*, Royal Society of Chemistry, London, 2017, pp. 535-564, http://pubs.rsc.org/en/content/ebook/978-1-78262-435-6#!divbookcontent;

Alexander Vaiserman, Oleh Lushchak, "Anti-aging drugs: where are we and where are we going?" in Alexander Vaiserman (Ed.), *Anti-aging Drugs: From Basic Research to Clinical Practice*, Royal Society of Chemistry, London, 2017, pp. 3-10, http://pubs.rsc.org/en/content/ebook/978-1-78262-435-6#!divbookcontent.

29. Liran I. Shlush, Karl L. Skorecki, Shalev Itzkovitz, Shiran Yehezkel, Yardena Segev, Hofit Shachar, Ron Berkovitz, Yochai Adir, Irma Vulto, Peter M. Lansdorp, Sara Selig, "Telomere elongation followed by telomere length reduction, in leukocytes from divers exposed to intense oxidative stress – implications for tissue and organismal aging," *Mechanisms of Ageing and Development*, 132(3), 123-130, 2011, http://www.sciencedirect.com/science/article/pii/S0047637411000224.

30. Vasilij N. Novoseltsev, Janna Novoseltseva, Anatoli I. Yashin, "A homeostatic model of oxidative damage explains paradoxes observed in earlier aging experiments: a fusion and extension of older theories of aging," *Biogerontology*, 2(2), 127-138, 2001, https://link.springer.com/article/10.1023/A:1011511100472.

31. John B. West, "Exciting Times in the Study of Permanent Residents of High Altitude," *High Altitude Medicine & Biology*, 12(1), 1, 2011, http://online.liebertpub.com/doi/abs/10.1089/ham.2011.12101;

Martin Burtscher, "Effects of Living at Higher Altitudes on Mortality: A Narrative Review," *Aging and Disease*, 5(4), 274-280, 2014, https://www.ncbi.nlm.nih.gov/pmc/articles/PMC4113517/;

Jay F. Storz, Hideaki Moriyama, "Mechanisms of Hemoglobin Adaptation to High Altitude Hypoxia," *High Altitude Medicine & Biology*, 9(2), 148-157, 2008, https://www.ncbi.nlm.nih.gov/pmc/articles/PMC3140315/;

Jean-Marie Robine, Fred Paccaud, "Nonagenarians and centenarians in Switzerland, 1860-2001: a demographic analysis," *Journal of Epidemiology and Community Health*, 59(1), 31-37, 2005, http://jech.bmj.com/content/59/1/31;

Alexander Leaf, *Youth in Old Age*, McGraw-Hill Book Company, New York, 1975;

Khatchik Muradian, "Atmosphere, Metabolism and Longevity," in Alexander M. Vaiserman, Alexey A. Moskalev, Elena G. Pasyukova (Eds.), *Life Extension: Lessons from Drosophila*, Dordrecht, Springer, 2015.

32. Khachik Muradian, "'Pull and push back' concepts of longevity and life span extension," *Biogerontology*, 14(6), 687-691, 2013, https://link.springer.com/article/10.1007%2Fs10522-013-9472-1;

Reuven Tirosh, "Ballistic Protons and Microwave-induced Water Solitons in Bioenergetic Transformations," *International Journal of Molecular Sciences*, 7(9), 320-345, 2006, http://www.mdpi.com/1422-0067/7/9/320.

33. Angela Navarrete-Opazo, Gordon S. Mitchell, "Therapeutic potential of intermittent hypoxia: a matter of dose," *American Journal of Physiology - Regulatory, Integrative and Comparative Physiology*, 307(10), R1181-1197, 2014, http://ajpregu.physiology.org/content/307/10/R1181.

34. Michael H. Bennett, Christopher French, Alexander Schnabel, Jason Wasiak, Peter Kranke, Stephanie Weibel, "Normal pressure oxygen therapy and hyperbaric oxygen therapy for migraine and cluster headaches," *The Cochrane Database of Systematic Reviews*, (12):CD005219, 2015, http://onlinelibrary.wiley.com/doi/10.1002/14651858.CD005219.pub3/full;

Aneesh B. Singhal, "A review of oxygen therapy in ischemic stroke," *Neurological Research*, 29(2), 173-183, 2007, http://www.tandfonline.com/doi/abs/10.1179/016164107X181815.

35. Konstantin Pavlovich Buteyko, *Metod Buteyko. Opyt Vnedrenia v Medizinskuyu Praktiku* (The Buteyko Method. The Experience of Application in Medical Practice), Patriot, Moscow, 1990, http://www.buteyko.ru/rus/index.shtml;

Vladimir K. Buteyko and Marina M. Buteyko, *The Buteyko Theory about a Key Role of Breathing for Human Health, Scientific Introduction to the Buteyko Therapy for Experts* (in Russian and English), Buteyko Co LTD, Voronezh, 2005, http://www.doctorbuteykodiscoverytrilogy.com/the-buteyko-theory-about-a-key-role-of-breathing-for-human-health.php;

Paul M. Macey, Mary A. Woo, Ronald M. Harper, "Hyperoxic Brain Effects Are Normalized by Addition of CO2," *PLoS Medicine*, 4(5), e173, 2007, https://doi.org/10.1371/journal.pmed.0040173.

36. Gennady G. Rogatsky, Edward G. Shifrin, Avraham Mayevsky, "Physiologic and biochemical monitoring during hyperbaric oxygenation," *Undersea and Hyperbaric Medicine*, 26(2), 111-122, 1999, https://www.researchgate.net/publication/12927497_Physiologic_and_biochemical_monitoring_during_hyperbaric_oxygenation_A_review.

37. Judith Sonn, Avraham Mayevsky, "Responses to Cortical Spreading Depression under Oxygen Deficiency," *The Open Neurology Journal*, 6, 6-17, 2012, https://www.ncbi.nlm.nih.gov/pmc/articles/PMC3367297/;

Greg Zaharchuk, Reed F. Busse, Guy Rosenthal, Geoffery T. Manley, Orit A. Glenn, William P. Dillon, "Noninvasive oxygen partial pressure measurement of human body fluids in vivo using magnetic resonance imaging," *Academic Radiology*, 13(8), 1016-24, 2006, http://www.sciencedirect.com/science/article/pii/S1076633206002704;

Nili Zarchin, Sigal Meilin, Joseph Rifkind, Avraham Mayevsky, "Effect of aging on brain energy-metabolism," *Comparative Biochemistry and Physiology*

Part A: Molecular & Integrative Physiology, 132(1), 117-120, 2002, http://www.sciencedirect.com/science/article/pii/S1095643301005372.
38. Ward Dean, "Biologic aging measurement: its rationale, history, and current status," in Arthur K. Balin (Ed.), *Human Biologic Age Determination*, Boca Raton FL, CRC Press, 1994, pp. 3-14;
Walter M. Bortz 4th, Walter M. Bortz 2nd, "How fast do we age? Exercise performance over time as a biomarker," *Journal of Gerontology A, Biological Sciences and Medical Sciences*, 51(5), M223-225, 1996, https://www.ncbi.nlm.nih.gov/pubmed/8808993;
Johannes H.G.M. van Beek, Thomas B.L. Kirkwood, James B. Bassingthwaighte, "Understanding the physiology of the ageing individual: computational modelling of changes in metabolism and endurance," *Interface Focus*, 6(2), 20150079, 2016, http://rsfs.royalsocietypublishing.org/content/6/2/20150079.
39. Kristine E. Ensrud, Susan K. Ewing, Peggy M. Cawthon, Howard A. Fink, Brent C. Taylor, Jane A. Cauley, Thuy-Tien Dam, Lynn M. Marshall, Eric S. Orwoll, Steven R. Cummings, and The Osteoporotic Fractures in Men (MrOS) Research Group, "A comparison of frailty indexes for the prediction of falls, disability, fractures, and mortality in older men," *Journal of the American Geriatrics Society*, 57(3), 492-498, 2009, https://www.ncbi.nlm.nih.gov/pmc/articles/PMC2861353/;
Linda P. Fried, Catherine M. Tangen, Jeremy Walston, Anne B. Newman, Calvin Hirsch, John Gottdiener, Teresa Seeman, Russell Tracy, Willem J. Kop, Gregory Burke, Mary Ann McBurnie, for the Cardiovascular Health Study Collaborative Research Group, "Frailty in older adults: evidence for a phenotype," *Journal of Gerontology A, Biological Sciences and Medical Sciences*, 56(3), M146–M156, 2001, http://www.sld.cu/galerias/pdf/sitios/gericuba/fenotipo_frailty.pdf.
40. Yang Guang, Dong Feng, Li Yuzhong, Liu Hui, "Theoretical and Experimental Evidence in Mixed Serum Samples as Natural Reference Materials for Measuring Activity of Biomacromolecules in Serum," *Clinical Laboratory*, 64, 04/2017, https://www.clin-lab-publications.com/article/2331;
Avraham Mayevsky, Efrat Barbiro-Michaely, "Shedding light on mitochondrial function by real time monitoring of NADH fluorescence: II: human studies," *International Journal of Clinical Monitoring and Computing*, 27(2), 125-145, 2013, https://link.springer.com/article/10.1007/s10877-012-9413-6.
41. Robert N. Butler, Richard Sprott, Huber Warner, Jeffrey Bland, Richie Feuers, Michael Forster, Howard Fillit, S. Mitchell Harman, Michael Hewitt, Mark Hyman, Kathleen Johnson, Evan Kligman, Gerald McClearn, James Nelson, Arlan Richardson, William Sonntag, Richard Weindruch, Norman Wolf, "Biomarkers of aging: from primitive organisms to

humans," *Journal of Gerontology A, Biological Sciences Medical Sciences*, 59, B560-567, 2004, https://www.researchgate.net/publication/8493491_Aging_The_Reality_B iomarkers_of_Aging_From_Primitive_Organisms_to_Humans;

Thomas Craig, Chris Smelick, Robi Tacutu, Daniel Wuttke, Shona H. Wood, Henry Stanley, Georges Janssens, Ekaterina Savitskaya, Alexey Moskalev, Robert Arking, João Pedro de Magalhães, "The Digital Ageing Atlas: integrating the diversity of age-related changes into a unified resource," *Nucleic Acids Research*, 43(Database issue), D873-878, 2015, https://academic.oup.com/nar/article-lookup/doi/10.1093/nar/gku843;

Georg Fuellen, Paul Schofield, Thomas Flatt, Ralf-Joachim Schulz, Fritz Boege, Karin Kraft, Gerald Rimbach, Saleh Ibrahim, Alexander Tietz, Christian Schmidt, Rüdiger Köhling, Andreas Simm, "Living Long and Well: Prospects for a Personalized Approach to the Medicine of Ageing," *Gerontology*, 62(4), 409-416, 2016, https://www.researchgate.net/publication/287212601_Living_Long_and_ Well_Prospects_for_a_Personalized_Approach_to_the_Medicine_of_Agei ng.

42. David Blokh, Ilia Stambler, "The application of information theory for the research of aging and aging-related diseases," *Progress in Neurobiology*, S0301-0082(15)30059-9, 2016, doi: http://dx.doi.org/10.1016/j.pneurobio.2016.03.005.

David Blokh, Ilia Stambler, "The use of information theory for the evaluation of biomarkers of aging and physiological age," *Mechanisms of Ageing and Development*, 163, 23-29, 2017, doi: http://dx.doi.org/10.1016/j.mad.2017.01.003.

David Blokh, Ilia Stambler, "Quantified Longevity Guide (QLG)," Comorbidity Detection Technologies, 2017, https://ec.europa.eu/eip/ageing/commitments-tracker/a3/quantified-longevity-guide-qlg_en, http://www.longevityisrael.org/comorbidity-detection.html, http://www.qlongevityguide.com/.

43. John N. Kheir, Laurie A. Scharp, Mark A. Borden, Edward J. Swanson, Andrew Loxley, James H. Reese, Katherine J. Black, ..., Francis X. McGowan Jr., "Oxygen gas-filled microparticles provide intravenous oxygen delivery," *Science Translational Medicine*, 4(140), 140ra88, 2012, https://www.researchgate.net/publication/228089270_Oxygen_Gas-Filled_Microparticles_Provide_Intravenous_Oxygen_Delivery;

Thad Henkel-Honke, Mark Oleck, "Artificial oxygen carriers: A current review," *AANA Journal*, 75(3), 205-211, 2007, https://www.aana.com/newsandjournal/Documents/henkelhanke205-211.pdf.

44. Winfred M. Phillips, "The artificial heart: history and current status," *Journal of Biomechanical Engineering*, 115(4B), 555-557, 1993,

http://biomechanical.asmedigitalcollection.asme.org/article.aspx?articleid=
1399644;
Andréia Cristina Passaroni, Marcos Augusto de Moraes Silva, Winston
Bonetti Yoshida, "Cardiopulmonary bypass: development of John Gibbon's
heart-lung machine," *The Brazilian Journal of Cardiovascular Surgery/Revista
Brasileira de Cirurgia Cardiovascular*, 30(2), 235-245, 2015,
https://www.ncbi.nlm.nih.gov/pmc/articles/PMC4462970/;
Emma J. Birks, Patrick D. Tansley, James Hardy, Robert S. George,
Christopher T. Bowles, Margaret Burke, Nicholas R. Banner, Asghar
Khaghani, Magdi H. Yacoub, "Left Ventricular Assist Device and Drug
Therapy for the Reversal of Heart Failure," *New England Journal of Medicine*,
355(18), 1873-1884, 2006,
http://www.nejm.org/doi/full/10.1056/NEJMoa053063.
45. Costin G.E., Birlea S.A., Norris D.A., "Trends in wound repair: cellular
and molecular basis of regenerative therapy using electromagnetic fields,"
Current Molecular Medicine, 12(1), 14-26, 2012,
http://www.eurekaselect.com/75862/article;
Oren M. Tepper, Matthew J. Callaghan, Edward I. Chang, Robert D.
Galiano, Kirit A. Bhatt, Samuel Baharestani, Jean Gan, Bruce Simon,
Richard A. Hopper, Jamie P. Levine, Geoffrey C. Gurtner,
"Electromagnetic fields increase in vitro and in vivo angiogenesis through
endothelial release of FGF-2," *FASEB Journal*, 18(11), 1231-1233, 2004,
https://www.ncbi.nlm.nih.gov/pubmed/15208265;
Robert O. Becker, Gary Selden, *The Body Electric. Electromagnetism and the
Foundation of Life*, Quill, New York, 1985.
46. Kristoffer Famm, Brian Litt, Kevin J. Tracey, Edward S. Boyden,
Moncef Slaoui, "Drug discovery: a jump-start for electroceuticals," *Nature*,
496(7444), 159-161, 2013,
https://www.ncbi.nlm.nih.gov/pmc/articles/PMC4179459/.
47. Michael W. Lee, Scott A. Deppe, Mary Ellen Sipperly, Roger R.
Barrette, Dan R. Thompson, "The efficacy of barbiturate coma in the
management of uncontrolled intracranial hypertension following
neurosurgical trauma," *Journal of Neurotrauma*, 11(3), 325-331, 1994,
http://online.liebertpub.com/doi/abs/10.1089/neu.1994.11.325;
Kees H. Polderman, "Application of therapeutic hypothermia in the ICU:
opportunities and pitfalls of a promising treatment modality," *Intensive Care
Medicine*, 30, 556-575, 2004,
https://link.springer.com/article/10.1007%2Fs00134-003-2151-y.
48. White D.P., Weil J.V., Zwillich C.W., "Metabolic rate and breathing
during sleep," *Journal of Applied Physiology*, 59(2), 384-391, 1985,
http://jap.physiology.org/content/59/2/384.long;
Kurt Kräuchi, Britta Gompper, Daniela Hauenstein, Josef Flammer,
Marlon Pflüger, Erich Studerus, Andy Schötzau, Selim Orgül, "Diurnal

blood pressure variations are associated with changes in distal-proximal skin temperature gradient," *Chronobiology International*, 29(9), 1273-1283, 2012, http://www.chronobiology.ch/wp-content/uploads/2014/11/krauchi__bloodpressure_2012.pdf.

49. Jill Waalen, Joel N. Buxbaum, "Is Older Colder or Colder Older? The Association of Age With Body Temperature in 18,630 Individuals," *Journal of Gerontology A, Biological Sciences and Medical Sciences*, 66A(5), 487-492, 2011, https://www.ncbi.nlm.nih.gov/pmc/articles/PMC3107024/.

50. Alexander Leonidovich Chizhevsky, "Ionizatsia vozdukha, kak fiziologicheski activniy factor atmosfernogo electrichestva. Experimentalnie issledovania (Air ionization as a physiologically active factor of atmospheric electricity. Experimental Studies), Doklad (Presentation), Kaluga, Russia, 1919, quoted in Alexander Chizhevsky, *Aeroionifikatsia v narodnom hozyaystve*, Stroyizdat, Moscow, 1989 (Aero-ionization in people's economy, 2nd edition, first published in 1960), https://en.wikipedia.org/wiki/Alexander_Chizhevsky;

Vanessa Perez, Dominik D. Alexander, William H. Bailey, "Air ions and mood outcomes: a review and meta-analysis," *BMC Psychiatry*, 13, 29, 2013, https://bmcpsychiatry.biomedcentral.com/articles/10.1186/1471-244X-13-29;

Elvis A.F. Martis, Ekta Shah, "Ozone therapy: A clinical review," *The Journal of Natural Science, Biology and Medicine*, 2(1), 66-70, 2011, https://www.ncbi.nlm.nih.gov/pmc/articles/PMC3312702/;

Reuven Tirosh, "Ballistic Protons and Microwave-induced Water Solitons in Bioenergetic Transformations," *International Journal of Molecular Sciences*, 7(9), 320-345, 2006, http://www.mdpi.com/1422-0067/7/9/320.

51. David B. Jarrett, Joel B. Greenhouse, Jean M. Miewald, Iva B. Fedorka, David J. Kupfer, "A reexamination of the relationship between growth hormone secretion and slow wave sleep using delta wave analysis," *Biological Psychiatry*, 27(5), 497-509, 1990, http://www.biologicalpsychiatryjournal.com/article/0006-3223(90)90441-4/pdf;

Eve Van Cauter, Laurence Plat, Martin B. Scharf, Rachel Leproult, Sonya Cespedes, Mireille L'Hermite-Balériaux, Georges Copinschi, "Simultaneous Stimulation of Slow-wave Sleep and Growth Hormone Secretion by Gamma-hydroxybutyrate in Normal Young Men," *Journal of Clinical Investigations*, 100(3), 745-753, 1997, https://www.ncbi.nlm.nih.gov/pmc/articles/PMC508244/.

52. Ladyslav V. Vyazovskiy, Kenneth D. Harris, "Sleep and the single neuron: the role of global slow oscillations in individual cell rest," *Nature Reviews Neuroscience*, 14, 443-451, 2013, http://www.nature.com/nrn/journal/v14/n6/abs/nrn3494.html.

53. Bryce A. Mander, Joseph R. Winer, Matthew P. Walker, "Sleep and Human Aging," *Neuron*, 94(1), 19-36, 2017, http://www.cell.com/neuron/fulltext/S0896-6273(17)30088-0;
Karine Spiegel, Rachel Leproult, Eve Van Cauter, "Impact of sleep debt on metabolic and endocrine function," *The Lancet*, 354(9188), 1435-1439, 1999, http://www.thelancet.com/journals/lancet/article/PIIS0140-6736(99)01376-8/fulltext;
Mark R. Zielinski, Dmitry Gerashchenko, Svetlana A. Karpova, Varun Konanki, Robert W. McCarley, Fayyaz S. Sutterwala, Robert E. Strecker, Radhika Basheer, "The NLRP3 inflammasome modulates sleep and NREM sleep delta power induced by spontaneous wakefulness, sleep deprivation and lipopolysaccharide," *Brain, Behavior, and Immunity*, 62, 137-150, 2017, https://www.ncbi.nlm.nih.gov/pubmed/28109896;
Lulu Xie, Hongyi Kang, Qiwu Xu, Michael J. Chen, Yonghong Liao, Meenakshisundaram Thiyagarajan, John O'Donnell, Daniel J. Christensen, Charles Nicholson, Jeffrey J. Iliff, Takahiro Takano, Rashid Deane, Maiken Nedergaard, "Sleep Drives Metabolite Clearance from the Adult Brain," *Science*, 342(6156), 373-3777, https://www.ncbi.nlm.nih.gov/pmc/articles/PMC3880190/;
Alice Park, "The Sleep Cure: The Fountain of Youth May Be Closer Than You Ever Thought," *TIME Health*, February 16, 2017, http://time.com/4672988/the-sleep-cure-fountain-of-youth/;
Vladimir M. Kovalzon, Tatyana V. Strekalova, "Delta sleep-inducing peptide (DSIP): a still unresolved riddle," *Journal of Neurochemistry*, 97(2), 303-309, 2006, http://onlinelibrary.wiley.com/doi/10.1111/j.1471-4159.2006.03693.x/full;
György Buzsáki, Andreas Draguhn, "Neuronal oscillations in cortical networks," *Science*, 304, 1926-1929, 2004, http://science.sciencemag.org/content/304/5679/1926.full;
Tarja Porkka-Heiskanen, Robert E. Strecker, Mahesh Thakkar, Alvhild A. Bjørkum, Robert W. Greene, Robert W. McCarley, "Adenosine: a mediator of the sleep-inducing effects of prolonged wakefulness," *Science*, 276, 1265-1268, 1997, https://www.ncbi.nlm.nih.gov/pmc/articles/PMC3599777/.
54. Lisa Marshall, Halla Helgadóttir, Matthias Mölle, Jan Born, "Boosting slow oscillations during sleep potentiates memory," *Nature*, 444, 610-613, 2006, http://www.nature.com/nature/journal/v444/n7119/abs/nature05278.html;
Massimini Marcello, Tononi Giulio, Huber Reto, "Slow waves, synaptic plasticity and information processing: insights from transcranial magnetic stimulation and high-density EEG experiments," *The European Journal of Neuroscience*, 29(9), 1761-1770, 2009, https://www.ncbi.nlm.nih.gov/pmc/articles/PMC2776746/;

Marcello Massimini, Fabio Ferrarelli, Steve K. Esser, Brady A. Riedner, Reto Huber, Michael Murphy, Michael J. Peterson, Giulio Tononi, "Triggering sleep slow waves by transcranial magnetic stimulation," *Proceedings of the National Academy of Sciences USA*, 104(20), 8496-8501, 2007, http://www.pnas.org/content/104/20/8496.full.

55. Tatiana-Danai Dimitriou, Magdalini Tsolaki, "Evaluation of the efficacy of randomized controlled trials of sensory stimulation interventions for sleeping disturbances in patients with dementia: a systematic review," *Clinical Interventions in Aging*, 12, 543-548, 2017, https://www.dovepress.com/evaluation-of-the-efficacy-of-randomized-controlled-trials-of-sensory--peer-reviewed-article-CIA;

Jessa Gamble, "Sleep and dreaming: Slumber at the flick of a switch," *New Scientist*, 2902, February 06, 2016, https://www.scribd.com/document/124630444/New-Scientist-Sleep-and-Dreaming-Slumber-at-the-Flick-of-a-Switch.

56. Eve Van Cauter, Laurence Plat, Martin B. Scharf, Rachel Leproult, Sonya Cespedes, Mireille L'Hermite-Balériaux, Georges Copinschi, "Simultaneous Stimulation of Slow-wave Sleep and Growth Hormone Secretion by Gamma-hydroxybutyrate in Normal Young Men," *Journal of Clinical Investigations*, 100(3), 745-753, 1997, https://www.ncbi.nlm.nih.gov/pmc/articles/PMC508244/;

James K. Walsh, Ellen Snyder, Janine Hall, Angela C. Randazzo, Kara Griffin, John Groeger, Rhody Eisenstein, Stephen D. Feren, Pam Dickey, Paula K. Schweitzer, "Slow Wave Sleep Enhancement with Gaboxadol Reduces Daytime Sleepiness During Sleep Restriction," *Sleep*, 31(5), 659-672 2008, https://www.ncbi.nlm.nih.gov/pmc/articles/PMC2398757/.

20. Resources for Longevity Promotion

Introduction

The field of longevity promotion is vast and ever expanding. It would be very difficult to provide a comprehensive list of resources that would help obtain a thorough grip of the field and instruct a potential longevity researcher and activist for further study and action. Yet, below is a short list of personal academic works that can provide some additional small gateway for further expansion. This list is admittedly and intentionally limited, and the readers are welcome to advise on improvements.[1]

Longevity Advocacy

1. Longevity Promotion: Multidisciplinary Perspectives[2]

This book considers the multidisciplinary aspects of longevity promotion, from the advocacy, historical, philosophical and scientific perspectives. The first part on longevity advocacy includes examples of pro-longevity campaigns, outreach materials, frequent debates and policy suggestions and frameworks that may assist in the promotion of research and development for healthy longevity. The second part on longevity history includes analyses of the definition of life-extensionism as a social and intellectual movement, the dialectics of reductionism vs. holism and the significance of the concept of constancy in the history of life extension research, an historical overview of evolutionary theories of aging, and a tribute to one of the founding figures of modern longevity science. The third part on longevity philosophy surveys the aspirations and supportive arguments for increasing healthy longevity in the philosophical and religious traditions of ancient Greece, India, the Middle East, in particular in Islam and Judaism, and the Christian tradition. Finally, the fourth part on longevity science includes brief discussions of some of the scientific issues in life extension research, in particular regarding some potential interventions to ameliorate degenerative aging, some methodological issues with diagnosing and treating degenerative aging as a medical condition, the application of information theory for aging and longevity research, some potential physical means for life extension, and some resources for further consideration. These discussions are in no way exhaustive, but are intended to simulate additional interest, consultation and study of longevity science and its social and cultural implications. It is hoped that this book will contribute to broadening, diversifying and strengthening the academic and public deliberation on the prospects of healthy life extension for the entire

314

population. The setting and careful consideration of a goal may be seen as a first step toward its accomplishment.

2. The critical need to promote research of aging and aging-related diseases to improve health and longevity of the elderly population[3]

Due to the aging of the global population and the derivative increase in aging-related non-communicable diseases and their economic burden, there is an urgent need to promote research on aging and aging-related diseases as a way to improve healthy and productive longevity for the elderly population. To accomplish this goal, we advocate the following policies: 1) Increasing funding for research and development specifically directed to ameliorate degenerative aging processes and to extend healthy and productive lifespan for the population; 2) Providing a set of incentives for commercial, academic, public and governmental organizations to foster engagement in such research and development; and 3) Establishing and expanding coordination and consultation structures, programs and institutions involved in aging-related research, development and education in academia, industry, public policy agencies and at governmental and supra-governmental levels.

3. Recognizing degenerative aging as a treatable medical condition: methodology and policy[4]

It is becoming increasingly clear that in order to accomplish healthy longevity for the population, there is an urgent need for the research and development of effective therapies against degenerative aging processes underlying major aging-related diseases, including heart disease, neurodegenerative diseases, type 2 diabetes, cancer, pulmonary obstructive diseases, as well as aging-related complications and susceptibilities of infectious communicable diseases. Yet, an important incentive for the research and development of such therapies appears to be the development of clinically applicable and scientifically grounded definitions and criteria for the multifactorial degenerative aging process (or "senility" using the existing ICD category), underlying those diseases, as well as for the safety and effectiveness of interventions against it. Such generally agreed definitions and criteria are currently absent. The devising of such criteria is important not only for the sake of their scientific value and their utility for the development of therapeutic solutions for the aging population, but also to comply with and implement major existing national and international programmatic and regulatory requirements. Some methodological

315

suggestions and potential pitfalls for the development of such criteria are examined.

4. Human life extension: opportunities, challenges, and implications for public health policy[5]

An analysis of possibilities of human life extension involves an extremely broad variety of questions regarding the opportunities, challenges and implications for the human society that such a prospect would raise. Still, despite the wide variety, the related questions may be categorized into several groups. The first group of questions may concern the feasibility of the accomplishment of life extension. Is it theoretically and technologically possible? What are our grounds for optimism? The second group concerns the desirability of the accomplishment of life extension for the individual and the society, provided it will some day become possible through scientific intervention. How then will life extension affect the perception of personhood? How will it affect the availability of resources for the population? The third group concerns normative action. Assuming that life extension is scientifically possible and socially desirable, and that its implications are either demonstrably positive or, in case of a negative forecast, they are amenable – what practical implications should these determinations have for public policy, in particular health policy and research policy, in a democratic society? Should we pursue the goal of life extension? If yes, then how? How can we make it an individual and social priority? Given the rapid population aging and the increasing incidence and burden of age-related diseases, on the pessimistic side, and the rapid development of medical technologies, on the optimistic side, these become vital questions of social responsibility.

5. The pursuit of longevity – The bringer of peace to the Middle East[6]

Despite the common apprehensions regarding the aging population, this work aims to argue, on both deontological and utilitarian moral grounds, that any increase in general life-expectancy will be beneficial for the Middle East, countering the common fears associated with this increase. A set of ethical arguments concerning increasing longevity is presented, from both the deontological and utilitarian perspective. A wide selection of economic, psychological, demographic and epidemiological literature and databases is analyzed to determine common correlates of extended longevity. On the deontological grounds, the value of extended longevity is derived from the value of life preservation, regardless of its term. On the utilitarian grounds, the value of extended longevity is demonstrated by its correlation with further human values, such as education level and

316

intellectual activity, economic prosperity, equality, solidarity and peacefulness. With the common apprehensions of stagnation and scarcity due to life extension found wanting, the pursuit of longevity by the population can be seen as a cross-cultural and cross-generational good. Though the current study mainly refers to sources and data relevant to the Middle East, a similar pro-longevity argument can be also made for other cultural contexts. In view of its numerous benefits, normatively, the goal of longevity should be set clearly and openly by the society, and actively pursued, or at least discussed, in academia, the political system and broader public.

6. Stop Aging Disease! ICAD 2014[7]

On November 1–2, 2014, there took place in Beijing, China, the first International Conference on Aging and Disease (ICAD 2014) of the International Society on Aging and Disease (ISOAD). The conference participants presented a wide and exciting front of work dedicated to amelioration of aging-related conditions, ranging from regenerative medicine through developing geroprotective substances, elucidating a wide range of mechanisms of aging and aging-related diseases, from energy metabolism through genetics and immunomodulation to systems biology. The conference further emphasized the need to intensify and support research on aging and aging-related diseases to provide solutions for the urgent health challenges of the aging society.

Longevity History and Philosophy

7. A History of Life-Extensionism in the Twentieth Century[8]

This book explores the history of life-extensionism in the 20th century. The term life-extensionism is meant to describe an ideological system professing that radical life extension (far beyond the present life expectancy) is desirable on ethical grounds and is possible to achieve through conscious scientific efforts. This work examines major lines of life-extensionist thought, in chronological order, over the course of the 20th century, while focusing on central seminal works representative of each trend and period, by such authors as Elie Metchnikoff, Bernard Shaw, Alexis Carrel, Alexander Bogomolets and others. Their works are considered in their social and intellectual context, as parts of a larger contemporary social and ideological discourse, associated with major political upheavals and social and economic patterns. The following national contexts are considered: France (Chapter One), Germany, Austria,

317

Romania and Switzerland (Chapter Two), Russia (Chapter Three), the US and UK (Chapter Four).

This work pursues three major aims. The first is to attempt to identify and trace throughout the century several generic biomedical methods whose development or applications were associated with radical hopes for life-extension. Beyond mere hopefulness, this work argues, the desire to radically prolong human life often constituted a formidable, though hardly ever acknowledged, motivation for biomedical research and discovery. It will be shown that novel fields of biomedical science often had their origin in far-reaching pursuits of radical life extension. The dynamic dichotomy between reductionist and holistic methods will be emphasized.

The second goal is to investigate the ideological and socio-economic backgrounds of the proponents of radical life extension, in order to determine how ideology and economic conditions motivated the life-extensionists and how it affected the science they pursued. For that purpose, the biographies and key writings of several prominent longevity advocates are studied. Their specific ideological premises (attitudes toward religion and progress, pessimism or optimism regarding human perfectibility, and ethical imperatives) as well as their socioeconomic conditions (the ability to conduct and disseminate research in a specific social or economic milieu) are examined in an attempt to find out what conditions have encouraged or discouraged life-extensionist thought. This research argues for the inherent adjustability of life-extensionism, as a particular form of scientific enterprise, to particular prevalent state ideologies.

The third, more general, aim is to collect a broad register of life-extensionist works, and, based on that register, to establish common traits and goals definitive of life-extensionism, such as valuation of life and constancy, despite all the diversity of methods and ideologies professed. This work will contribute to the understanding of extreme expectations associated with biomedical progress that have been scarcely investigated by biomedical history.

8. The unexpected outcomes of anti-aging, rejuvenation and life extension studies: an origin of modern therapies[9]

The search for life-extending interventions has been often perceived as a purely academic pursuit, or as an unorthodox medical enterprise, with little or no practical outcome. Yet, in fact, these studies, explicitly aiming to prolong human life, often constituted a formidable, though hardly ever acknowledged, motivation for biomedical research and discovery. At least several modern biomedical fields have originated directly from rejuvenation and life extension research: (1) Hormone replacement therapy was born in

318

Charles-Edouard Brown-Sequard's rejuvenation experiments with animal gland extracts (1889). (2) Probiotic diets originated in Elie Metchnikoff's conception of radically prolonged "orthobiosis" (c. 1900). (3) The development of clinical endocrinology owed much to Eugen Steinach's "endocrine rejuvenation" operations (c. 1910s-1920s). (4) Tissue transplantations in humans (allografts and xenografts) were first widely performed in Serge Voronoff's "rejuvenation by grafting" experiments (c. 1910s-1920s). (5) Tissue engineering was pioneered during Alexis Carrel's work on cell and tissue immortalization (c. 1900-1920). (6) Cell therapy (and particularly human embryonic cell therapy) was first widely conducted by Paul Niehans for the purposes of rejuvenation as early as the 1930s. Thus, the pursuit of life extension and rejuvenation has constituted an inseparable and crucial element in the history of biomedicine. Notably, the common principle of these studies was the proactive maintenance of stable, long-term homeostasis of the entire organism.

9. Has aging ever been considered healthy?[10]

The current research topic inquires: "Should we treat aging as a disease?" Yet, in this inquiry, the question "Can aging be considered a disease?" is secondary, while the more primary question really must be "Is aging treatable?" Paradoxically, the answer given to the second question largely determines the answer to the first. The perceived unchangeable, and hence untreatable, nature of aging is the root cause for many subsequent rationalizations, even to the point of claiming the desirability of aging-derived suffering and death. This is a well recognized psychological phenomenon sometimes referred to as "apologism" (Gruman, 1966) or even "deathism," a ramification of the "sour grapes syndrome," vilifying something that we think we cannot attain, while accepting as "good" or "healthy" something that we believe is inevitable for us (such as degenerative aging). Yet, I argue that, historically, medical tradition has always recognized the morbid character of aging and endeavored to fight it. The rationalizations of aging as "natural," "justified," or "healthy" could never entirely prevail.

10. Life extension – a conservative enterprise? Some fin-de-siècle and early twentieth-century precursors of transhumanism[11]

The beginning of the modern period in the pursuit of radical human enhancement and longevity can be traced to *fin-de-siècle*/early twentieth-century scientific and technological optimism and therapeutic activism. The works of several authors of the period – Fedorov, Stephens, Bogdanov, Nietzsche and Finot – reveal conflicting ideological and social pathways

319

toward the goals of human enhancement and life extension. Each author represents a particular existing social order, and his vision of human advancement may be seen as a continuation and extension of that order. Therefore, the pursuit of life extension may be considered a fundamentally conservative (or conservationist) enterprise.

11. Elie Metchnikoff – the founder of longevity science and a founder of modern medicine: In honor of the 170th anniversary[12]

The years 2015-2016 mark a double anniversary – the 170th anniversary of birth and the 100th anniversary of death – of one of the greatest Russian scientists, a person that may be considered a founding figure of modern immunology, aging and longevity science – Elie Metchnikoff (May 15, 1845 – July 15, 1916). At this time of the rapid aging of the world population and the rapid development of technologies that may ameliorate degenerative aging processes, Metchnikoff's pioneering contribution to the search for anti-aging and healthspan-extending means needs to be recalled and honored.

12. On the history of life-extension research: Does the whole have parts?[13]

This presentation will explore the history of life-extension research in the 20th century. I will argue that the search for life-extension has often constituted a formidable, though hardly ever acknowledged, source for biomedical research and discovery, in such diverse fields as endocrinology (Steinach, 1910s-1920s); probiotic diets (Metchnikoff, 1900s); blood transfusion (Bogdanov, 1920s), systemic immunotherapy (Bogomolets, 1930s-1940s) and cell therapy, including human embryonic cell therapy (Niehans, 1930s-1950s). This presentation will briefly recapitulate some of the biomedical interventions (actual or potential) which were investigated as possible means for life-extension over the century. A taxonomy will be suggested between reductionist/therapeutic and holistic/hygienic approaches to potential life-extending interventions. Both approaches sought to achieve biological equilibrium and constancy of internal environment, yet emphasized diverging means and diverging perceptions of what constitutes equilibrium and constancy. The reductionist approach saw the human body as a machine in need of repair and internal adjustment and equilibration, seeking to achieve material homeostasis by eliminating damaging agents and introducing biological replacements, in other words, working by subtraction and addition toward balance. The holistic approach, in contrast, focused on the equilibration of the organism as a unit within the environment, strongly emphasizing the direct sustaining and revitalizing power of the mind and hygienic regulation of behavior. In the holistic approach, internal equilibrium was sought not so much through calibrating intrusions, but through resistance to intrusions. The apparent relative weight of each approach in public discourse will be shown to change with time, in several western countries, reflecting the initial hopes, disappointments and reactions to those disappointments in a variety of scientific programs.

13. Heroic Power in Thomas Carlyle and Leo Tolstoy[14]

This paper explores two opposed paradigmatic approaches to heroic power: Thomas Carlyle's versus Leo Tolstoy's. In *On Heroes, Hero Worship and the Heroic in History* (1840), Carlyle argues for its crucial importance, whereas in *War and Peace* (1869), Tolstoy denies its very possibility. Carlyle's heroic model attributes to the hero (the leader) a high degree of mastery and control over social and political circumstances, whereas Tolstoy's a-heroic model implies a small degree of personal mastery and much greater constraints on the individual leader. Both models achieved prominence in the wake of the Napoleonic Wars, which brought the role of the individual (hero) in history to the forefront of intellectual and political debate throughout Europe. The two models are shown as parts of and important links in long-established traditions; they are internally coherent yet totally contradictory of each other. The comparison of these opposed perceptions of heroic figures in history suggests that they might originate in an ambivalent, polarized perception of power and mastery, and in the sense of individual insecurity in the face of historical upheavals. Probably the most important implication of the two models regards their attitudes toward death. Carlyle's heroic model justifies fighting, and even dying for a heroic cause and under the leadership of a hero. In Tolstoy's a-heroic model, on the contrary, death is never glorious, never good, never attractive.

Longevity Science

14. The application of information theory for the research of aging and aging-related diseases[15]

This article reviews the application of information-theoretical analysis, employing measures of entropy and mutual information, for the study of aging and aging-related diseases. The research of aging and aging-related diseases is particularly suitable for the application of information theory methods, as aging processes and related diseases are multi-parametric, with continuous parameters coexisting alongside discrete parameters, and with the relations between the parameters being as a rule non-linear. Information theory provides unique analytical capabilities for the solution of such problems, with unique advantages over common linear biostatistics. Among the age-related diseases, information theory has been used in the study of neurodegenerative diseases (particularly using EEG time series for diagnosis and prediction), cancer (particularly for establishing individual and combined cancer biomarkers), diabetes (mainly utilizing mutual information to characterize the diseased and aging states), and heart disease (mainly for the analysis of heart rate variability). Few works have employed information theory for the analysis of general aging processes and frailty, as underlying determinants and possible early preclinical diagnostic measures for aging-related diseases. Generally, the use of information-theoretical analysis permits not only establishing the (non-linear) correlations between diagnostic or therapeutic parameters of interest, but may also provide a theoretical insight into the nature of aging and related diseases by establishing the measures of variability, adaptation, regulation or homeostasis, within a system of interest. It may be hoped that the increased use of such measures in research may considerably increase diagnostic and therapeutic capabilities and the fundamental theoretical mathematical understanding of aging and disease.

15. The use of information theory for the evaluation of biomarkers of aging and physiological age[16]

The present work explores the application of information-theoretical measures, such as entropy and normalized mutual information, for research of biomarkers of aging. The use of information theory affords unique methodological advantages for the study of aging processes, as it allows evaluating non-linear relations between biological parameters, providing the precise quantitative strength of those relations, both for individual and multiple parameters, showing cumulative or synergistic effect. Here we illustrate those capabilities utilizing a dataset on heart disease, including diagnostic parameters routinely available to physicians. The use of information-theoretical methods, utilizing normalized mutual information, revealed the exact amount of information that various diagnostic parameters or their combinations contained about the persons' age. Based on those exact informative values for the correlation of measured parameters with age, we constructed a diagnostic rule (a decision tree) to evaluate physiological age, as compared to chronological age. The present data illustrated that younger subjects suffering from heart disease showed characteristics of people of higher age (higher physiological age). Utilizing information-theoretical measures, with additional data, it may be possible to create further clinically applicable information-theory-based markers and models for the evaluation of physiological age, its relation to age-related diseases and its potential modifications by therapeutic interventions.

16. Information theoretical analysis of aging as a risk factor for heart disease[17]

We estimate the weight of various risk factors in heart disease, and the particular weight of age as a risk factor, individually and combined with other factors. To establish the weights we use the information theoretical measure of normalized mutual information that permits determining both individual and combined correlation of diagnostic parameters with the disease status. The present information theoretical methodology takes into account the non-linear correlations between the diagnostic parameters, as well as their non-linear changes with age. Thus it may be better suited to analyze complex biological aging systems than statistical measures that only estimate linear relations. We show that individual parameters, including age, often show little correlation with heart disease. Yet in combination, the correlation improves dramatically. For diagnostic parameters specific for heart disease the increase in the correlative capacity thanks to the combination of diagnostic parameters, is less pronounced than for the less specific parameters. Age shows the highest influence on the presence of disease among the non-specific parameters and the combination of age with other diagnostic parameters substantially improves the correlation with the disease status. Hence age is considered as a primary "metamarker" of aging-related heart disease, whose addition can improve diagnostic capabilities. In the future, this methodology may contribute to the development of a system of biomarkers for the assessment of biological/physiological age, its influence on disease status, and its modifications by therapeutic interventions.

17. Estimation of heterogeneity in diagnostic parameters of age-related diseases[18]

The heterogeneity of parameters is a ubiquitous biological phenomenon, with critical implications for biological systems functioning in normal and diseased states. We developed a method to estimate the level of objects set heterogeneity with reference to particular parameters and applied it to type II diabetes and heart disease, as examples of age-related systemic dysfunctions. The Friedman test was used to establish the existence of heterogeneity. The Newman-Keuls multiple comparison method was used to determine clusters. The normalized Shannon entropy was used to provide the quantitative evaluation of heterogeneity. There was obtained an estimate for the heterogeneity of the diagnostic parameters in healthy subjects, as well as in heart disease and type II diabetes patients, which was strongly related to their age. With aging, as with the diseases, the level of heterogeneity (entropy) was reduced, indicating a formal analogy between these phenomena. The similarity of the patterns in aging and disease suggested a kind of "early aging" of the diseased subjects, or alternatively a "disease-like" aging process, with reference to these particular parameters. The proposed method and its validation on the chronic age-related disease samples may support a way toward a formal mathematical relation between aging and chronic diseases and a formal definition of aging and disease, as determined by particular heterogeneity (entropy) changes.

18. Applying information theory analysis for the solution of biomedical data processing problems[19]

The use of information-theoretical methods can be highly valuable for the solution of biomedical data processing problems. Some of the problems that can be solved by those methods include: The assessment of the influence of diagnostic parameters, biomarkers and risk factors, on the emergence of disease; the discretization of diagnostic parameters; the analysis of a combined influence of a group of parameters; the partition of a group of diagnostic parameters according to the amount of diagnostic information contained in those parameters; the analysis of the parameters' heterogeneity or variability and more. To illustrate the solution of those problems, we use a data base on diabetes patients. There are grounds to believe that an increasing application of information-theoretical methodologies in biomedical research will lead to significant practical dividends for diagnosis and therapy.

19. The information-theory analysis of Michaelis-Menten constants for detection of breast cancer[20]

The Michaelis-Menten constants (K(m) and V(max)) operated by the Information Theory were employed for detection of breast cancer. The rate of enzymatic hydrolysis of fluorescein diacetate (FDA) in live peripheral blood mononuclear cells (PBMC), derived from healthy subjects and breast cancer (BC) patients, was assessed by measuring the fluorescence intensity (FI) in individual cells under incubation with either the mitogen phytohemagglutinin (PHA) or with tumor tissue, as compared to control. The data were processed by the Information Theory to determine the parameters and test conditions, which can best discriminate between the different groups. The normalized mutual information (uncertainty coefficient) was used as the measure of correlation/discrimination. An estimated general correlation was established between the K(m)/V(max) parameters and the examined patterns in the different bioassays. The information-theoretical analysis revealed the relative diagnostic value of each parameter. It was found that K(m) and V(max) as individual parameters show relatively low correlations with the presence or absence of disease, yet in combination often provide a good diagnostic measure. Based on the relative diagnostic values of each parameter, a diagnostic decision making rule was constructed. The diagnostic rule provided correct diagnosis for 37 out of 40 subjects.

20. Hyperbaric oxygenation for resuscitation and therapy of elderly patients with cerebral and cardio-respiratory dysfunction[21]

Hyperbaric oxygenation (HBO) therapy has been gaining an increasing recognition as a versatile therapeutic approach. This article reviews the application of hyperbaric oxygenation as a method for resuscitation and therapy of elderly patients with cerebral and cardio-respiratory dysfunction, in acute as compared to chronic impairments. The vital role of proper dosage of HBO therapy to ensure both the efficacy and safety of the treatment is emphasized. We argue that in the acute stages of brain and cardiorespiratory impairment, the adequate hyperbaric oxygen dose is the most important condition for obtaining maximum therapeutic effect, due to the powerful anti-hypoxic capabilities of this method. In contrast, during the chronic course of such impairments, there is an increased importance of safe dosing for the prevention of oxygen intoxication. Further dosage adjustments need to be made for the elderly as compared to younger patients, while examining and taking into consideration long term therapy effects. Some potential geroprotective mechanisms of HBO therapy are considered, that may be analogous to other geroprotective medications.

References and notes

1. See additional resources at the author's personal sites:
Longevity for All http://www.longevityforall.org/resources/;
Longevity History http://www.longevityhistory.com;
Longevity Israel http://www.longevityisrael.org/;
https://www.linkedin.com/in/ilia-stambler-5099977/;
https://www.researchgate.net/profile/Ilia_Stambler;
https://www.facebook.com/ilia.stambler.
2. Ilia Stambler, *Longevity Promotion: Multidisciplinary Perspectives*, Longevity History, 2017, http://www.longevityhistory.com.
3. Kunlin Jin, James W. Simpkins, Xunming Ji, Miriam Leis, Ilia Stambler, "The critical need to promote research of aging and aging-related diseases to improve health and longevity of the elderly population," *Aging and*

Disease, 6(1), 1-5, 2015, http://www.aginganddisease.org/EN/10.14336/AD.2014.1210. Along with English, the text of this article is available in full and partial translations in 12 languages: http://www.longevityforall.org/the-critical-need-to-promote-research-of-aging-around-the-world/.

4. Ilia Stambler, "Recognizing degenerative aging as a treatable medical condition: methodology and policy," *Aging and Disease*, 8(5), 2017, http://www.aginganddisease.org/EN/10.14336/AD.2017.0130.

5. Ilia Stambler, "Human life extension: opportunities, challenges, and implications for public health policy," in Alexander Vaiserman (Ed.), *Anti-aging Drugs: From Basic Research to Clinical Practice*, Royal Society of Chemistry, London, 2017, pp. 535-564, http://pubs.rsc.org/en/content/ebook/978-1-78262-435-6#!divbookcontent, http://www.longevityforall.org/wp-content/uploads/2016/04/LONGEVITY-PROMOTION.pdf.

6. Ilia Stambler, "The pursuit of longevity – The bringer of peace to the Middle East," *Current Aging Science*, 6, 25-31, 2014, http://www.eurekaselect.com/122295/article, http://www.ifa-fiv.org/wp-content/uploads/2013/11/Ilia-Stambler-1100-Lapis-B.pdf

7. Ilia Stambler, "Stop Aging Disease! ICAD 2014," *Aging and Disease*, 6(2), 76-94, 2015, http://www.aginganddisease.org/EN/10.14336/AD.2015.0115.

8. Ilia Stambler, *A History of Life-Extensionism in the Twentieth Century*, Longevity History, 2014, http://www.longevityhistory.com/.

9. Ilia Stambler, "The unexpected outcomes of anti-aging, rejuvenation and life extension studies: an origin of modern therapies," *Rejuvenation Research*, 17, 297-305, 2014, http://online.liebertpub.com/doi/abs/10.1089/rej.2013.1527.

10. Ilia Stambler, "Has aging ever been considered healthy?" *Frontiers in Genetics. Genetics of Aging*, 6, 00202, 2015, http://journal.frontiersin.org/article/10.3389/fgene.2015.00202/full.

11. Ilia Stambler, "Life extension – a conservative enterprise? Some fin-de-siecle and early twentieth-century precursors of transhumanism," *Journal of Evolution and Technology*, 21, 13-26, 2010, http://ieet.org/index.php/IEET/more/stambler20100328, http://jetpress.org/v21/stambler.htm, http://jetpress.org/v21/stambler.pdf.

12. Ilia Stambler, "Elie Metchnikoff – the founder of longevity science and a founder of modern medicine: In honor of the 170th anniversary," *Advances in Gerontology*, 28(2), 207-217, 2015 (Russian), 5(4), 201-208, 2015 (English), https://link.springer.com/article/10.1134/S2079057015040219, http://www.longevityforall.org/170th-anniversary-of-elie-metchnikoff-the-founder-of-gerontology-may-15-2015/,

http://www.gersociety.ru/news/news_209.html,
http://www.gersociety.ru/information/uspexi/.
13. Ilia Stambler, "On the history of life-extension research: Does the whole have parts?" *Sixth SENS Conference (SENS6). Reimagine Aging*, Queens' College – Cambridge UK, September 3-7, 2013, proceedings at *Rejuvenation Research*, 16, S41, 2013, http://www.sens.org/videos/history-life-extension-research-does-whole-have-parts-ilia-stambler, https://www.youtube.com/watch?v=EoBkf8rEGOo.
14. Ilia Stambler, "Heroic Power in Thomas Carlyle and Leo Tolstoy," *The European Legacy*, 11(7), 737-751, December 2006.
This article is based on Ilia Stambler, *Heroism and Heroic Death in Nineteenth Century Literature*, MA Thesis, English Department, Bar Ilan University, Israel, 2001, http://life-extension-history.blogspot.co.il/2017/04/heroism-and-heroic-death-in-19c.html, also at http://www.longevityhistory.com/.
The article was republished in the monograph: Ilia Stambler, "Heroic Power in Thomas Carlyle and Leo Tolstoy," in David S. Bell (Ed.), *Political Leadership, SAGE Library of Political Science*, SAGE Publications Ltd, 2011.
Though not directly related to scientific life extension, it examines the debates regarding the value of individual human life (any life) against the glorification of death (any death, under whatever circumstances).
15. David Blokh, Ilia Stambler, "The application of information theory for the research of aging and aging-related diseases," *Progress in Neurobiology*, S0301-0082(15)30059-9, 2016, doi: http://dx.doi.org/10.1016/j.pneurobio.2016.03.005.
16. David Blokh, Ilia Stambler, "The use of information theory for the evaluation of biomarkers of aging and physiological age," *Mechanisms of Ageing and Development*, 163, 23-29, 2017, doi: http://dx.doi.org/10.1016/j.mad.2017.01.003.
17. David Blokh, Ilia Stambler, "Information theoretical analysis of aging as a risk factor for heart disease," *Aging and Disease*, 6, 196-207, 2015, http://www.aginganddisease.org/EN/10.14336/AD.2014.0623.
18. David Blokh, Ilia Stambler, "Estimation of heterogeneity in diagnostic parameters of age-related diseases," *Aging and Disease*, 5, 218-225, 2014, http://www.aginganddisease.org/EN/10.14336/AD.2014.0500218, https://www.youtube.com/watch?v=uaTNRJW36cg.
19. David Blokh, Ilia Stambler, "Applying information theory analysis for the solution of biomedical data processing problems," *American Journal of Bioinformatics*, 3(1), 17-29, 2015, http://thescipub.com/abstract/10.3844/ajbsp.2014.17.29, http://thescipub.com/PDF/ajbsp.2014.17.29.pdf.
20. David Blokh, Ilia Stambler, Elena Afrimzon, Yana Shafran, Eden Korech, Judith Sandbank, Ruben Orda, Naomi Zurgil, Mordechai Deutsch, "The information-theory analysis of Michaelis–Menten constants for

detection of breast cancer," *Cancer Detection and Prevention*, 31, 489-498, 2007, doi: http://dx.doi.org/10.1016/j.cdp.2007.10.010.

The method developed in this work was presented in the monograph: Pedro Jose Gutierrez Diez, Irma H. Russo, Jose Russo, *The Evolution of the Use of Mathematics in Cancer Research*, Springer, New York, 2012.

21. Gennady G. Rogatsky, Ilia Stambler, "Hyperbaric oxygenation for resuscitation and therapy of elderly patients with cerebral and cardio-respiratory dysfunction," *Frontiers In Bioscience* (Scholar Edition), 9, 230-243, June 1, 2017, http://www.bioscience.org/2017/v9s/af/484/2.htm, https://www.bioscience.org/special-issue-details?editor_id=1746, https://www.ncbi.nlm.nih.gov/pubmed/28410116.